Early Clinical Diagnosis

How a Text book should be written:

'He doth, as if your journey should lie through a fair vineyard, at the first give you a cluster of grapes, that, full of taste, you may long to pass further. He beginneth not with obscure definitions, which must blur the margent with interpretations and load the memory with doubtfulness; but he cometh to you with words set in delightful proportions, either accompanied with, or prepared for, the well-enchanting skill of music.'

How a Text book is usually written:

'When a man was reading a long essay, and gave a glimpse of a page at the end of the book with no writing on it, Diogenes said, "Courage, I see land."'

Samson Wright, *Applied Physiology*
Eighth Edition (1945) Oxford University Press,
London.

Early Clinical Diagnosis

Gerald Sandler

MD, FRCP
Consultant Physician,
Barnsley District General Hospital

and

John Fry

OBE, MD, FRCS, FRCGP
General Practitioner,
Beckenham, Kent

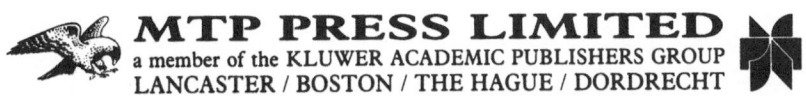

MTP PRESS LIMITED
a member of the KLUWER ACADEMIC PUBLISHERS GROUP
LANCASTER / BOSTON / THE HAGUE / DORDRECHT

Published in the UK and Europe by
MTP Press Limited
Falcon House
Lancaster, England

British Library Cataloguing in Publication Data

Sandler, Gerald
   Early clinical diagnosis.
   1. Diagnosis
   I. Title   II. Fry, John, *1922–*
   616.07′5   RC71
ISBN-13: 978-94-010-8340-9   e-ISBN-13: 978-94-009-4147-2
DOI: 10.1007/978-94-009-4147-2

Published in the USA by
MTP Press
A division of Kluwer Boston Inc
190 Old Derby Street
Hingham, MA 02043, USA

Library of Congress Cataloging in Publication Data

Sandler, Gerald, 1928–
   Early clinical diagnosis.

   Includes index.
   1. Diagnosis.   2. Symptomatology.   3. Medical
history taking.   I. Fry, John.
II. Title.   [DNLM: 1. Diagnosis—outlines.
WB 18 S217e]
RC71.S185   1985   616.07′5   85–21706

Contents

Preface

Why yet another book on clinical diagnosis?

The profusion of medical text books for students and young postgraduates is known to all of us, and so also is the time-consuming and frequently frustrating search in these books for the relevant facts we need, so often submerged in a mass of information which we do not really require. The traditional textbook that most clinicians have used in their training may well be written in the leisurely, discursive and unstructured style much loved by our teachers of old, but perhaps out of place in modern medical education where knowledge is so rapidly expanding and time available for its assimilation rapidly contracting.

It is with these considerations in mind that we felt it would be useful to provide a clear, concise, easily readable and well-illustrated book on the essentials of clinical diagnosis.

Each chapter deals with a medical problem commonly encountered in daily clinical practice and begins with a list of the possible causes and a practical perspective of their prevalence in general practice and in hospital practice; the age distribution and the clinical significance of the various disorders is also pointed out. The major part of the chapter is concerned with the diagnostic approach to the particular problem and emphasizes the importance of symptoms and signs in reaching the correct diagnosis, as well as the value and limitation of the investigational approach to the diagnosis.

The book emphasizes the fundamental clinical skills of history-taking and clinical examination in diagnosis, so frequently and mistakenly subordinated to the investigational approach which is often disappointing in the limited diagnostic help which it does provide.

As a general physician and as a general practitioner we have combined our 60 physician-years of experience to encompass the widest possible views of clinical medicine.

In writing this book we have each learnt much from the other and we believe that our readers likewise will share our enthusiasm in helping to restore the art of clinical skills to the process of early diagnosis.

1986   *Gerald Sandler*
                                                                        John Fry

Acknowledgements

G.S: 'I am greatly indebted to my secretary, Christine Green, for typing the manuscript. I would also like to sincerely thank my understanding wife, Ella, who continues to have inexhaustible patience with my writing and with the inevitable neglect that it entails.'

J.F: 'I too am indebted to my typists Mildred Lucas and Jill Bremberg and to my wife Joan who now accepts my out-of-hours occupation: writing.'

We both dedicate our book to our past, present and future patients who have taught us much on Early Clinical Diagnosis.

1 Chest Pain

Introduction

Chest pain is one of the commonest presenting symptoms and has a wide spectrum of significance. At one end it may be life-threatening and even rapidly fatal, at the other end a minor self-limiting nuisance. Accurate assessment and diagnosis are necessary if lives are to be saved and anxiety relieved.

Causes of chest pain

The most frequent causes are:

Cardiovascular	• angina
	• myocardial infarction
	• pericarditis
	• dissecting aneurysm
Pulmonary	• pleurisy – infection infarction
	• spontaneous pneumothorax
Gastro-oesophageal	• acid regurgitation
	• peptic ulcer
	• oesophageal spasm
	• gall bladder disease
Chest wall	• muscular
	• herpes zoster
	• costo-chondritis
	• cervical spondylosis
'Functional'	• no organic cause found

1

Chest pain – spectrum of significance

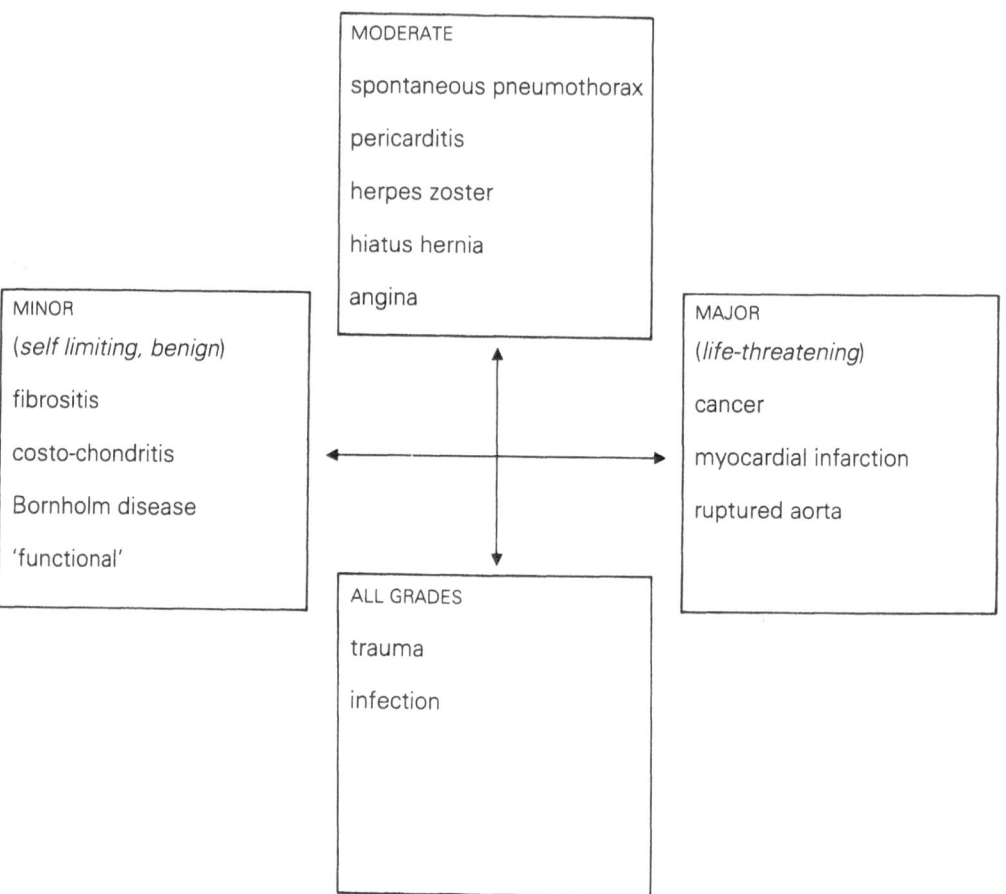

MODERATE

spontaneous pneumothorax

pericarditis

herpes zoster

hiatus hernia

angina

MINOR

(*self limiting, benign*)

fibrositis

costo-chondritis

Bornholm disease

'functional'

MAJOR

(*life-threatening*)

cancer

myocardial infarction

ruptured aorta

ALL GRADES

trauma

infection

Frequency

In a general practice of 2500 patients annual prevalence may be about one new case of chest pain per week to assess and treat.

Annual prevalence of conditions presenting as chest pain in a general practice of 2500 patients	
Cardiovascular	
myocardial infarction	3–5
angina	5–10
ruptured aorta	1 in 7 years
pericarditis	1 in 15 years
Respiratory	
infection (pleurisy/pneumonia)	5–10
pulmonary infarction	1–2
lung cancer	1 in 5 years
spontaneous pneumothorax	1 in 5 years
Gastrointestinal	
hiatus hernia/oesophagitis	2–3
Skin	
herpes zoster	2–3
Musculoskeletal	
'fibrositis/neuralgia'	5–10
trauma	5–10
Tietze's syndrome	1–2
clicking rib	1–2
Bornholm disease	1–2
No discoverable cause (NAD)	10–20

Age incidence

The relative prevalence of possible conditions in different age groups helps in diagnosis.

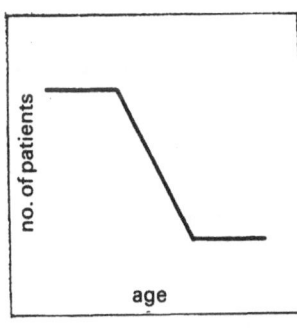

- spontaneous pneumothorax
- pleurisy
- trauma
- musculoskeletal
- costo-chondritis (Tietze)
- fibrositis
- clicking rib
- (functional)

3

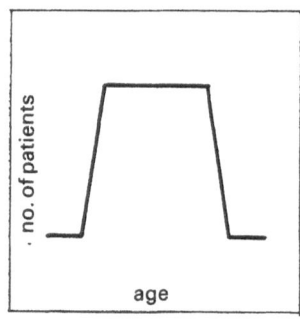

- myocardial infarction
- angina
- pleurisy
- hiatus hernia
- cancer
- (functional)

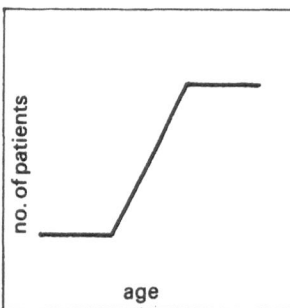

- cancer
- pleurisy
- herpes zoster
- myocardial infarction/angina
- ruptured aorta

Diagnostic approach

History

The diagnosis of chest pain should be made on the basis of the history.

The features of the chest pain should be assessed in a regular and orderly sequence

- site
- character
- radiation
- precipitation
- relief
- associated symptoms

The application of this approach to the diagnosis of the chest pain is shown in the tables:

- cardiovascular causes – Table 1.1
- pulmonary causes – Table 1.2
- gastro-oesophageal causes – Table 1.3
- chest wall causes – Table 1.4
- functional chest pain – Table 1.5

Table 1.1 Chest pain assessment in cardiovascular disease

	Angina	Myocardial infarction	Pericarditis	Dissecting aneurys
Site	deep retrosternal	deep retrosternal	surface sternal	front of chest (proximal aorta)
Character	constricting	constricting	aching	tearing
Radiation	left arm frequent right arm uncommon throat lower jaw	similar to angina	left arm occasional right arm rare throat rare	front to back of chest down back to abdomen
Precipitation	exertion anxiety heavy meals cold wind	often in bed rare on exertion	lying flat deep breath coughing	severe exertion or strain
Relief	rest nitrates	potent analgesic	sitting up	potent analgesic
Associated symptoms	strangling in throat	nausea/vomiting sweating breathlessness faintness angor animi	sometimes pleuritic pain	shock circulatory collapse mono/hemi-plegia

Table 1.2   *Chest pain assessment in respiratory disease*

	Pleurisy	Spontaneous pneumothorax
Site	lateral chest	lateral chest
Character	stabbing	stabbing
Radiation	basal pleurisy → shoulder tip	—
Precipitation	deep breathing coughing	deep breathing coughing
Relief	shallow breathing	shallow breathing

Associated symptoms	infective
	  cough
	  purulent sputum
	  recent cold/flu
	embolism
	  cough
	  haemoptysis
	  recent immobilization
	  recent operation
	    (especially pelvic)
		breathlessness
		  severe in tension
		  pneumothorax

Table 1.3   *Chest pain assessment in gastro-oesophageal disease*

	Acid regurgitation	Peptic ulcer	Oesophageal spasm	Gall bladder disease

Site	epigastric	epigastric
		right
		  hypochondrium
			deep in
			  chest
				right
				  hypochondrium

Character	burning	gnawing	squeezing	constant ache or colicky

Radiation	sternum
	throat
		through to back
		  (D.U.)
			—	below right
				  scapula
				tip of right
				  shoulder

Precipitation	eating
	lying
	bending
		eating
		  G.U. – $\frac{1}{2}$ h
		  D.U. – 2–3 h
			—	fatty food

Relief	standing antacids	antacids	anti- spasmodics	—

Associated symptoms	water-brash	vomiting
		  (especially
		  pyloric
		  stenosis)
			dysphagia	flatulent
				dyspepsia

Table 1.4   *Pain assessment in chest wall disorders*

	Muscular	*Herpes zoster*	*Costo-chondritis (Tietze's syndrome)*	*Cervical spondylosis*
Site	periscapular intercostal	dermatome on chest wall	over costo-chondral junctions	upper chest (C4)
Character	ache	severe lancinating	ache	deep ache
Radiation	shoulder/arm	affected nerve root	submammary	shoulder/arm
Precipitation	physical effort coughing deep breathing	contact with chicken pox	lifting and straining	neck movements
Relief	rest heat	potent analgesic	analgesics	immobilization of neck (collar)
Associated symptoms	limitation of movement shoulder/arm local tenderness over muscle	vesicular rash in dermatome (pain precedes rash)	local swelling and tenderness over joints	paraesthesiae in nerve root distribution

Table 1.5   *Characteristics features of functional chest pain*

Site	can be anywhere in the chest but often in left submammary area
Character	sharp, stabbing continuous
Radiation	usually no radiation may be referred down arms
Precipitation	anxiety tension depression
Relief	by reassurance psychotropic drugs
Associated symptoms	palpitations deep breathing tremor agitation/anxiety depression

Clinical examination (Fig. 1.1)

Cardiovascular disease

angina	• of very limited value
	• may show evidence of arteriosclerosis
myocardial infarction	• examination more helpful
dissecting aneurysm	• absent femoral pulses may be diagnostic
pericarditis	• friction rub diagnostic

Pulmonary disease

a silent hyper-resonant chest is diagnostic of pneumothorax

a friction rub is diagnostic of pleurisy which may be due to

pulmonary infarction	• haemoptysis
	• recent immobilization
	• recent operation
	• recent leg vein thrombosis
	• contraceptive pill
pulmonary infection	• cough
	• purulent sputum
	• rhonchi/crepitations in lungs

Gastro-oesophageal disease	• epigastric tenderness but non-specific

Chest wall disease

tender costo-chondral junctions → costo-chondritis

rash of herpes zoster

restricted painful neck movement ± crepitus → cervical spondylosis

Investigation

Cardiovascular disease

Angina

electrocardiogram (ECG) of little diagnostic value – may show evidence of previous ischaemic damage: frequently entirely normal

exercise ECG – of more value in diagnosing ischaemic chest pain: S-T depression occurring during exercise indicates ischaemia but the change is only of diagnostic value *if accompanied by the identical pain of which the patient complains*

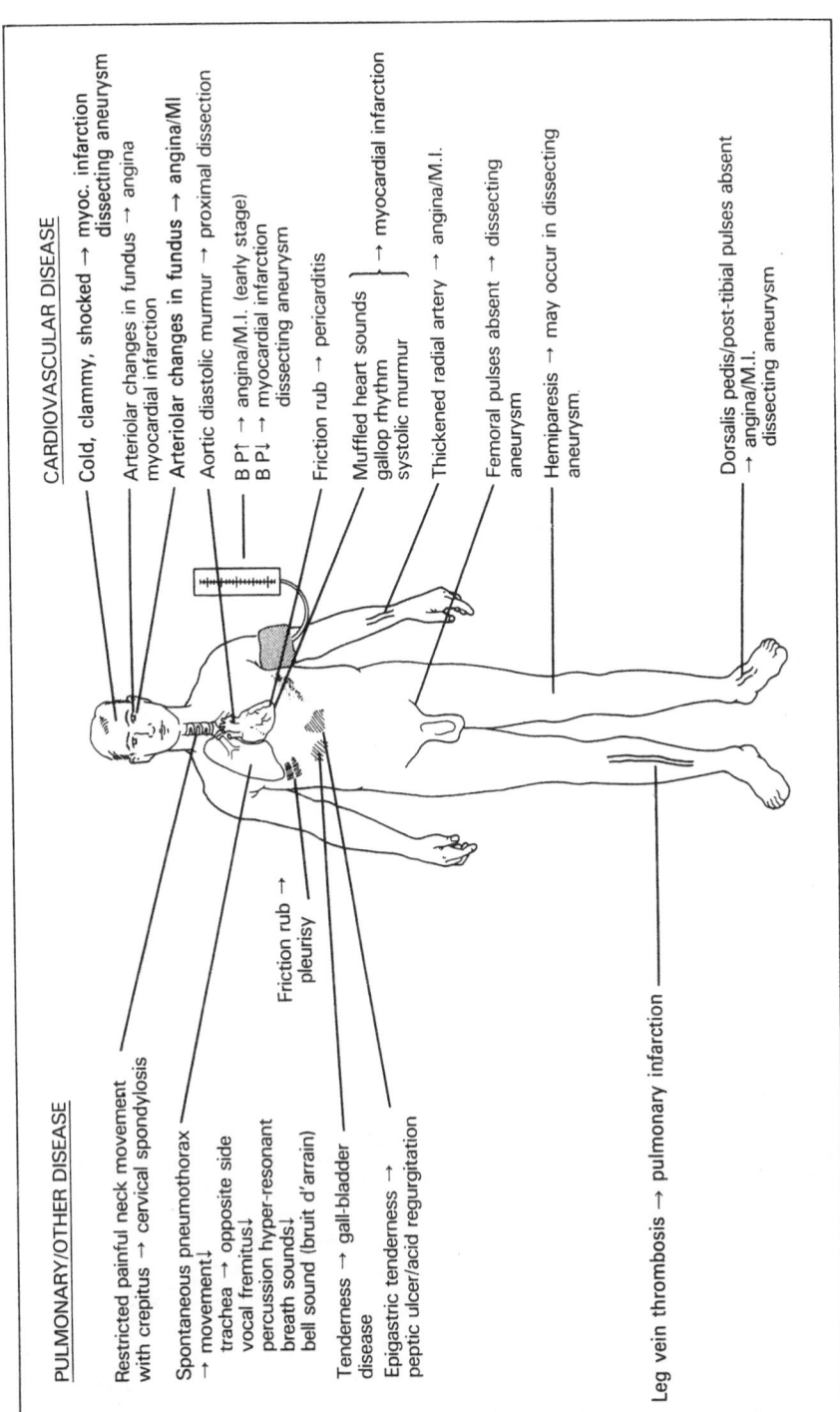

CARDIOVASCULAR DISEASE

Cold, clammy, shocked → myoc. infarction
dissecting aneurysm

Arteriolar changes in fundus → angina
myocardial infarction

Arteriolar changes in fundus → angina/MI

Aortic diastolic murmur → proximal dissection

B P↑ → angina/M.I. (early stage)
B P↓ → myocardial infarction
dissecting aneurysm

Friction rub → pericarditis

Muffled heart sounds
gallop rhythm } → myocardial infarction
systolic murmur

Thickened radial artery → angina/M.I.

Femoral pulses absent → dissecting
aneurysm

Hemiparesis → may occur in dissecting
aneurysm

Dorsalis pedis/post-tibial pulses absent
→ angina/M.I.
dissecting aneurysm

PULMONARY/OTHER DISEASE

Restricted painful neck movement
with crepitus → cervical spondylosis

Spontaneous pneumothorax
→ movement↓
trachea → opposite side
vocal fremitus↓
percussion hyper-resonant
breath sounds↓
bell sound (bruit d'arrain)

Tenderness → gall-bladder
disease

Epigastric tenderness →
peptic ulcer/acid regurgitation

Friction rub →
pleurisy

Leg vein thrombosis → pulmonary infarction

Fig. 1.1   *Possible findings on examination in a patient with chest pain*

9

chest X-ray – of no diagnostic value in angina, but suggests an adverse prognosis if the heart is enlarged

blood lipids – elevated blood lipids are of limited and non-specific help in angina, merely indicating a susceptibility to arteriosclerosis. No justification for their routine measurement in angina unless the patient is young – under 40 years – when their therapeutic reduction may, theoretically, be of potential benefit

coronary arteriography – definitive investigation: it is usually indicated in young patients (arbitrarily < 40 years), and in anginal patients intractable to medical treatment who may require bypass surgery or angioplasty

Myocardial infarction

electrocardiogram – mandatory in suspected infarction: some findings may be conclusive. The changes which occur (Figs. 1.2a, 1.2b) are:

- Q or QS waves
- ST elevation
- T inversion

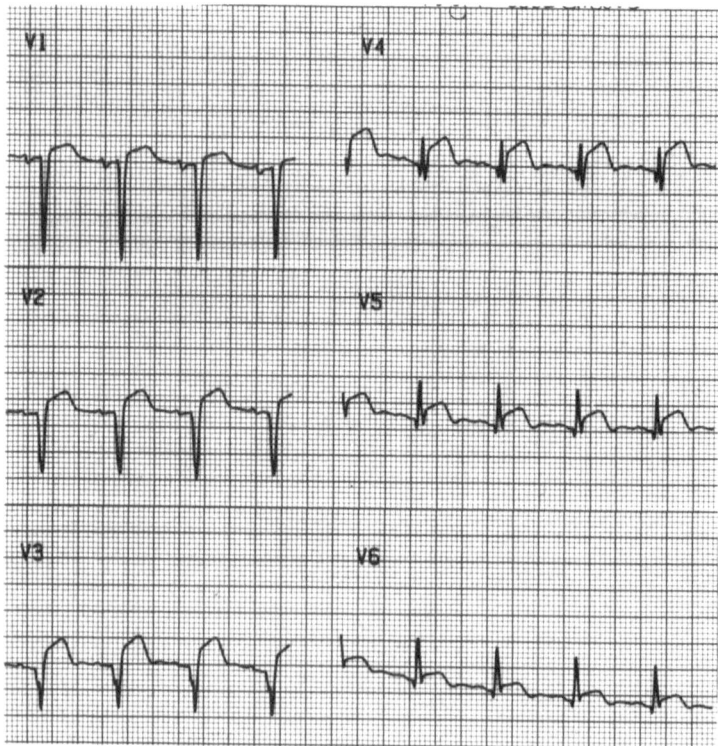

Fig. 1.2a *ECG in anterior myocardial infarction showing QS waves and ST elevation in leads V1–V3 with smaller Q waves and ST elevation in V4–V6*

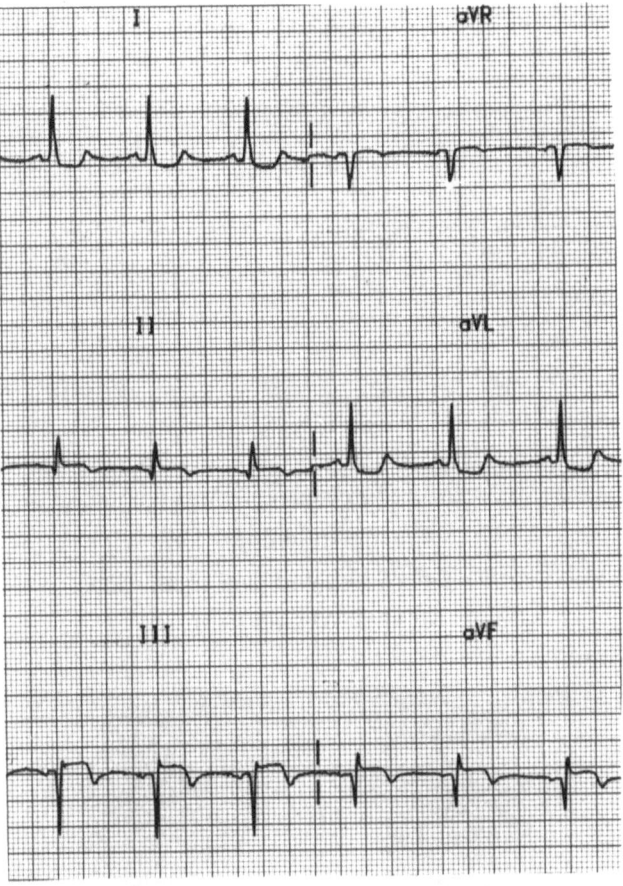

Fig. 1.2b *ECG in inferior myocardial infarction showing QS waves, ST elevation and T inversion in leads III, aVF*

cardiac enzymes – necessary in suspected myocardial infarction. The enzymes assessed are:

Cardiac enzymes in myocardial infarction

Enzyme	Time of increase	Normal range (*International units*)
Creatine phosphokinase (CPK)	Within 4 h	24–195
Glutamic oxaloacetic transaminase (SGOT)	12 h – 3 days	13–42
Lactic dehydrogenase (LDH)	24 h – 7 days	240–525

chest X-ray – limited diagnostic help. It may show changes of complicating left ventricular failure, so frequent after severe myocardial infarction (Fig. 1.3):

- congestion upper lobe veins
- basal pulmonary shadowing
- bilateral hilar flare

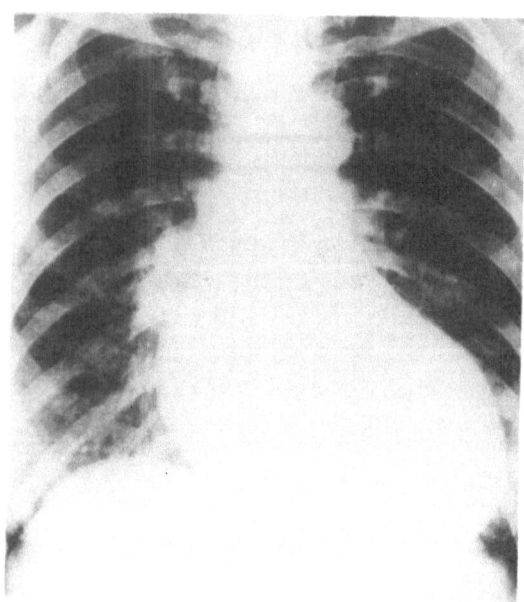

Fig. 1.3 *Chest X-ray showing 'boot-shaped' heart in left ventricular enlargement*

Pericarditis

electrocardiogram – may show diagnostic changes in pericarditis with S–T elevation, concave upwards, over the affected part of the heart (Fig. 1.4).

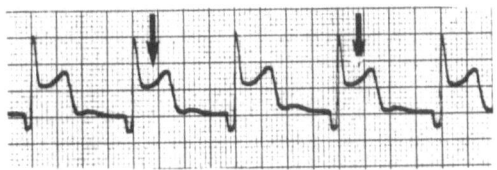

Fig. 1.4   *ECG in pericarditis showing ST elevation, concave upwards (arrowed)*

chest X-ray and *echocardiogram* – only of value if a pericardial effusion is suspected:

- apex beat difficult to feel
- heart enlarged (percussion)
- heart sounds distant
- pulsus paradoxus

Dissecting aneurysm

chest X-ray – necessary to show widening of the mediastinal shadow

abdominal X-ray – may show widening of the shadow of the abdominal aorta

angiography – definitive investigation

Respiratory disease

Pleurisy

chest X-ray – of no diagnostic help in uncomplicated pleurisy but may show evidence of underlying pulmonary infection if there is associated pneumonia or broncho-pneumonia. If a pulmonary embolism has caused the pleurisy, a peripheral wedge-shaped shadow may be evident (Fig. 1.5)

sputum examination – of little value in pulmonary infection since culture is frequently negative and the result is often available too late to influence treatment: however, if the infection is resistant to initial empirical antibiotic treatment, sputum culture may give guidance on further antibiotics

lung scan – useful diagnostic test in pulmonary infarction when it may show the typical localized area of reduced perfusion with blood but normal ventilation with air

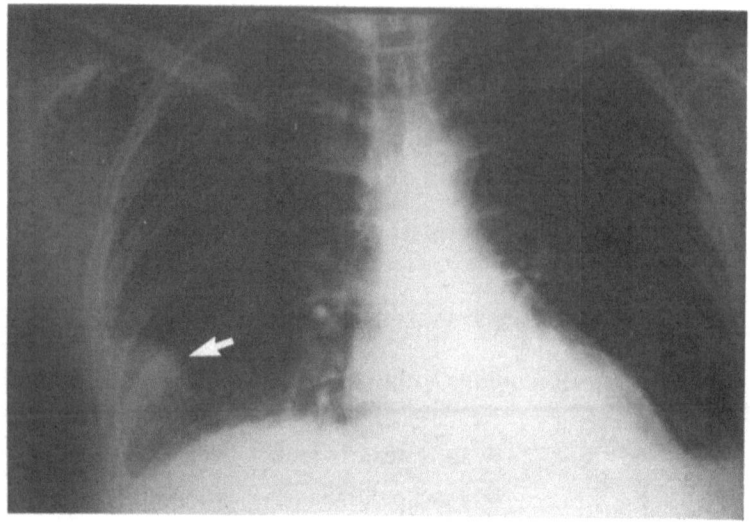

Fig. 1.5 *Chest X-ray showing shadow at right base (arrowed) due to pulmonary embolism*

Spontaneous pneumothorax

chest X-ray – an essential test to diagnose this condition and the findings are pathognomonic (Fig. 1.6)

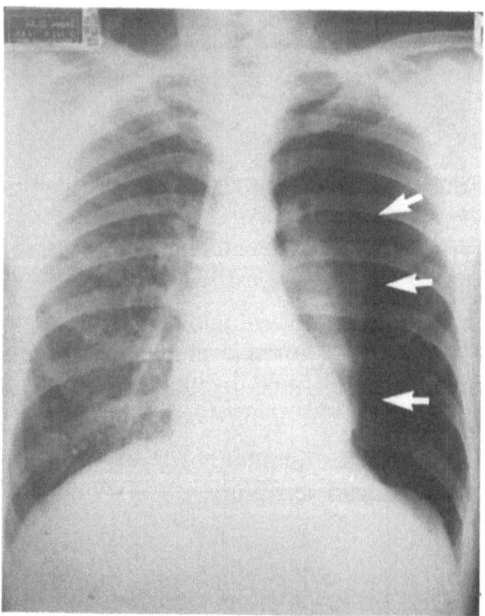

Fig. 1.6 *Chest X-ray showing a collapsed left lung (arrowed) due to pneumothorax*

Gastro-oesophageal disease

gastro-oesophageal regurgitation – best seen by barium studies with the patient tipped head down: a hiatus hernia may be found (Fig. 1.7)

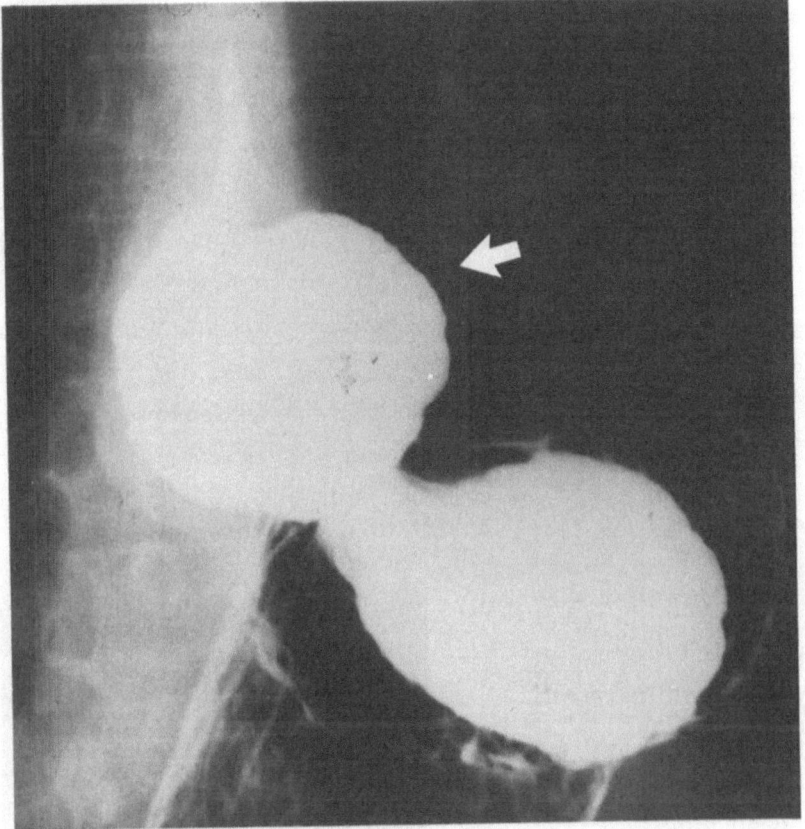

Fig. 1.7   *Barium meal showing large hiatus hernia (arrowed)*

peptic ulcer – gastric and duodenal ulcers are diagnosed by *barium meal* and/or *endoscopy*. The relative merits of the two tests are shown in the table

oesophageal spasm – *barium studies* are unlikely to help in diagnosis unless oesophageal spasm, with accompanying pain, occurs fortuitously during the X-ray examination

gall bladder disease
- cholecystography
- percutaneous cholangiography
- ultrasound

Comparison of barium meal and gastroscopy in the diagnosis of peptic ulcer

	Barium meal	Gastroscopy
Advantages	simple inexpensive widely available	accurate reliable distinguishes benign from malignant ulcer biopsy possible can assess healing of ulcer can control bleeding – diathermy laser

Disadvantages	may miss ulcer (10–30%)
	poor differentiation between
	  benign and malignant
	    ulcers
		not readily available
		uncomfortable
		
		complications:
		  perforated oesophagus
		  perforation of ulcers

Chest wall disease

- muscular pain – no relevant tests

- herpes zoster – no relevant tests

- costo-chondritis – X-ray of the affected joints is unlikely to show any abnormality and there are no other relevant tests

Cervical spondylosis – X-ray of the cervical spine may show spondylosis (Fig. 1.8) but this is very common in *asymptomatic* middle-aged and elderly patients so its presence does not necessarily indicate a causal relationship

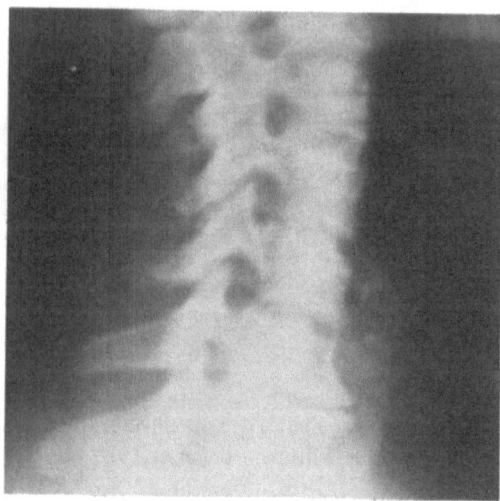

Fig. 1.8 *Neck X-ray showing cervical spondylosis*

Functional chest pain

Tests will all be negative, but they are often a necessary part of successful management to convince the patient that everything possible has been done and that all is well. An ECG is the most important test from this point of view and a chest X-ray will also help to reassure.

Pitfalls in diagnosis

General

- Major causes of chest pain may be misinterpreted as 'functional' in anxious individuals.
- Instant diagnosis is dangerous – careful attention to history is important.
- It is disastrous to have a patient die following an initial diagnosis of 'functional chest pain'.
- Minor abnormalities in ECG should not lead to an erroneous 'organic' diagnosis when the true one is 'functional'.

Angina

- A patient with objective evidence of myocardial ischaemia on the ECG may, and often does, have co-existing functional (non-organic) chest pain.
- A patient with a long history of functional (non-organic) chest pain may develop true anginal pain. Therefore each episode of chest pain must be assessed on its own merits in as unbiased a manner as possible.
- Basing the diagnosis of angina on so-called relief of the pain with glyceryl trinitrate is only acceptable if the pain relief occurs within 1–3 minutes: very often the 'relief' is accepted uncritically by the doctor without enquiring on its rapidity.

Pulmonary disease

- The absence of clinical evidence of deep vein thrombosis does not exclude pulmonary embolism in a patient with suspected pulmonary infarction, since clinical evidence is lacking in at least 50% of established cases of deep vein thrombosis. Always enquire if woman is taking 'the Pill'.
- A normal chest X-ray and white count does not exclude pulmonary infection; the best guide is the colour of the sputum, but even this is inconclusive.
- Spontaneous pneumothorax is often forgotten in the differential diagnosis of sudden pleuritic pain: a silent hyper-resonant lung is the clue but chest X-ray is necessary for the confirmation.

Gastro-oesophageal disease

- In oesophageal spasm rapid relief of the chest pain with glyceryl trinitrate may falsely suggest angina.
- Gall bladder disease may co-exist with angina: it may produce chest pain simulating angina or may trigger off an authentic attack of angina.
- Belching terminating chest pain does not necessarily indicate a gastro-oesophageal cause of the pain, since it may sometimes occur when an attack of angina is ending – the mechanism is unknown.
- Finding gastro-oesophageal reflux on barium meal examination does not necessarily indicate that chest pain is due to this cause, since it is often found in asymptomatic individuals.

Chest wall disease

- Radiological evidence of cervical spondylosis does not necessarily mean that it is the cause of the chest pain since many asymptomatic middle-aged or older individuals will have this X-ray finding. Clinical evidence of restricted movement and precipitation of pain are more important in diagnosis.
- Herpes zoster is often forgotten as an acute cause of left-sided chest pain, especially in older patients: the diagnostic clue is the localization of the chest pain to the dermatome. Appearance of rash clinches diagnosis.

Useful practical points in dealing with chest pain

- Consider differential diagnoses of likely causes and diagnose firmly on the basis of history if possible – clinical examination usually offers little help.
- Make sure that the most serious conditions are considered first.
- Consider tests only when they give a definite answer not obtainable on history and examination alone. Don't order a test unless you have a specific question to answer.
- The most important diagnosis to consider is angina but remember functional chest pain is probably the most frequently encountered.
- With acute prolonged ischaemic-type pain consider hospital admission.
- With doubtful chronic chest pain try effects of nitroglycerine and/or antacids and re-assess.
- Always explain the condition and treatment expectations simply and clearly to the patient – especially important in functional chest pain.
- Functional chest pain

  probably the most likely type of chest pain

  diagnosis should be made confidently more on positive symptoms than on a lengthy process of exclusion

  management should be strong explanatory reassurance rather than with medication or restriction of normal activities

Case challenge

A 39-year-old carpenter presented at night with a gradual onset over several hours of increasingly severe epigastric and retrosternal pain. The pain radiated through to his back but also down the left arm which he described as feeling heavy. He felt sick but had not vomited. There was a past history of a vagotomy for duodenal ulcer 15 years earlier and he had been subject to occasional bouts of indigestion and heartburn since, usually relieved promptly by antacids. He also had a neck injury at work 5 years earlier since when he had suffered with pain at the back of his neck, sometimes associated with aching in the left shoulder and tingling in the lateral fingers of the left hand.

He smoked 15–20 cigarettes daily since he was 15 years old. He drank 3 to 4 pints of beer on average each week.

The findings on clinical examination are shown in Fig. 1.9.

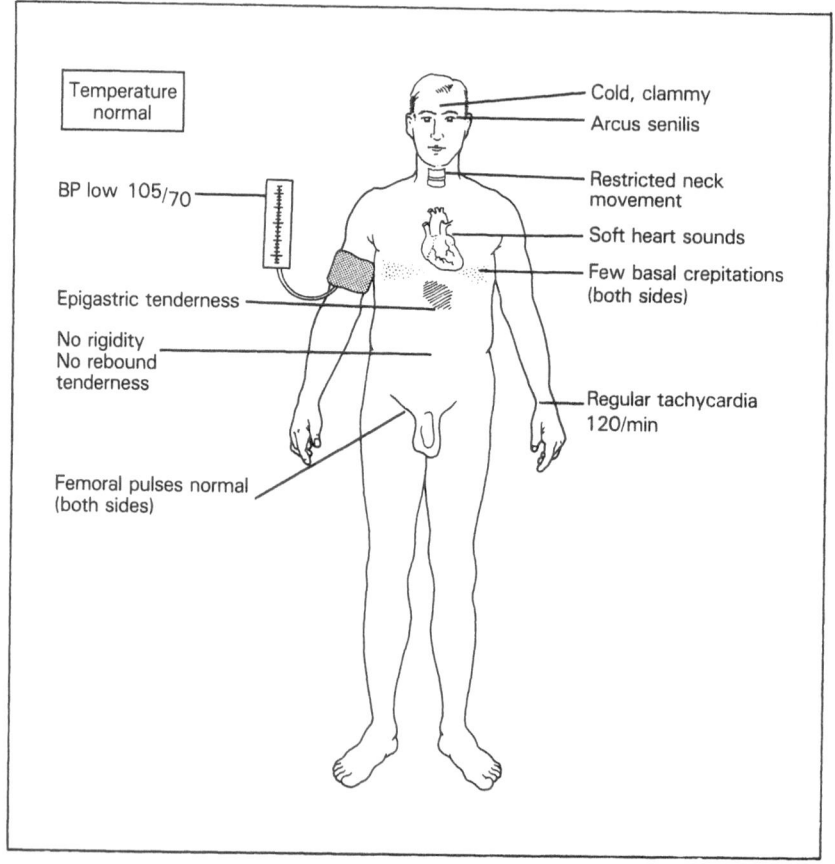

Fig. 1.9 *Examination findings on case challenge*

Questions

Give four possible diagnoses
How would you differentiate them?
What would you do at midnight
  to establish the diagnosis?
  to manage the patient?
What would you do the next morning?

Possible diagnoses

- peptic ulcer disease
- cervical spondylosis
- myocardial infarction
- dissecting aneurysm

Chest pain

Peptic ulcer disease

For   history
- past history of peptic ulcer
- recurrent indigestion
- radiation through to back – suggests penetrating duodenal ulcer

           exam
- epigastric tenderness

Against   history
- radiation of pain down left arm – in practice this is *very* uncommon in peptic ulcer

           exam
- cold, clammy skin with low blood pressure and tachycardia if associated with peptic ulcer would mean either bleeding or perforation – there was no other evidence of either condition

Tests
- gastroscopy is the best test
- barium meal if gastroscopy not available

Cervical spondylosis

For   history
- previous neck injury – may predispose to spondylosis
- neck pain radiating to shoulder and some fingers only very suggestive of nerve root compression due to cervical spondylosis

           exam
- restricted neck movement

Against   history
- heaviness in an arm is virtually never due to root irritation from cervical spondylosis
- nausea is not a symptom of spondylosis

           exam
- the signs of shock are not a feature of spondylosis

Tests
- neck X-ray is not helpful since spondylosis is often present in asymptomatic individuals

Myocardial infarction (MI)

For   history
- retrosternal pain radiating down left arm
- heaviness in arm is highly suggestive of ischaemic pain
- nausea common in MI
- long-term smoker

	exam	• signs of shock (cold, clammy, low BP, tachycardia)
		• soft heart sounds
		• basal crepitations – left ventricular failure frequent in MI
		• arcus senilis – indicates premature arteriosclerosis
Against	history	• radiation of pain through to the back is uncommon (but does occur)
	exam	• epigastric tenderness rarely occurs (but could be due to co-existent peptic ulcer)
Tests		• ECG
		• cardiac enzyme levels

Dissecting aneurysm of the aorta

For	history	• retrosternal pain radiating through to the back
	exam	• signs of shock common in dissection
Against	history	• no radiation of pain down back into legs
	exam	• normal femoral pulses
		• no hypertension – frequent in dissection
Tests		• chest X-ray – widened mediastinum
		• abdominal X-ray – widened aortic shadow
		• angiography – definitive test

What would you do at midnight?

To establish the diagnosis:

ask some pertinent questions about the pain

nature of pain	• tight/constricting → myocardial infarction
	• tearing → dissecting aneurysm
	• burning/nagging → peptic ulcer

radiation down back into legs → dissecting aneurysm

associated $\left. \begin{array}{l} \text{sweating/vomiting} \\ \text{faintness/dyspnoea} \end{array} \right\}$ → myocardial infarction

past history – previous angina → myocardial infarction

 ᶦly history – premature cardiovascular disease → myocardial infarction

Chest pain

look for relevant findings

arteriosclerosis
- premature arcus senilis
- thickened radial/brachial arteries
- reduced/absent foot pulses
- thickened retinal arteries

findings of myocardial infarction
- muffled heart sounds and/or gallop rhythm
- basal pulmonary crepitations

absent/asymmetrical femoral pulses → dissecting aneurysm

epigastric tenderness → peptic ulcer

To manage the patient

at midnight

if suspicious of myocardial infarction and within 3 hours of onset of pain – admit to hospital.

if suspicious of myocardial infarction but over 3 hours from onset and no complications
- keep at home
- relieve pain with effective analgesic
- reassure
- review next day

if dissecting aneurysm – admit urgently

if not myocardial infarction from history/examination
- reassure
- simple analgesic
- review next day

if peptic ulcer
- give antacids
- review next day

next morning

MI still doubtful – arrange ECG

MI definite – check for
complications
- heart failure
- shock
- arrhythmias

if present – consider hospital admission

if absent – consider home/hospital treatment on basis
of criteria listed previously

peptic ulcer likely
- continue antacids
- consider H_2-blockers but arrange barium meal or endoscopy first if readily available – otherwise treat anyway

no clear diagnosis – further review in due course

Actual diagnosis:
myocardial infarction

Treatment

Patient admitted to hospital as an emergency. The only complications were minor:

some ventricular ectopic beats – not treated as they were not
- multifocal
- in runs
- R-on-T

pericarditis – treated with aspirin

subsequent course uneventful

referred for coronary arteriography within 3 weeks of discharge – found to have 3-vessel disease

treated by coronary artery bypass grafting which is considered to improve prognosis in
- multivessel disease
- left main stem disease

2 Diarrhoea

Introduction

Because of the variability of normal bowel action the diagnosis of diarrhoea should be based on two requirements:

- increased frequency of bowel action
- softer, more fluid stools

Causes

Acute diarrhoea

gastro-enteritis
- salmonella
- *E. coli*
- staphylococci
- campylobacter

dysentery
- shigella
- amoebiasis

toxaemia – pseudomembranous colitis (*C. difficile*)

Chronic diarrhoea

inflammatory
- ulcerative colitis
- Crohn's disease

carcinoma of colon

diverticulitis

malabsorption states

irritable bowel syndrome

ischaemic colitis

fibrocystic disease

endocrine
- thyrotoxicosis
- diabetes
- Addison's disease

metabolic
- amyloidosis

drugs
- magnesium-containing antacids
- antibiotics
- digitalis
- guanethedine
- excessive purgatives

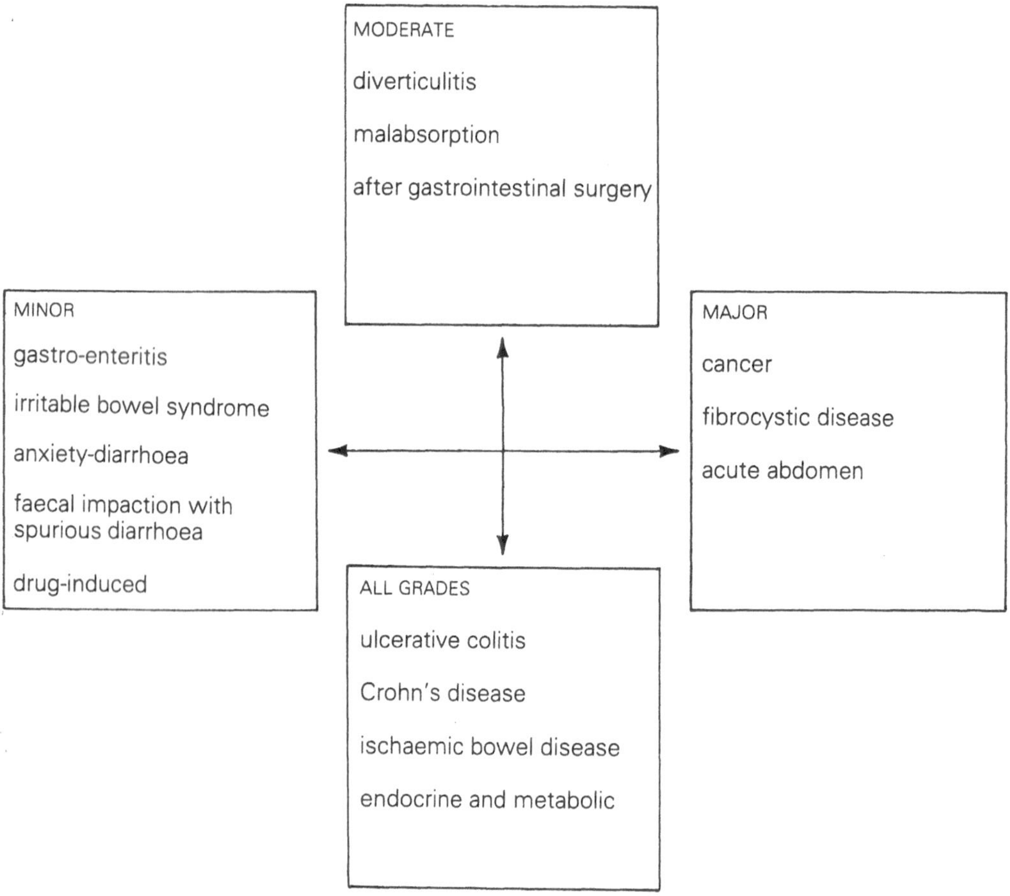

MODERATE

diverticulitis

malabsorption

after gastrointestinal surgery

MINOR

gastro-enteritis

irritable bowel syndrome

anxiety-diarrhoea

faecal impaction with
spurious diarrhoea

drug-induced

MAJOR

cancer

fibrocystic disease

acute abdomen

ALL GRADES

ulcerative colitis

Crohn's disease

ischaemic bowel disease

endocrine and metabolic

Table 2.1 *Spectrum of clinical significance
of the various types of diarrhoea*

Prevalence

The prevalence of the various types of diarrhoea in a general practice of 2500 patients is shown in Table 2.2.

Table 2.2   *Annual prevalence of conditions presenting as 'diarrhoea' in a general practice of 2500 persons*

Acute intestinal infections	125
'Irritable bowel syndrome'	50
Iatrogenic drug reactions	10
Diverticular disease	10
Faecal impaction	4
Colitis	3
Cancer	1
Fibrocystic disease	1
Less than 1 per year	
Acute abdomen	2 in 3 years
Coeliac disease and other malabsorption disorders	1 in 2 years
Crohn's disease	1 in 5 years
Ischaemic bowel disease	1 in 7 years

Age incidence

The distribution of the various conditions causing diarrhoea according to the age group in which they usually present is shown in Table 2.3.

Table 2.3   *Age incidence of different types of diarrhoea*

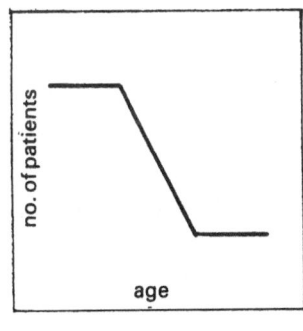

- acute gastro-enteritis
- coeliac disease
- fibrocystic disease
- intussusception

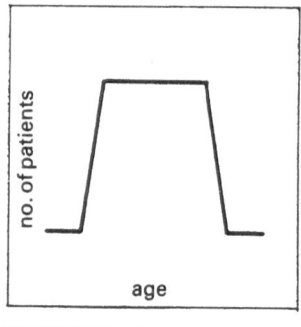

- irritable bowel syndrome
- ulcerative colitis
- Crohn's disease
- steatorrhoea
- after gastrointestinal surgery
- drug-induced, e.g. antacids

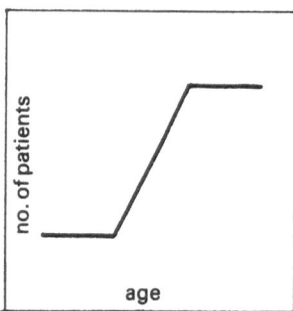

- cancer
- diverticular disease
- faecal impaction
- drug-induced, e.g. laxative
  digoxin

Diagnostic approach

Diarrhoea may present as an *acute* condition, usually self-limiting and lasting only a few days, or as a *chronic* condition in which there are either prolonged or recurrent episodes of diarrhoea lasting for weeks, months or years.
Both acute and chronic presentations may occur in children and in adults.

A systematic approach to diagnosis involves:

- enquiring about the past history including the taking of any drugs
- the nature of the current symptoms – gastrointestinal, other
- clinical examination
- deciding whether any investigations are necessary, and if so, which
- management decisions

History

Past history

recent travel abroad → acute gastro-enteritis

unusual food in last 72 hours → food poisoning (*E. Coli, Staphylococci, Salmonella*)

recent domicile in
   tropical country →   • dysentery

                        • parasites

28

shared diarrhoea after same meal → food poisoning

recent antibiotic treatment → pseudo-membranous colitis (*C. difficile*)

drug taking →
- digoxin (especially in elderly)
- magnesium-containing antacids
- laxatives (especially in elderly)
- guanethedine (for hypertension)

previous surgery →
- post-gastrectomy diarrhoea
- ileal resection with malabsorption

previous illnesses →
- diabetes
- renal disease
- chronic suppuration, especially bronchiectasis (amyloidosis)
- rheumatoid arthritis (amyloidosis)

family history of
diarrhoea →
- coeliac disease (in children)
- ulcerative colitis
- Crohn's disease

Current symptoms

nature of the stools

frequency/timing of diarrhoea

tenesmus

associated abdominal pain

The nature of the stools

volume
- small → inflammatory or neoplastic bowel disease
- large → malabsorption, laxative abuse

consistency
- liquid and uniform → small bowel disease
- loose with bits of faeces → colonic disease
- pale, bulky, offensive → malabsorption
- pellets or ribbons → irritable bowel syndrome

blood
- profuse bright-red → colonic carcinoma
- with mucus or muco-pus → ulcerative colitis, Crohn's disease

mucus only → irritable bowel syndrome

Frequency and timing of diarrhoea

the frequency of the diarrhoea gives an indication of the severity of the condition and is also relevant to the development of excessive fluid and electrolyte loss.

the timing of the diarrhoea is significant in that nocturnal diarrhoea is almost invariably of organic origin.

Tenesmus

the presence of tenesmus suggests a rectal or lower colonic cause for the diarrhoea, and in particular carcinoma: incontinence may also occur if the disease is low in the rectum and involves the internal anal sphincter.

Abdominal pain

the site of abdominal pain indicates whether the small or large bowel are likely to be involved.

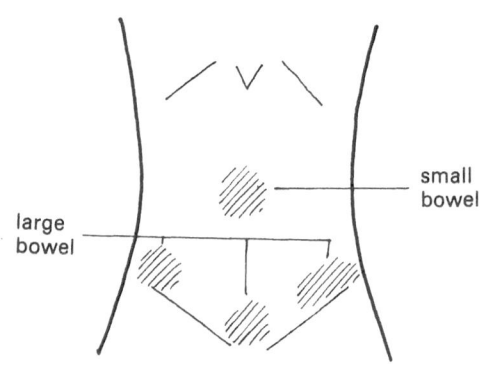

Symptoms in other systems

ulcerative colitis	● painful small joints
Crohn's disease	● pain/stiffness in back
	● painful eyes
	● skin – tender lumps
	ulcers

Endocrine/metabolic disease

diabetes	● thirst
	● polyuria
	● loss of weight
thyrotoxicosis	● heat intolerance
	● sweating
	● nervousness and tremors
	● loss of weight

Diarrhoea

Addison's disease	• excessive fatigue
	• postural dizziness
	• darkening of the skin
uraemia	• previous kidney disease
	• polydipsia
	• hiccups
	• easy bruising
	• muscle twitching
	• paraesthesiae
amyloidosis	• oedema due to nephrotic syndrome
	• breathlessness due to heart failure
	• paraesthesiae due to polyneuropathy
scleroderma	• difficulty in swallowing
	• attacks of cold white fingers
	• painful joints
	• thickening of the skin
carcinoid syndrome	• flushing
	• wheezing

Clinical examination

The extent of examination depends on the presenting clinical picture:

• acute diarrhoea of a few hours/days onset in an adult does not require detailed examination.

• acute diarrhoea and vomiting in an infant/child requires a general examination of chest, ears and abdomen.

• persistent diarrhoea may require very detailed systematic examination and investigation.

Examination should involve	• abdomen – including rectal examination
	• ears, throat and lungs – especially in children
	• eyes
	• joints and spine
	• peripheral nervous system
	• skin

31

Abdominal findings which may be of help are shown in Fig. 2.1.

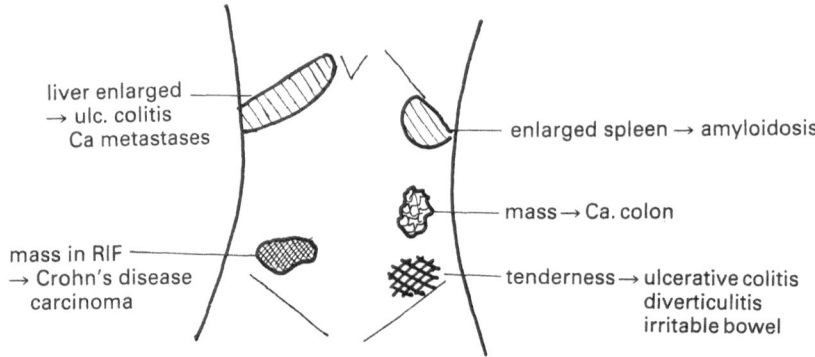

Fig. 2.1   *Abdominal findings in diarrhoea*

ano-rectal exam

Crohn's disease
- perianal bluish discolouration
- anal skin tags
- perianal induration
- abscess
- fistula

cancer of rectum
- mass felt

extra-abdominal findings

general
- cachexia and marked weight loss → carcinoma of colon
- sighing respiration → uraemia
- anaemia → malabsorption, uraemia
- goitre → thyrotoxicosis

skin (including throat)
eyes and ears
musculo-skeletal
neurological
cardiovascular
} Fig. 2.2

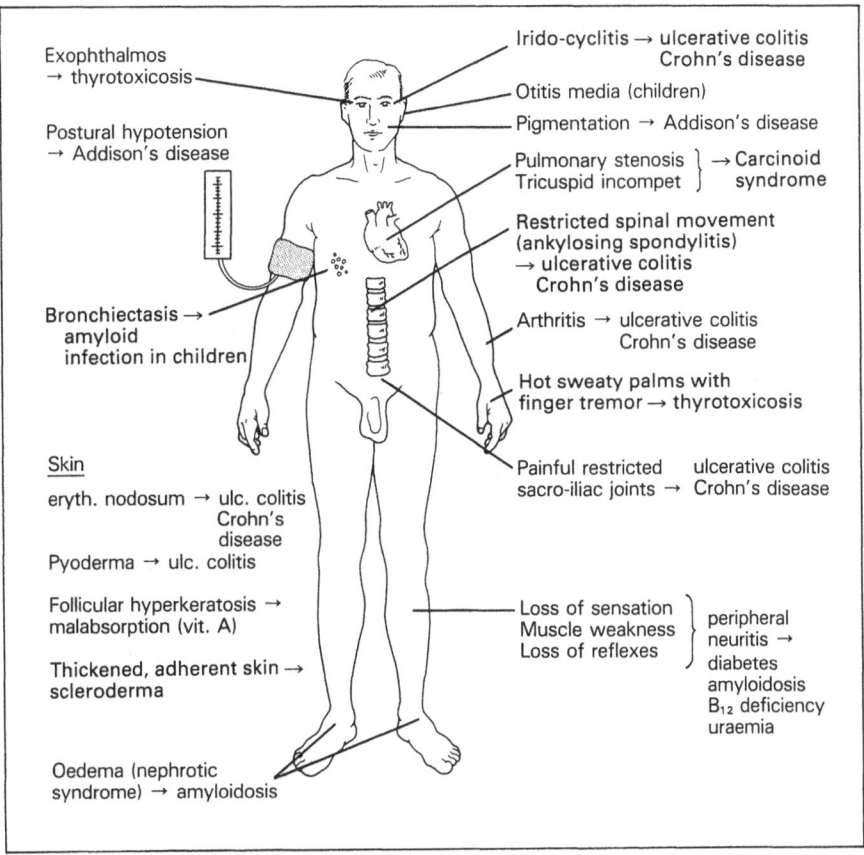

Fig. 2.2 *Extra-abdominal findings of diagnostic help in diarrhoea*

Investigation

Faeces

for *pathogens* – only of value if specific organisms are suspected

- salmonella (enteric fever)
- shigella or entamoeba (dysentery)
- *Giardia lamblia*

In 95% of patients with acute gastro-enteritis no organism is isolated.

occult blood – helpful in	• carcinoma colon
	• inflammatory disease
fat content	• increased in malabsorption

Urine

limited value

- sugar → diabetes
- salmonella → enteric fever
- increased excretion of 5HIAA → carcinoid (a very rare cause of diarrhoea)

Blood tests

acute diarrhoea

- salmonella cultured
- haemagglutination tests for amoebiasis

chronic diarrhoea

- microcytic anaemia → chronic blood loss
- macrocytic anaemia → malabsorption
- hypocalcaemia ⎫
- hypoalbuminaemia ⎭ → malabsorption
- abnormal liver function → ulcerative colitis
  Crohn's disease
- raised blood sugar → diabetes
- reduced serum cortisol → Addison's disease
- abnormal thyroid tests → thyrotoxicosis

Endoscopy – very helpful in chronic diarrhoea for

- visualization of diseased mucosa
- biopsy

procto-sigmoidoscopy

- carcinoma – blood or mucus with normal mucosa
- ulcerative colitis mild – uniform hyperaemia with contact bleeding

  severe – mucosal ulceration with blood or muco-pus
- Crohn's disease – patchy mucosal oedema with linear ulceration ('cobblestones')
- diverticulitis – diverticulae with mucosal inflammation and muco-pus

- laxative abuse (especially senna) – dark brown stains on rectal mucosa (melanosis coli)

colonoscopy – not for routine use in chronic diarrhoea but is helpful in certain circumstances:

- differentating ulcerative colitis and Crohn's disease
- assessment of extent of bowel disease prior to surgery
- to detect carcinoma in long-standing ulcerative colitis
- to biopsy proximal lesion suspicious of carcinoma

Radiology

plain X-ray abdomen – of limited value – may show an outline of ragged ulcerated mucosa in a dilated air-filled segment of bowel in ulcerative colitis.

barium enema

mandatory in chronic diarrhoea

double contrast techniques (barium and air in bowel) give better diagnostic results.

the barium enema findings which are of diagnostic help are –

ulcerative colitis (Fig. 2.3)
- rectum usually involved
- generalized granular outline
- complete loss of haustration
- diffuse shallow ulceration
- pseudo-polyps

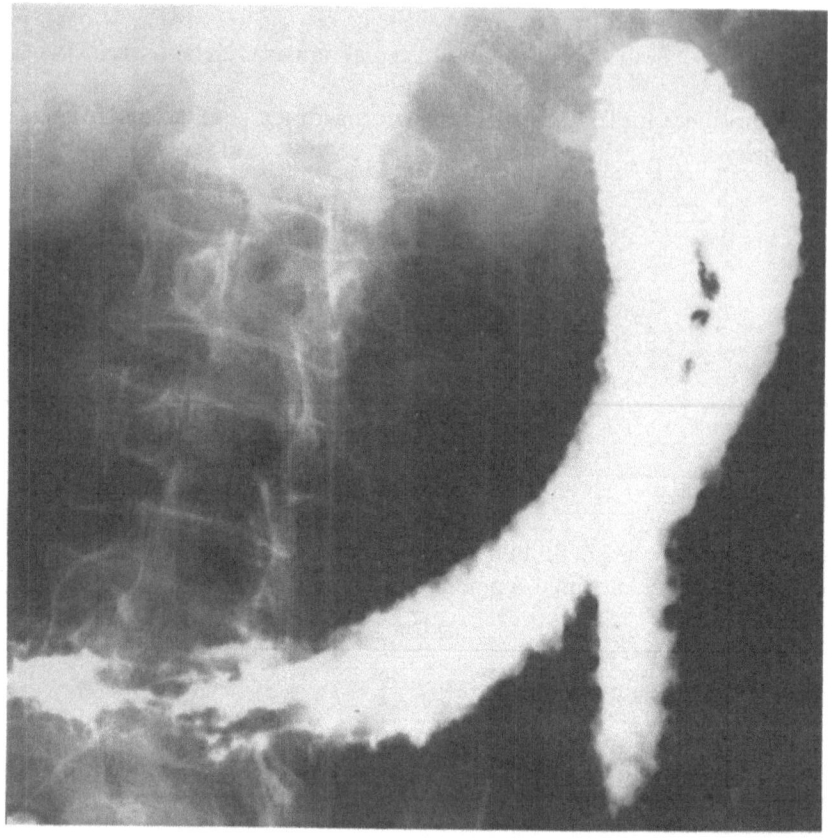

Fig. 2.3 *Barium enema showing ulcerative colitis with a ragged mucosa and loss of haustration*

Crohn's disease (Fig. 2.4)	• irregular segmented pattern ('cobblestone')
	• deep linear ulceration
	• terminal ileum narrow and irregular
	• fistulae common, also strictures
	• incomplete haustral loss
carcinoma (Fig. 2.5)	• polypoid filling defect
	• stricture
diverticulitis	• diverticulae
ischaemic colitis	• 'thumbprinting'
	• fibrous strictures
polyposis	• multiple polyps

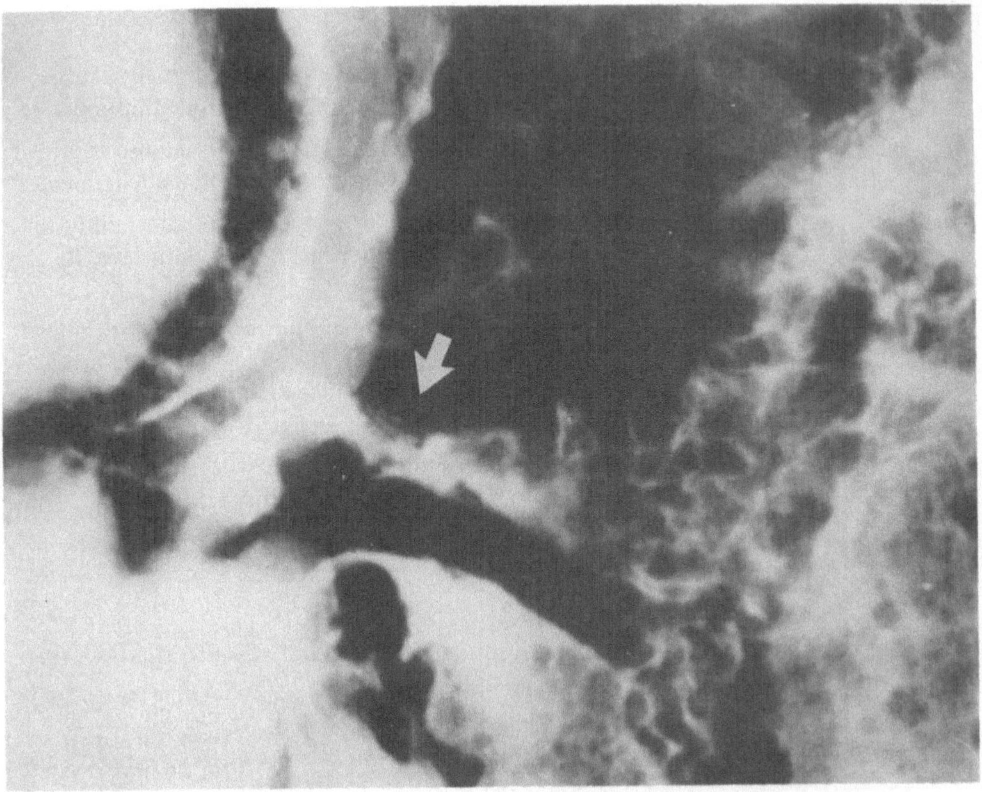

Fig. 2.4 *Small bowel enema showing narrowing and irregularity of the terminal ileum in Crohn's disease*

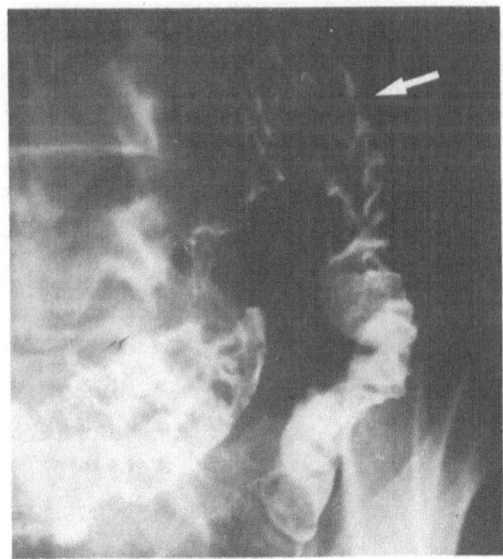

Fig. 2.5 *Barium enema showing filling defect in hepatic flexure of colon due to carcinoma (arrowed)*

Specific conditions

Acute gastro-enteritis

- constitutional symptoms usually present – fever, malaise, muscle aching, nausea and vomiting.
- recent travel abroad especially in countries with poor hygiene may indicate 'traveller's diarrhoea'.
- similar symptoms in a member of the family or other individual sharing a meal indicates food poisoning.
- clinical examination should be directed to dehydration, especially in the elderly, and to bradycardia, rose spots and splenomegaly indicating enteric fever.
- stool cultures not usually necessary unless salmonella, shigella or amoebiasis suspected.
- notify District Medical Officer if an outbreak of food poisoning or enteric fever is suspected.

Pseudo-membranous colitis

- most frequent after ampicillin – also clindamycin
- usually 7 days after drug started – may be up to 3 weeks
- stools watery and bloody: perforation may occur
- stools must be examined for *Clostridium difficile* and its toxin (found in 95% of patients)
- may subside 1 to 3 weeks after drug discontinued
- if severe requires urgent hospital admission for rehydration and vancomycin

Irritable bowel syndrome

- more frequent in younger women (20–40 years)
- vague abdominal pain in varying sites
- 'rumbling', abdominal distension and flatulence frequent
- both constipation and diarrhoea occur
- stools pellet-like or ribbon-like often with mucus
- barium enema is necessary to exclude organic disease and *to reassure the patient*
- added bran and high residue diet may help

Diverticulitis	• predominantly in middle-aged or elderly, both sexes
	• local pain and tenderness in left iliac fossa
	• constipation and diarrhoea both occur
	• rectal bleeding may occur
	• may present as acute abdomen (left-sided) or subacute obstruction
	• urinary symptoms may develop
	• barium enema is the most useful diagnostic test
Cancer	• the most common malignancy of the alimentary tract
	• previous history of long-standing ulcerative colitis or familial polyposis highly relevant
	• right-sided tumours usually produce diarrhoea and left-sided tumours produce obstruction
	• recent change in bowel habit is the diagnostic clue
	• tenesmus suggests a rectal carcinoma
	• rectal examination mandatory in all suspected cases but 25% of growths are beyond examining finger
	• sigmoidoscopy reveals 50% of the tumours
	• barium enema should be carried out and may show tumours beyond sigmoidoscopic reach but the caecum is difficult to visualize
	• colonoscopy is the best diagnostic method for proximal growths
Malabsorption	• Causes

	Intestinal	– surgery	gastrectomy
			ileal resection
		inflammation	Crohn's disease
			tuberculosis
			scleroderma
		infiltration	malignancy
			amyloidosis

               coeliac disease and idiopathic
               steatorrhoea

pancreatic – chronic pancreatitis

               fibrocystic disease

vascular   – chronic mesenteric ischaemia

endocrine – diabetes

               Addison's disease

               hypoparathyroidism

- The diagnostic feature is pale, bulky, offensive stools which are difficult to flush away
- multiple deficiencies may be present with their clinical manifestations

  anaemia (iron, B 12, folate)

  bleeding (vitamin K)

  tetany (low calcium)

  rickets/osteomalacia (vitamin D, calcium)

  dry skin (vitamin A)

  sore tongue and mouth (vitamin B)

  oedema (low serum albumin)

- tests

  barium studies of the small bowel are necessary

  tests of malabsorption of iron, vitamins, calcium, fat and carbohydrate are required

  pancreatic function tests may be required

  biopsy of the small intestinal mucosa may be diagnostic of coeliac disease, sprue and idiopathic steatorrhoea

Ulcerative colitis

- predominantly in young adults (20–40 years)
- systemic symptoms frequent in exacerbations (fever, malaise and loss of weight)
- frequent stools with blood-stained mucus or muco-pus
- abdominal examination shows tenderness over descending colon
- *extra-abdominal manifestations* (Fig. 2.6)

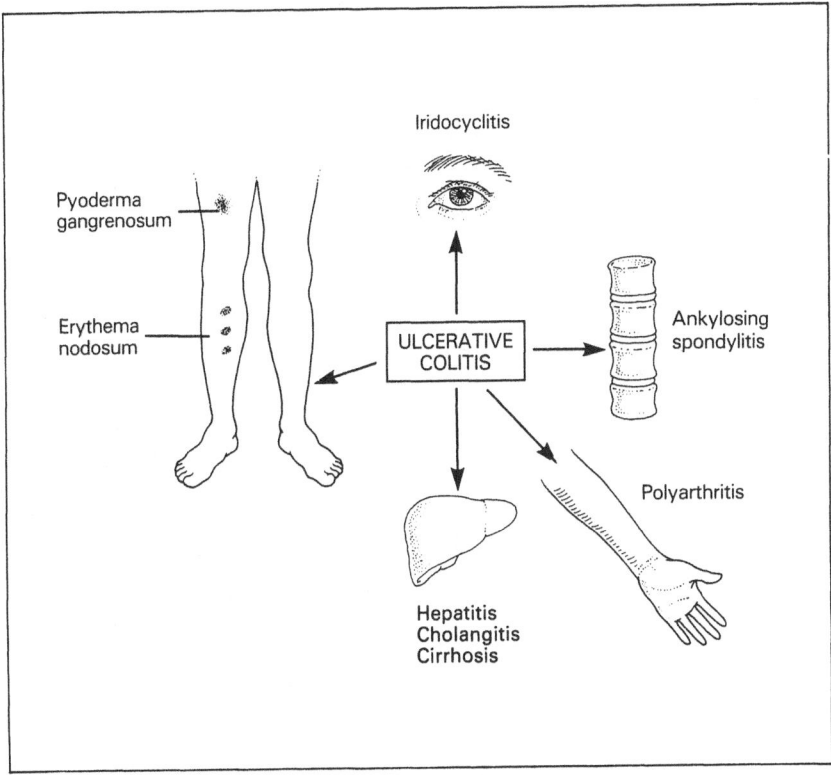

Fig. 2.6   *Extra-abdominal manifestations of ulcerative colitis*

- procto-sigmoidoscopy necessary for diagnosis
    - hyperaemia/oedema
    - red granular mucosa
    - contact bleeding
    - ulcerated mucosa
    - spontaneous bleeding
- barium enema necessary to indicate extent of the disease
    - shallow ulceration
    - loss of haustral patterns
    - uniform shortening and constriction
    - pseudopolyps
- increasing risk of carcinoma in pancolitis of 10 years standing

Crohn's disease

- predominantly young adults (20–40 years)
- may present as acute appendicitis
- recurrent diarrhoea with blood-stained stools and passage of mucus but less than ulcerative colitis
- abdominal pain usually central or right iliac fossa
- clinical signs –

  mass in right iliac fossa

  perianal findings (see p. 32)

  systemic complications similar to ulcerative colitis – eyes, joints, spine, skin, liver
- small bowel enema essential for diagnosis

  terminal ileum narrow and irregular

  segmental involvement

  cobblestone appearance

  deep transverse linear fissures

  strictures

  sinuses

  fistulae
- differentiation from ulcerative colitis

  radiological

  histology most helpful
- prognosis less favourable than ulcerative colitis with both medical and surgical treatment.

Mesenteric ischaemia

- the typical symptoms of atherosclerotic obstruction of the superior mesenteric artery are recurrent post-prandial colicky peri-umbilical pain, 15 to 30 minutes after eating, with diarrhoea
- inferior mesentery artery obstruction is usually acute with severe left sided abdominal pain and bloody diarrhoea.

- clinical examination may show a systolic murmur over the central abdomen due to aortic atheroma, together with other evidence of generalized arteriosclerosis

  premature arcus senilis

  thickened radial artery

  tortuous brachial artery

  reduced or absent foot pulses

  narrowed irregular fundal arterioles with arterio-venous nipping

- barium examination may show 'thumb-printing'
- the only definitive test is aortography and selective angiography of the mesenteric vessels.

Pitfalls in diagnosis

Acute diarrhoea

- Acute appendicitis, tonsillitis, otitis media or bronchitis in children may present with acute diarrhoea.
- Retrocaecal appendicitis in adults may also present with acute diarrhoea.
- Spurious diarrhoea in the elderly may mask faecal impaction.
- Failure to consider acute ischaemic colitis in an elderly patient with acute diarrhoea and bloody stools.
- Failure to enquire for – and search for evidence of – any drugs which may have precipitated the diarrhoea e.g. antibiotics, iron, colchicine.

Chronic diarrhoea

- Laxative abuse and digoxin therapy are easily forgotten especially in the elderly.
- A young patient with vague abdominal pain, mild diarrhoea, normal sigmoidoscopy and normal barium enema may easily be a missed Crohn's disease – a small bowel enema should always be considered in these patients.
- The association of anxiety and diarrhoea should not automatically lead to a diagnosis of functional diarrhoea unless the patient has been fully investigated with sigmoidoscopy and barium studies of both the small and large intestine.
- The psychological state of a patient with ulcerative colitis should not necessarily be considered the cause of the disease – it may well be the result.
- The possibility of carcinoma developing in long-standing extensive ulcerative colitis should always be remembered and the patient considered for colonoscopy.
- Although clinical and radiological features suggest a definite diagnosis of either ulcerative colitis or Crohn's disease, the differentiation between the two conditions may still be, and often is, wrong.

Useful practical points

Acute diarrhoea

- No detailed investigation necessary for first few days.
- Stool examination for ova, parasites and bacteria can be done if facilities are conveniently available.
- Supportive or anti-bacterial treatment not usually necessary except in the debilitated and the elderly.
- Correction of fluid and electrolyte loss required in elderly or debilitated:

    orally at home if possible

    intravenously if severe or oral replacement unfeasible – requires hospital admission
- Hospital admission is considered if:

    diarrhoea not settling

    increasing dehydration

    elderly or debilitated with severe attack

    further investigations required, e.g. enteric fever

    severe attack of pseudo-membranous colitis
- Notify DMO if food poisoning or enteric fever suspected.

Chronic diarrhoea

- Full general medical assessment necessary and not just the alimentary system, especially to detect systemic complications of ulcerative colitis/Crohn's disease.
- Don't forget diabetes as a cause of chronic diarrhoea, or other endocrine causes such as thyrotoxicosis and Addison's disease.
- Laboratory examination of the stool is only necessary if chronic infection with shigella, entamoeba, *Giardia lamblia* is suspected as a cause of the chronic diarrhoea.
- Sigmoidoscopy is required in all cases.
- Barium studies are necessary in all cases:

    large bowel for colonic lesions

    small bowel enema if Crohn's disease suspected.
- Colonoscopy is required if there is a doubtful radiological finding of malignancy.
- Malabsorption studies are mandatory if the stools are pale, bulky, offensive and difficult to flush away.
- Mild ulcerative colitis/Crohn's disease can be managed at home with Salazopyrin and steroid enemas: severe attacks need to be admitted to hospital.

Patient challenge

A 37-year-old housewife presented with a long history of vague abdominal pain in various locations associated with a lot of flatulence and 'rumbling': more recently the pain seemed to concentrate in the right iliac fossa. She had always been constipated but over the last few months her bowels have been loose and she had noticed blood-streaking of the stools. She was also losing weight but thought this was due to a reducing diet she was trying to follow.

She had a past history of anxiety and was taking tranquillizers. She also admitted to heavy periods which she associated with some low backache which had come on over the past year. In the family history her sister had died of carcinoma of the colon at 45 years of age.

Examination

The examination findings are shown in Fig. 2.7.

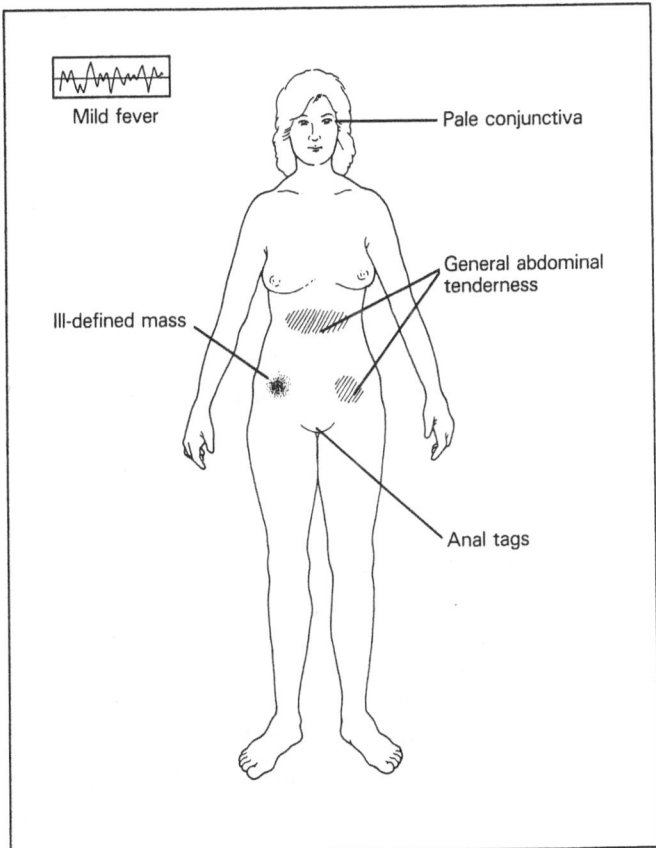

Fig. 2.7 *Examination findings on case challenge*

Questions   Suggest three possible diagnoses
                             What tests would you do to differentiate?

Diagnoses   The three likely diagnoses are:

- irritable bowel syndrome

- carcinoma of the colon

- Crohn's disease

Irritable bowel syndrome

For   history   • long history vague abdominal pain

                          • flatulence, rumbling

                          • constipation

                          • past history of anxiety

               exam   • general abdominal tenderness

Against   history   • rectal bleeding (does not occur in irritable bowel)

               exam   • mass in right iliac fossa

Tests   • barium studies and/or procto-sigmoidoscopy – of
                            no diagnostic help but highly desirable to reassure
                            the patient

Carcinoma of colon

For   history   • family history cancer colon

                          • recent rectal bleeding

                          • recent weight loss

               exam   • mass in right iliac fossa

                          • anaemia

Against   history   • long history

                          • reducing diet may have caused weight loss

                          • menorrhagia may have caused anaemia

               exam   • nil

Tests   • sigmoidoscopy for distal carcinoma

                          • barium enema for proximal carcinoma

                          • colonoscopy to be sure of the caecum

Crohn's disease

For	history	• recurrent abdominal pain
		• bloodstained stools
		• weight loss
		• backache and stiffness (ankylosing spondylitis)
	exam	• fever
		• anaemia
		• mass in right iliac fossa
		• anal tags
Against	history	• flatulence and rumbling unusual
		• diet may have caused weight loss
		• menorrhagia may have caused anaemia
	exam	• nil
Tests		• small bowel enema most useful
		• biopsy anal tag – non-caseating granuloma with giant cells
		• colonoscopy with mucosal biopsy
		• (sigmoidoscopy, barium enema less helpful)

Actual diagnosis:

The patient was found to have Crohn's disease in the small bowel enema which showed segmental narrowing (skip lesions), some deep ulcers and involvement of the terminal ileum and caecum accounting for the mass in the right iliac fossa.

Treatment and course

The patient was treated initially with Salazopyrin 1 g qds without much benefit. Her condition in fact became worse with severe abdominal pain and an increase in bloody diarrhoea. She was admitted to hospital and treated with a combination of oral and rectal steroids and improved considerably. However, the improvement was not maintained when she was taken off the prednisolone and required maintenance prednisolone 7.5 mg/day when her abdominal pain and diarrhoea remained under control.

3 Low Backache

Introduction

The human back's vulnerability is the result of our two-legged posture and propulsion.

Because of its anatomical structure it is the lower back that is particularly prone to strains, injuries and disease.

Causes of backache

Mechanical	• prolapsed intervertebral disc
	• fractures of the spine
	• osteochondritis (Scheuermann's disease)
	• congenital, e.g. lumbar sacralization
Degenerative	• osteoarthritis of the spine
	• spinal stenosis
	• Paget's disease
Inflammatory	• ankylosing spondylitis
	• infections – tuberculosis
	pyogenic
Neoplastic – Bone	
primary benign	• osteoma
	• haemangioma
	• cysts
malignant	• myeloma
	• reticulosis

Secondary	• lung
	• breast
	• kidney
	• thyroid
	• prostate
	• spinal cord tumours
Metabolic	• osteomalacia, rickets
	• osteoporosis
	• hyperparathyroidism
Referred pain	
gastrointestinal	• duodenal ulcer
	• carcinoma pancreas
	• gall bladder disease
	• carcinoma colon
genito-urinary	• renal disease
	• salpingitis/cervicitis
	• tumours
Psychosomatic	• anxiety
	• depression
	• compensation neurosis

Grades of severity

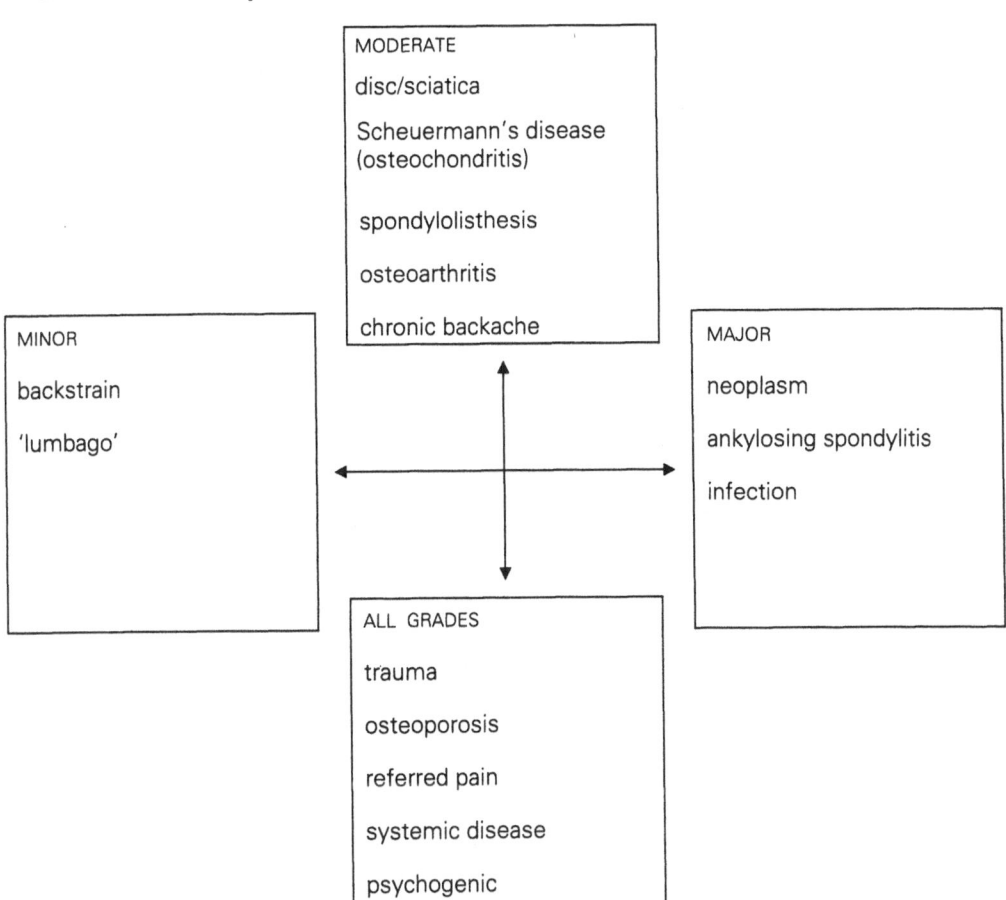

Frequency

Annual prevalence of low backache in a general practice of 2500 persons	
Acute Backstrain 'Lumbago'	50
Disc-sciatica	10
Chronic backache	25
Osteoporosis	5
Trauma (fractures)	2
Ankylosing spondylitis	2
Systemic disease – referred pain	2
Neoplasm Scheuermann's disease Spondylolisthesis	< 1

Age incidence

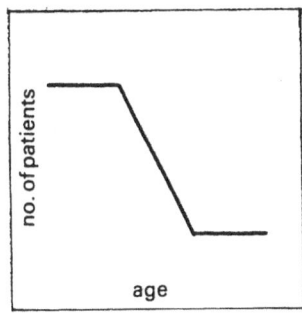

- Scheuermann's disease
- ankylosing spondylitis
- spondylolisthesis
- osteomalacia/rickets
- trauma (fractures)
- prolapsed disc

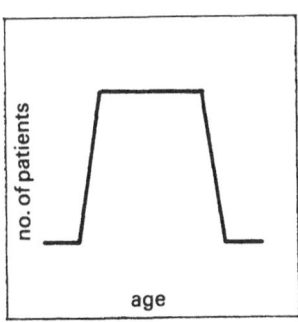

- acute back strain
- lumbago
- chronic back
- disc-sciatica
- osteoarthritis

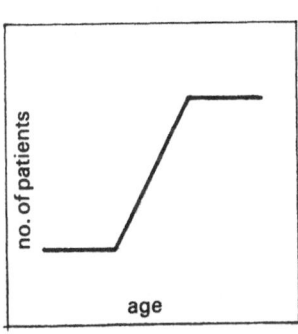

- osteoporosis
- neoplasms
- Paget's disease
- polymyalgia rheumatica
- osteoarthritis

Diagnostic approach

History

Duration – recurrent long-standing pain is likely to be of benign origin.
A sudden onset of acute back pain, especially in the elderly is likely to be due to organic disease.

Location – lumbar backache is the common site and the cause is usually benign. Acute pain in the dorsal spine is likely to be more serious and may indicate malignancy, especially in the elderly.

Radiation – radiation down the leg indicates nerve root irritation and the most likely cause is a prolapsed intervertebral disc.
The distribution of the radiated pain indicates the nerve root affected (Fig. 3.1).

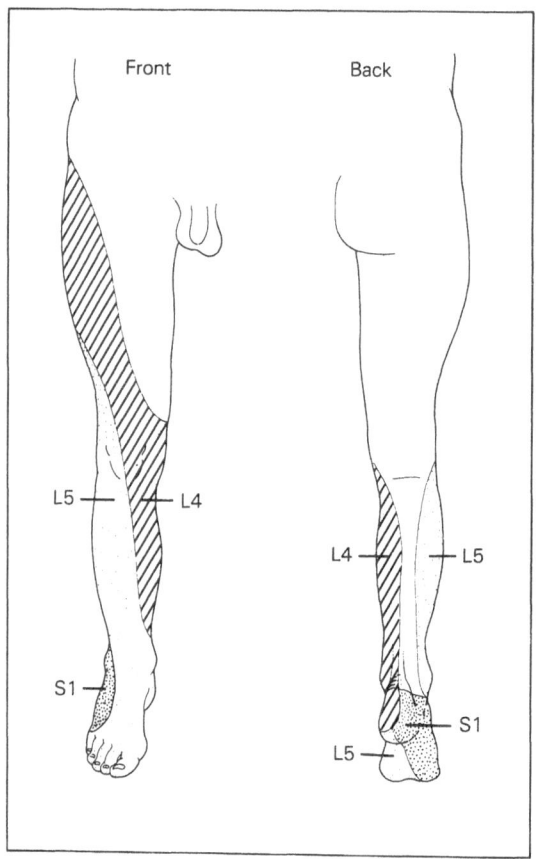

Fig. 3.1   *Radiation of pain in disc lesions at L4, L5, S1*

Precipitation – the diagnostic value of aggravating factors is:

   worse with movement →   • mechanical pain

                        • degenerative pain

   worse after resting → inflammatory pain

   worse on prolonged sitting → prolapsed disc

worse with prolonged standing → ·prolapsed disc

worse with coughing → prolapsed disc

worse in morning → ankylosing spondylitis

worse at night →
- neoplastic disease
- systemic disease

Relief – in general, mechanical causes of pain are better with rest while systemic and neoplastic causes are worse with rest

Associated symptoms – the importance of constitutional and other symptoms is shown in Fig. 3.2.

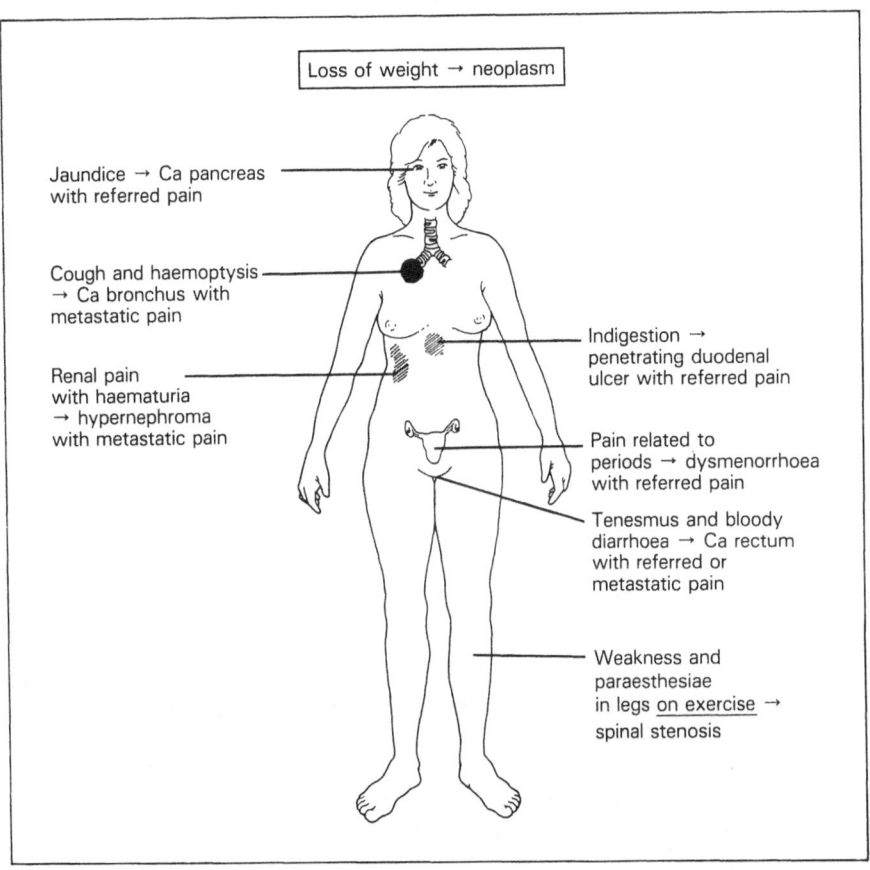

Fig. 3.2 *Value of associated symptoms in diagnosing back pain*

Examination

Back

posture
  loss of lumbar lordosis → disc lesion, inflammatory condition
  scoliosis (due to protective muscle spasm) → disc lesion
tenderness over spine → inflammation or neoplasm
restricted movement
  touching toes →
  - prolapsed disc
  - osteoarthritis
  lateral flexion
  - *one side* →
      disc lesion
      osteoarthritis
  - *both sides* → ankylosing spondylitis

Legs

restricted straight leg
raising
  - supine → L5/S1 lesion
  - prone → L4 lesion
impaired reflexes
  - knee jerk → L4 lesion
  - ankle jerk → S1 lesion
muscle power
  - weakness plantar flexion → S1 lesion
  - wasting of glutei → S1 lesion
  - weakness foot dorsiflexion → L5 lesion
  - weakness of quadriceps → L4 lesion

skin sensation – the impairment of light touch and pin-prick sensation related to the different nerve root involvement is shown in Fig. 3.1.

A particular sensory abnormality which should always be sought and is often forgotten is involvement of the *cauda equina* which produces loss of perineal sensation (S4): the most frequent cause is spinal stenosis due to ingrowth of osteophytes narrowing the spinal canal.

Table 3.1 summarizes the neurological differentation on clinical examination between L4, L5 and S1, the most frequent nerve roots affected by discs.

Table 3.1 *Clinical features of L4, L5 and S1 lesions*

	Pain	Weakness	Sensory impairment	Reflex reduced
L4	lateral thigh medial calf	dorsiflexion foot extension knee	medial leg	knee-jerk
L5	buttock back of thigh lateral leg	extension of hip flexion knee dorsiflexion foot	lateral calf dorsal and medial foot	usually none
S1	buttock back of thigh calf	flexion knee plantar flexion	lateral foot heel sole of foot	ankle-jerk

General and abdominal examination

The findings which might be relevant in the diagnosis of back pain are shown in Fig. 3.3.

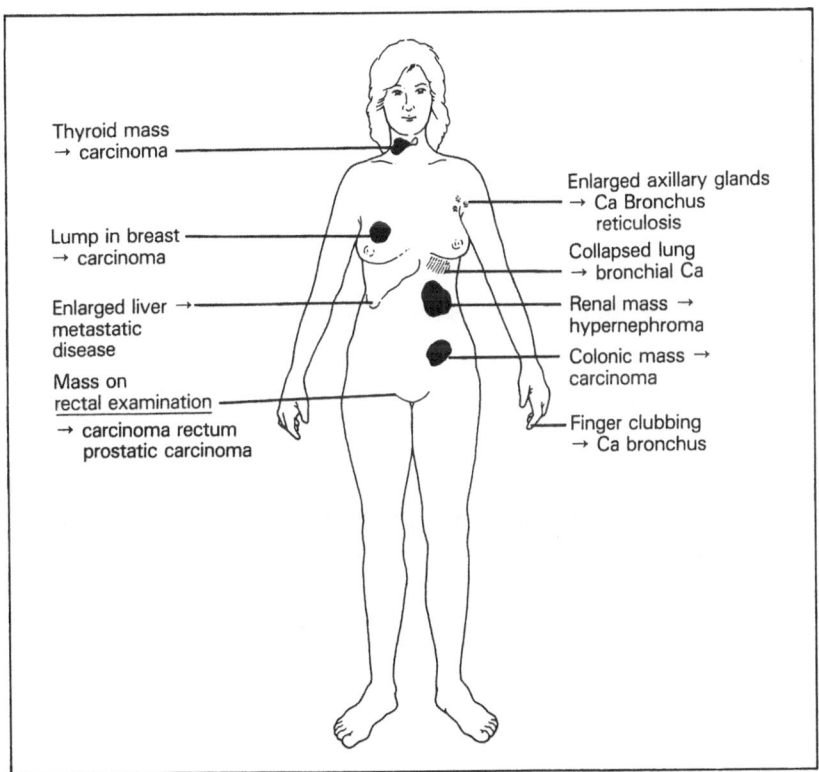

Fig. 3.3 *General signs of value in diagnosing back pain*

A summary of the main differentiating points between mechanical and systemic causes of back pain is shown in Table 3.2.

Table 3.2 *Differentiation between mechanical and systemic causes of backache*

	Mechanical	Systemic
Pain	worse on movement	worse at rest and at night
	worse with straining/coughing/ sneezing	
	intermittent	persistent and progressive
	unilateral buttock/leg pain	bilateral leg pain
Associated symptoms	none	constitutional, e.g. fever, weight loss
Examination	unilateral restriction of straight leg raising	bilateral restriction of straight leg raising
	unilateral root signs	bilateral root signs
	local spinal tenderness rare	local spinal tenderness frequent
		local tumour mass may be felt

Investigation

Radiology

plain X-ray spine

seldom helpful – not necessary as routine because

- it is normal in most cases of prolapsed intervertebral discs
- it does not show early metastatic disease
- osteoarthritic and spondylotic changes are often present in asymptomatic individuals

if pain severe and persistent, spinal X-rays are necessary and may show significant abnormalities (Fig. 3.4)

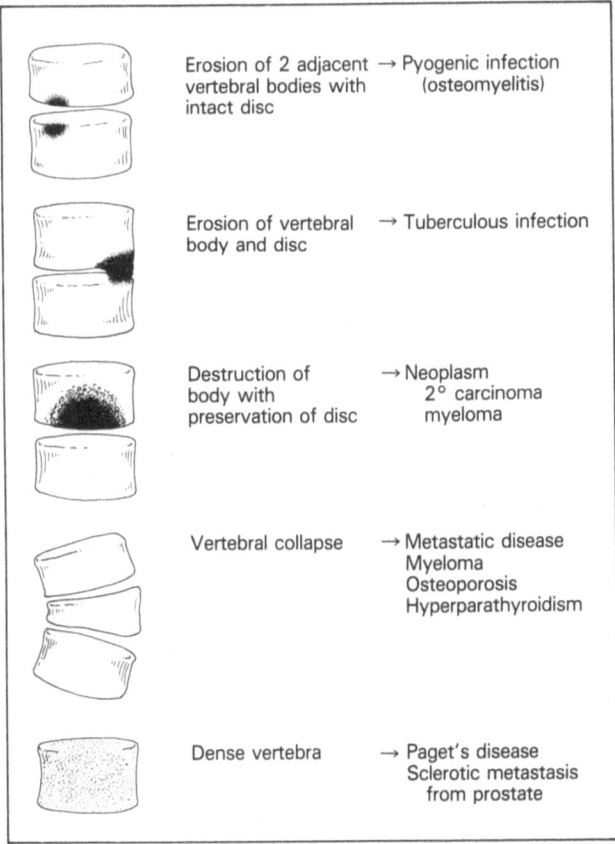

Fig. 3.4 *Diagnostic changes in plain X-ray of the spine in patients with back pain*

myelography – indications:

- a clinically diagnosed disc lesion with no improvement after 6 weeks strict bed rest
- surgery is being considered for recurrent back trouble interfering with life and/or work
- increasing neurological signs
- cauda equina pressure e.g. acute retention
- cause of persistent back pain not known

radiculography
This test in which dye is injected into the subarachnoid space to outline the nerve roots is a more accurate test for diagnosing disc lesions and other causes of back pain if the level of the lesion is known.

CT scan

This may well turn out to be the most useful test for investigation of back pain but is as yet still being researched and in any case is not generally available.

- *Technetium-99 bone scan*
  Useful in the diagnosis of metastatic deposits in the spine.

Blood tests

ESR ↑ indicates inflammatory or neoplastic disease

Serum *calcium/phosphate/alkaline phosphatase* – helpful in diagnosing hyperparathyroidism and in distinguishing osteoporosis and osteomalacia

	Calcium	Phosphate	Alkaline phosphatase
Osteoporosis	normal	normal	normal
Osteomalacia	normal or ↓	↓	↑

In Paget's disease serum calcium and phosphate are normal while the alkaline phosphatase is very high.

Serum *acid phosphatase* – this is high in carcinoma of prostate

Other tests

urine examination – Bence Jones protein indicates myelomatosis

sternal marrow – may help in the diagnoses of myelomatosis, reticulosis or carcinomatosis

Specific conditions

Backstrain – lumbago
- the usual cause is a prolapsed disc
- fairly sudden onset
- often precipitated by trauma e.g. lifting, twisting, bending
- low back pain
- back stiffness
- difficulties in movement particularly flexion and extension of the spine
- pain may radiate to buttocks or groins

- SLR normal
- can walk with difficulty
- investigations unnecessary
- usually settles with rest in a couple of weeks
- often recurs – a spinal support may be helpful

Sciatica

- the usual cause is a disc lesion
- fairly sudden onset
- may be related to definable cause (often minor)
- radiation of pain down leg to foot – the distribution depends on the nerve root involved (see Fig. 3.1)
- pains in leg may be worse than in back
- SLR limited
- ankle reflex diminished
- beware of bowel–bladder dysfunction if cauda equina is involved (urgent assessment indicated and ?surgery)
- investigations – only in specialist unit
- surgery may be required for cases not responding to rest, or in which there are repeated recurrences

Chronic low backache

- considerable functional disability
- persistent – recurrent
- pain may be referred down leg(s)
- painful, stiffness, limited movements
- SLR – reflexes variable
- X-rays show narrowing of disc spaces and osteophytosis – often present in asymptomatic individuals so its clinical significance is uncertain
- a compensation claim for work or accidental injury may be a contributory factor in the persistence of the pain
- depression and other emotional disturbances may be associated

Ankylosing spondylitis
- persistent low backache in young male adult
- stiff spine with progressive kyphosis
- the clinical features are shown in Fig. 3.5
- often associated anxiety/depression (beware of missed diagnosis)
- X-rays – characteristic sacro-iliac changes of sacro-iliitis
- ESR raised +
- HLA-B 27 antigen usually present
- progressive if untreated

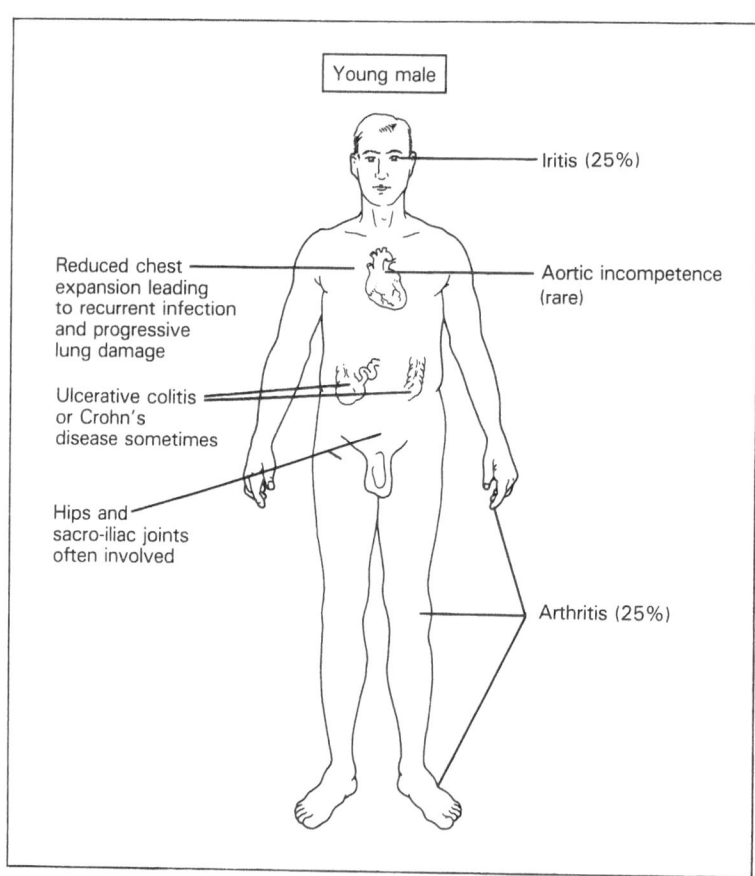

Fig. 3.5 *Clinical features of ankylosing spondylitis*

Osteoporosis

- F > M
- frequently postmenopausal
- almost inevitable ageing process in both sexes but occurs later in men than women
- loss of height
- kyphosis
- not all osteoporotic spines cause pain
- pain more prominent in upper lumbar and thoracic regions
- dull ache with episodes of severe acute pain if compression fractures
- X-rays – bone density not radiologically changed until 50% of mineralized bone is lost
- blood – serum calcium/phosphate and alkaline phosphatase normal

Neoplasms

- beware of new backache in the over 50s with no past history of back problems
- vague onset
- variable pain – may be very severe
- frequently at night in bed
- most often secondary neoplasms – the common primary sites are shown in Fig. 3.6
- multiple nerve root involvement may occur
- constitutional signs frequent e.g. fever, anorexia, loss of weight
- diagnosis made on X-ray of the spine but confirmation can be obtained with a radioactive scan (technetium-99)
- if myeloma suspected the relevant tests are:

    urine for Bence Jones protein

    very high ESR (> 100 mm/h)

    electrophoresis for abnormal M-protein

    bone marrow examination for myeloma cells

    X-ray of the skull often shows a distinctive appearance (Fig. 3.7)

63

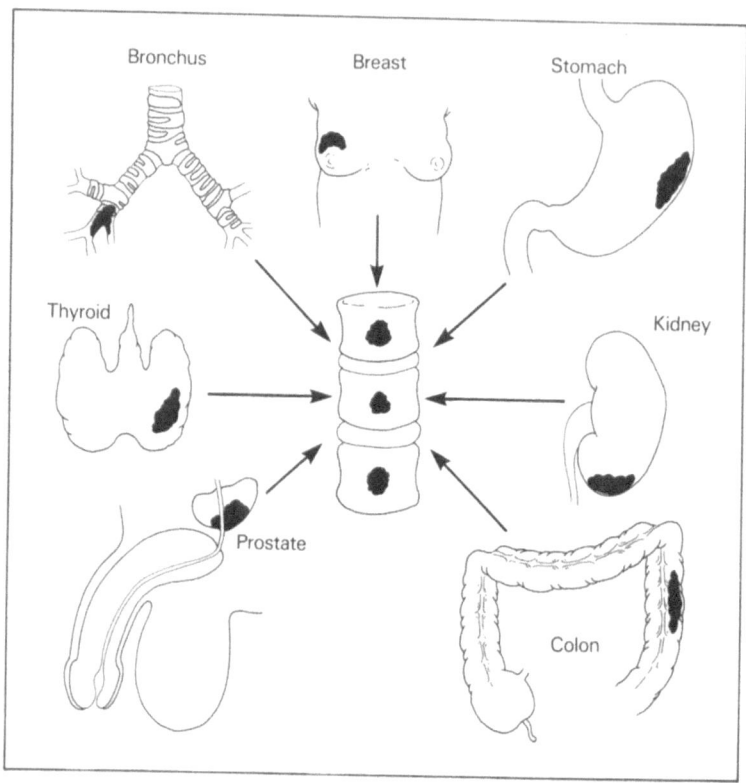

Fig. 3.6   *Common primary carcinoma metastasing to spine*

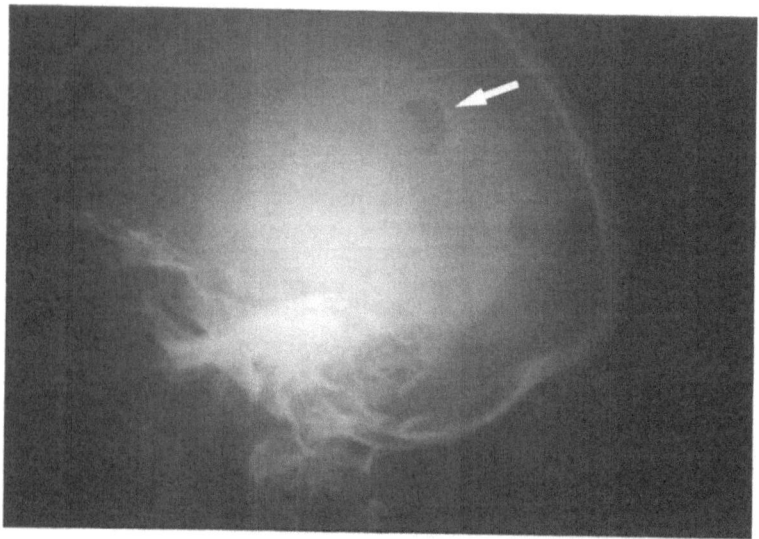

Fig. 3.7   *X-ray of skull showing filling defects (arrowed) due to myeloma*

Spinal stenosis

- usually caused by protrusion of osteophytes narrowing the spinal canal, but may rarely be congenital
- blood supply to cauda equina may be affected leading to weakness, numbness or burning in the lower limbs on exertion and relieved by rest. May be confused with intermittent claudication but the differentiation is shown in Table 3.3
- long history of backache frequent
- may lead to bowel and bladder symptoms from involvement of the cauda equina
- best detected by myelography

Table 3.3 *Differentiation of spinal stenosis and intermittent claudication*

Spinal stenosis	Intermittent claudication
Foot pulses present	Foot pulses absent
Pain mainly in back and thighs	Pain mainly in calves
Walking produces weakness as well as pain	Walking produces pain only
Pain eased by flexing spine	Pain relieved only on resting
Walking uphill produces less symptoms than downhill	Walking uphill aggravates the pain
Bowel and bladder symptoms may be present	No bowel or bladder symptoms

Pitfalls in diagnosis

- It may be very difficult to assess degree of pain and incapacity in a workman with back pain when no signs are present especially if compensation is involved.
- Any elderly patient with a new onset of back pain should have the spine X-rayed to exclude metastases.
- Spinal metastasis may simulate a disc lesion.
- Enquiry for urinary and bowel symptoms is often forgotten in assessing backache – they may be highly relevant in aetiology of the backache and also as a complication, especially in spinal stenosis.
- Spinal stenosis may be easily mistaken for intermittent claudication, especially if only pain is involved – the presence of good foot pulses should suggest the correct diagnosis.
- A tumour of the spinal cord is often forgotten as a cause of 'sciatica'
- A retroverted or prolapsed uterus is a very rare cause of severe or persistent backache.

Useful practical points

- Back pain in childhood or adolescence is uncommon and may be serious.
- Sudden onset of acute mid-dorsal pain in an elderly patient is often due to neoplastic disease – metastasis and myeloma are the commonest types.
- Chronic back pain may be a manifestation of discontent either at work or at home without any other psychiatric symptoms evident.
- Observation of the natural spinal movement of a patient with backache during the consultation may be helpful in deciding the cause.

Case challenge

A 55-year-old car salesman complained of the gradual development of aching in the lower lumbar region over a period of several weeks and more recently the pain had spread to the lateral side of his left thigh and medial side of the left leg. The pain was worse on straining or coughing and had started to keep him awake at night. He had suffered with two previous attacks of 'lumbago' in the last 5 years but the pain had

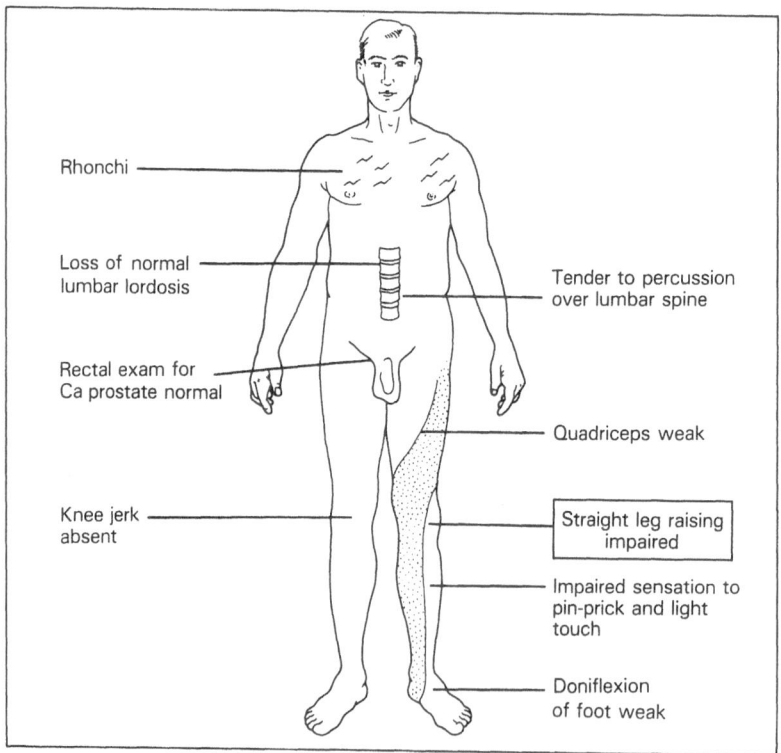

Fig. 3.8   *Clinical findings in case challenge*

never gone down his leg before. He drank fairly heavily and smoked 25 cigarettes a day for the past 40 years and had a chronic 'smoker's cough' as a result. He had lost weight over the last few weeks.

The examination findings are shown in Fig. 3.8.

Questions	What is the main differential diagnosis?
	What nerve root is involved?
	What tests would you carry out?

Possible diagnoses

- sciatica due to prolapsed intervertebral disc
- nerve root irritation due to neoplastic disease of the spine

Prolapsed intervertebral disc

For	history	• typical distribution of pain
		• worse on straining
		• 2 previous attacks
	exam	• SLR reduced
		• signs of root involvement
Against	history	• pain progressive over several weeks
		• not relieved by rest in bed
		• previous lumbago not associated with sciatica
	exam	• nil
Tests		• myelography
		• radiculography
		• CT scan if available

Neoplasm of the spine

For	history	• heavy smoker
		• pain worse at night
		• loss of weight
	exam	• tender over lumbar spine
Against	history	• nil
	exam	• nil

Tests

X-ray of the spine	• vertebral collapse
	• metastasis
	• myeloma
if metastasis	• chest X-ray for cancer bronchus
	• barium studies for cancer stomach or colon
	• IVP for cancer kidney or other renal disease
	• thyroid scan for carcinoma
	• blood tests

                acid phosphatase for cancer prostate

                ESR for myeloma

                electrophoresis for myeloma M-protein

            • urine test for Bence Jones protein (myeloma)

            • blood urea – renal disease including carcinoma

Which nerve root?

the pointers are	• pain lateral thigh, medial leg
	• sensory impairment medial leg
	• weak knee extension and foot dorsiflexion
	• absent knee jerk

these indicate L4 involvement (Fig. 3.1)

Actual diagnosis:
Carcinoma of lung with metastases in L4–L5 bodies

The diagnosis was made by
- X-ray spine → metastases
- chest X-ray → hilar lesion
- bronchoscopy/biopsy → anaplastic carcinoma

Treatment and course

Surgery is not feasible with hilar lesions. Radiotherapy for lung lesion was not considered necessary since there was no mechanical compression and no lung pain. Local radiotherapy was given to the metastatic deposits in his back to ease the pain. He survived only 4 months.

4 Multiple Painful Joints (Polyarthritis)

Introduction

Joints are target organs for a number of distinct disease processes

Clinical manifestations of painful joint swellings result from many varied causes

They can affect all ages

They present fascinating diagnostic challenges for the clinician

Causes (classification)

Degenerative
- osteoarthritis

Inflammatory
- sero-positive rheumatoid arthritis (80%)
- sero-negative rheumatoid arthritis (20%)
- ankylosing spondylitis
- psoriatic
- Reiter's syndrome
- Behçet's syndrome

Collagen disease
- systemic lupus erythematosus (SLE)
- polyarteritis nodosa (PAN)
- scleroderma
- mixed connective tissue disease
- giant cell arteritis

Nutritional
- scurvy
- rickets

Metabolic	• gout
	• pseudogout (pyrophosphate crystals)
	• sarcoid
	• amyloid
	• Mediterranean fever
	• familial hypercholesterolaemia
Infective	• rheumatic fever
	• viral (rubella, mumps, chicken pox, hepatitis, glandular fever)
	• infective endocarditis
	• bacterial (gonococcal, meningococcal, tuberculosis, brucellosis)
Blood diseases	• haemophilia
	• sickle cell disease
	• leukaemia
	• thalassaemia
Anaphylactoid	• Henoch–Schönlein
	• drug/serum sickness
Neoplasms	• hypertrophic pulmonary osteoarthropathy
	• lymphoma

Grades of severity

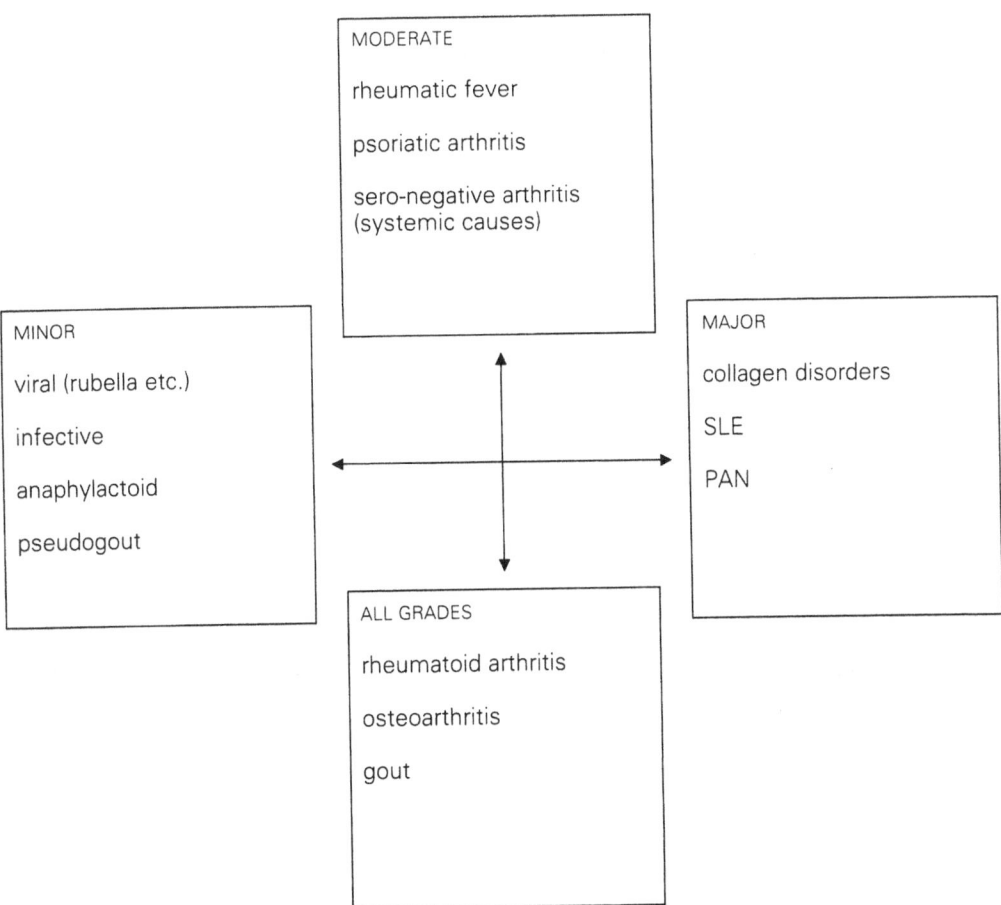

MODERATE

rheumatic fever

psoriatic arthritis

sero-negative arthritis
(systemic causes)

MINOR

viral (rubella etc.)

infective

anaphylactoid

pseudogout

MAJOR

collagen disorders

SLE

PAN

ALL GRADES

rheumatoid arthritis

osteoarthritis

gout

Note: 'rheumatism' accounts for one third of all severe disability in the community.

Frequency

Annual prevalence of polyarthritis in
a general practice population of 2500

---

osteoarthrosis	60
rheumatoid arthritis	13
gout	5
psoriatic	2
other sero-negative arthritis	1

less than 1 per year

infective and viral	1 in 3 years
anaphylactoid	1 in 5 years
collagen disease	1 in 10 years
rheumatic fever	1 in 20 years

Age incidence

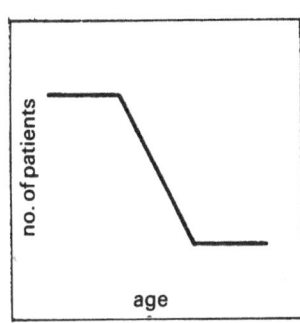

- Still's disease
- Henoch–Schönlein
- rheumatic fever
- glandular fever
- leukaemia
- haemophilia
- scurvy
- osteomyelitis
- post-viral, e.g. rubella

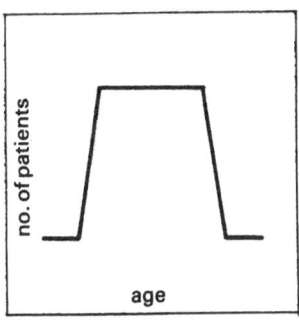

- rheumatoid arthritis
- sero-negative arthritis e.g. ankylosing spondylitis
- psoriatic
- collagen disorders
- viral e.g. hepatitis B, glandular fever
- systemic e.g. ulcerative colitis, Crohn's disease

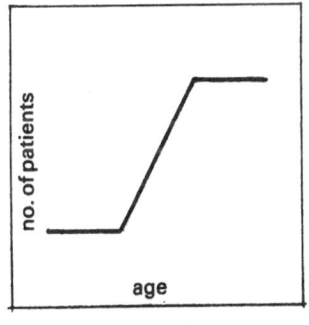

- osteoarthrosis
- gout
- pseudogout

Diagnostic approach

History

Onset

    acute polyarthritis

- rheumatic fever
- rubella
- viral hepatitis

- gonococcal
- brucellosis

chronic polyarthritis
- rheumatoid arthritis
- osteoarthrosis
- gout
- psoriasis
- collagen disease
- Reiter's disease
- systemic disease

Distribution – some helpful diagnostic features are shown in Fig. 4.1

Duration of joint pain – migratory or flitting joint pains are a distinctive feature of:
- rheumatic fever
- other infective and post-infective polyarthritis ·
- collagen disorders

rheumatoid arthritis is distinguished by the chronicity of the joint pains

Age and sex incidence

the age incidence of polyarthritis is shown on page 73

sex incidence

females
- rheumatoid arthritis
- systemic lupus erythematosus

males
- ankylosing spondylitis
- gout
- Reiter's disease
- polyarteritis nodosa
- giant cell arteritis

Family history may be relevant in some conditions:

74

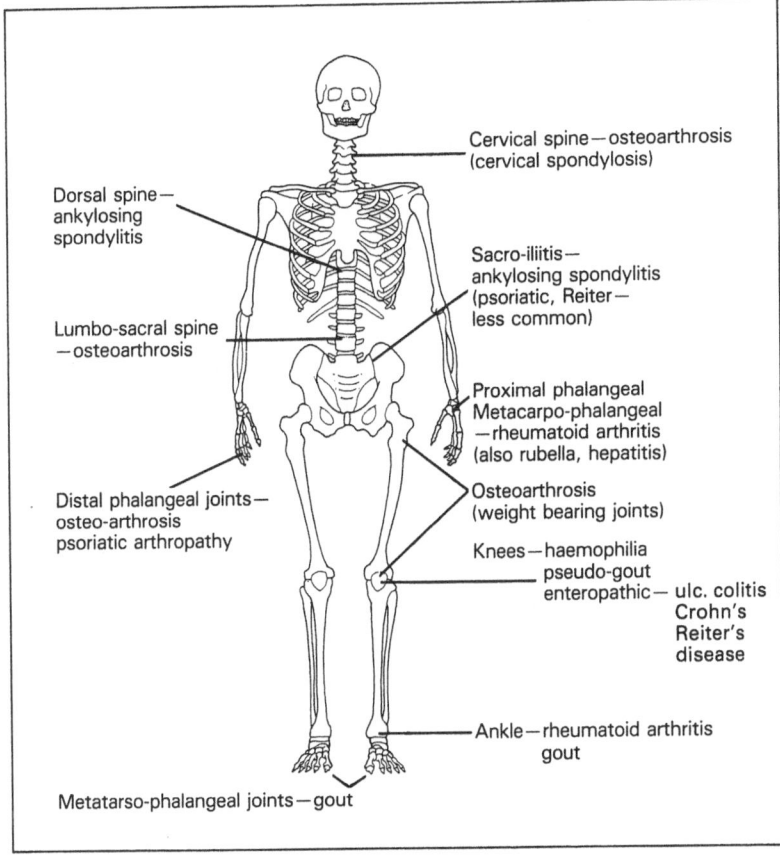

Fig. 4.1 *Joints affected in different conditions*

- rheumatoid arthritis
- ankylosing spondylitis
- enteropathic arthropathy
- collagen disorders
- psoriasis
- gout
- pseudogout (pyrophosphate arthropathy)
- haemophilia

the familial association in the first four conditions may either be with the arthritis itself or with other auto-immune diseases

Diurnal variation

    worse in the morning
- rheumatoid arthritis
- ankylosing spondylitis

    worse in the evening
- osteoarthrosis

Aggravation/relief
- worse after rest → rheumatoid arthritis
- worse after use → osteoarthrosis
- better with rest → infective arthritis

Association with other auto-immune disease – indicates auto-immune origin:
- pernicious anaemia
- Hashimoto's thyroiditis
- rheumatoid arthritis
- other collagen disorders
- ulcerative colitis
- Crohn's disease
- hypoparathyroidism

Associated symptoms – the presence of symptoms other than those due to arthritis may help to establish its cause

    painful eyes →
- enteropathic arthritis
- rheumatoid arthritis
- Reiter's disease
- ankylosing spondylitis

    pleuritic chest pain →
- rheumatoid arthritis
- systemic lupus erythematosus

    cold white fingers →
- rheumatoid arthritis
- scleroderma

    diarrhoea →
- ulcerative colitis/Crohn's disease
- amyloidosis

    sore throat →
- rheumatic fever
- glandular fever

    painful micturition →
- Reiter's disease
- gonorrhoea

    temporal headache →
- giant cell arteritis

asthma ⎫
paraesthesiae ⎬ → • polyarteritis nodosa
limb weakness ⎭

skin rashes → • psoriasis

• rheumatic fever

• rubella

mouth ulcers → • Behçet's syndrome

jaundice → • hepatitis B

Disability

a simple functional grading is helpful in assessing severity and response to treatment

   in the home • getting in/out of bed

• washing/bathing

• dressing

• coping with stairs

• coping with housework

   in the community • getting out of the house

• ability to shop

• ability to work

grading of incapacity can be based on ability to perform these tasks

completely independent at home and work

independent with some aids/appliances

partially dependent (help in dressing/toilet)

completely dependent (confined to bed/wheelchair)

Examination

Joints – a systematic examination must be carried out

   redness → • septic joint

• gouty joint

• rheumatic fever

   tenderness → • indicates disease activity

swelling →	• fluid
	• bony → osteoarthrosis
	• soft tissue → synovial tissue involved
	• bursae → repeated trauma
range of movement	• passive
	• active
limitation due to	• pain
	• effusion
	• muscle spasm
	• joint deformity
	• muscle contracture
crepitus	• fine → rheumatoid
	• coarse → osteoarthrosis

joint deformity

local muscle wasting → severe disease

pattern of joint
involvement

- • small joints (symmetrical) → rheumatoid
- • big toe → gout
- • lower > upper limbs → Reiter's disease
- • weight-bearing joints → osteoarthrosis
- • sacro-iliac joints

  ankylosing spondylitis

  psoriasis

  Reiter's disease

Other systems – the signs which may be of diagnostic help are shown in Fig. 4.2.

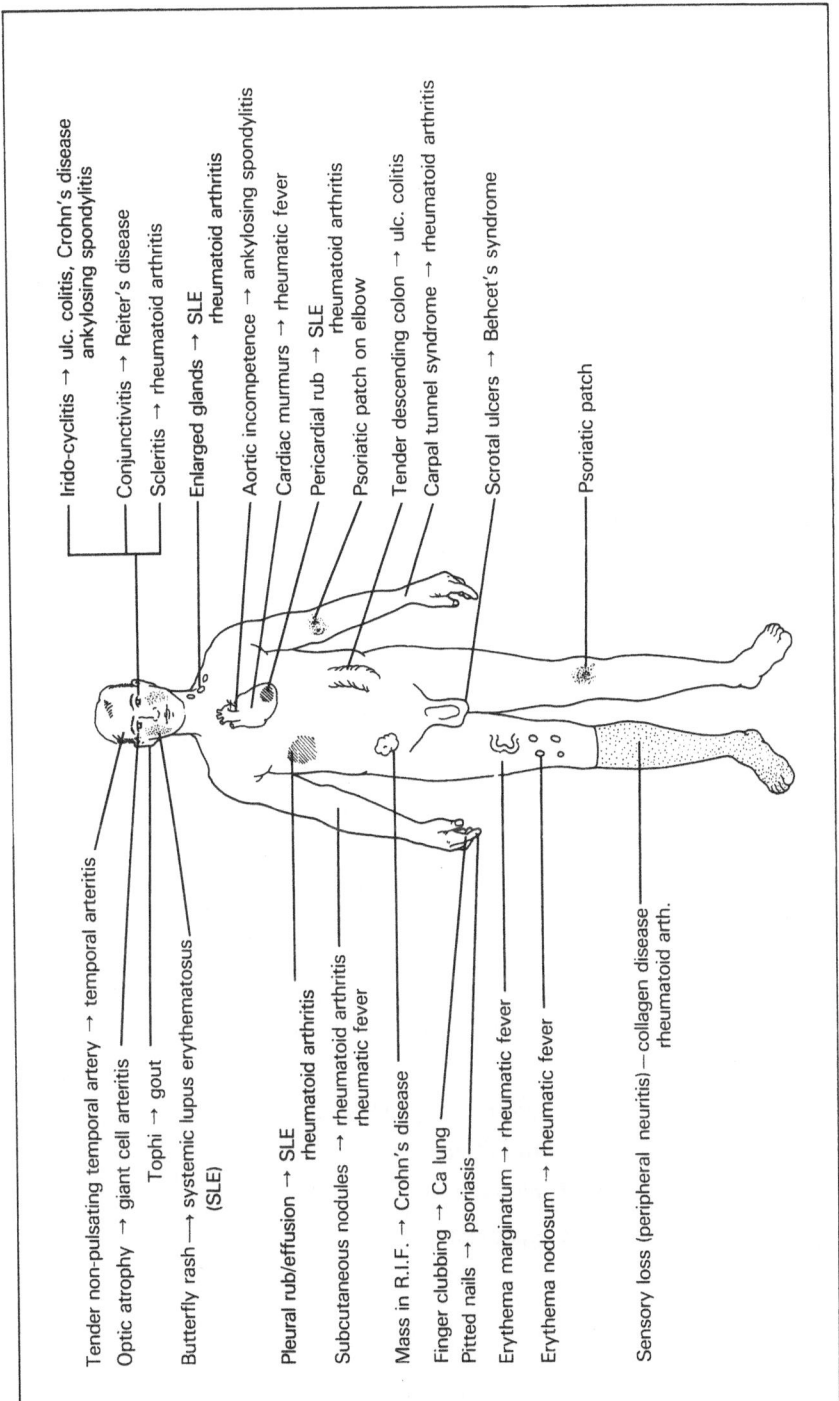

Fig. 4.2 *Signs of diagnostic help in polyarthritis*

Investigations

Radiology

plain X-ray

the conditions in which a plain X-ray picture of the affected joints gives diagnostic help are shown below:

Type of arthritis	Joints affected	X-ray changes
Rheumatoid arthritis	proximal interphalangeal metacarpophalangeal metatarsophalangeal	juxta-articular osteoporosis erosions joint margins joint destruction
Psoriatic	distal interphalangeal joints interphalangeal	erosions joint margins 'pencil-in-cup' appearance
Ankylosing spondylitis	thoraco-lumbar spine sacro-iliac	'bamboo' spine erosions marginal sclerosis
Gout	metatarsophalangeal	lateral marginal 'punched-out' erosions
Pseudogout	knees	pyrophosphate crystals in articular cartilage
Osteoarthrosis	lumbo-sacral spine cervical spine hips knees	loss of joint space marginal osteophytes joint sclerosis

some typical changes are shown in Figs. 4.3 a–d

arthrography – this is of limited value in the diagnosis of polyarthritis. The indications for this type of X-ray examination are shown:

knee
- injury to meniscus
- tears of the ligaments
- popliteal cysts

hip
- check prosthesis
- synovial disease

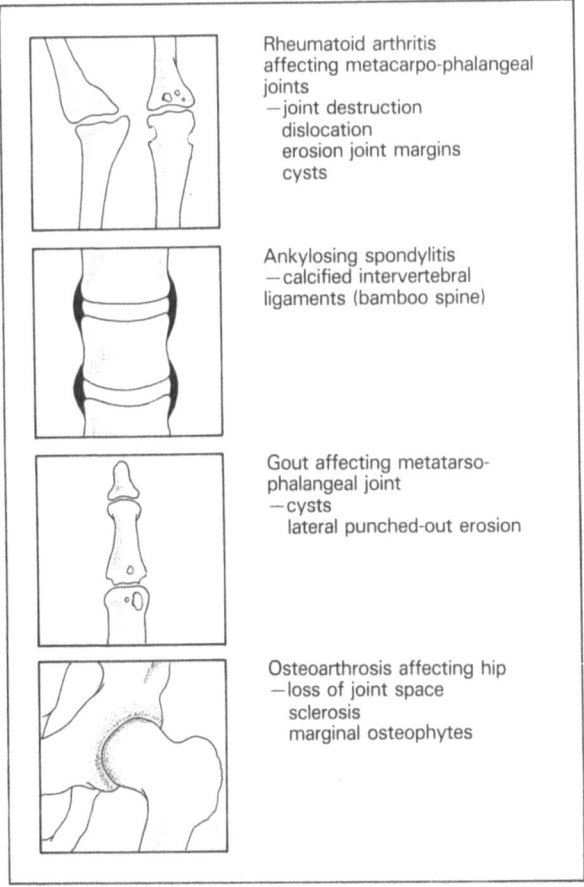

Rheumatoid arthritis
affecting metacarpo-phalangeal
joints
—joint destruction
 dislocation
 erosion joint margins
 cysts

Ankylosing spondylitis
—calcified intervertebral
ligaments (bamboo spine)

Gout affecting metatarso-
phalangeal joint
—cysts
 lateral punched-out erosion

Osteoarthrosis affecting hip
—loss of joint space
 sclerosis
 marginal osteophytes

Fig. 4.3   *Typical changes in plain X-ray*

shoulder

- rotator cuff tears
- adhesive capsulitis
- dislocation
- synovial disease
- biceps tendon injuries

other joints

- mainly for ligament injury

Blood tests

Evidence of inflammation

white blood count

high
- infection
- gout
- juvenile polyarthritis

low
- SLE
- Felty's syndrome
- drug sensitivity e.g. gold

ESR
- sensitive marker especially in RA
- non-specific
- affected by packed cell volume (anaemia)

plasma viscosity – good marker unaffected by
- age
- sex
- packed cell volume

acute phase proteins
– other proteins:
- C-reactive protein usual
- haptoglobin
- anti-trypsin
- caeruloplasmin

normal values
- WBC 4×10^9–10×10^9/litre
- ESR males up to 20 mm/h
  females up to 30 mm/h
- plasma viscosity 1.5–1.7 centipoises
- C-reactive protein 0–20 μg/ml

Immunology

Types of test
- rheumatoid factor
- antinuclear antibodies
- DNA binding tests
- HLA typing
- other antibody tests

Rheumatoid factor

    present
- rheumatoid arthritis (80%)
- chronic juvenile arthritis (15%)
- SLE (40%)
- scleroderma (30%)
- polyarteritis nodosa (30%)

    absent
- psoriasis
- ankylosing spondylitis
- enteropathic arthritis

Antinuclear antibodies
- SLE (99%)
- severe rheumatoid arthritis (30%)
- Felty's syndrome (60–80%)
- juvenile polyarthritis with iridocyclitis
- scleroderma

DNA binding test – has replaced LE test
- SLE – virtually invariable
- rheumatoid arthritis (20%)
- polyarteritis nodosa (20%)
- infective endocarditis
- chronic active hepatitis
- sarcoidosis

HLA typing
- ankylosing spondylitis (almost all) – B27
- rheumatoid arthritis – DR4, DW4
- psoriatic arthritis – B27, BW38
- Reiter's disease – B27
- Sjögren's syndrome – DW3

Anti-lymphocyte antibodies – occurs especially in SLE and may contribute to thrombocytopenia

Antibodies to infection
- anti-streptolysin titre in rheumatic fever
- brucella agglutination test
- virus infections: rubella

    mumps

    Coxsackie

    Monospot in glandular fever

    hepatitis B
- gonococcal fixation test

Biochemistry

urea/creatinine ↑
- connective tissue disease
- gout

uric acid ↑
- gout

calcium – increase
- hyperparathyroidism
- sarcoidosis

decrease
- connective tissue disease

alkaline phosphatase ↑
- rheumatoid arthritis
- bone infections
- Paget's disease

Analysis of synovial fluid

	Inflammatory	Septic	Crystal	Osteo-arthrosis
Appearance	cloudy yellow	cloudy green	cloudy yellow	clear yellow
Viscosity	low	low	low	high
Clotting	yes	yes	sometimes	no
Cells – total WBC/mm³ polymorphs (%)	2000–75 000 > 50	>100 000 > 75	200–2000 < 25	200–2000 < 25
Crystals	–	–	uric acid pyrophosphate	–
Organisms	–	present	–	–
Complement (CH50)	low in rheumatoid arthritis	normal	normal	normal

Arthroscopy/biopsy of synovial membrane

Indications
- diagnosis of tuberculosis
- diagnosis of synovial tumours

Specific conditions

Rheumatoid arthritis (RA) (Fig. 4.4)

- F>M
- onset may be sudden or gradual
- may be in single joint at first but soon involves others symmetrically
- usual joints (in order): hands
  knees
  wrists
  ankles
  feet
  jaw
  neck
  elbows

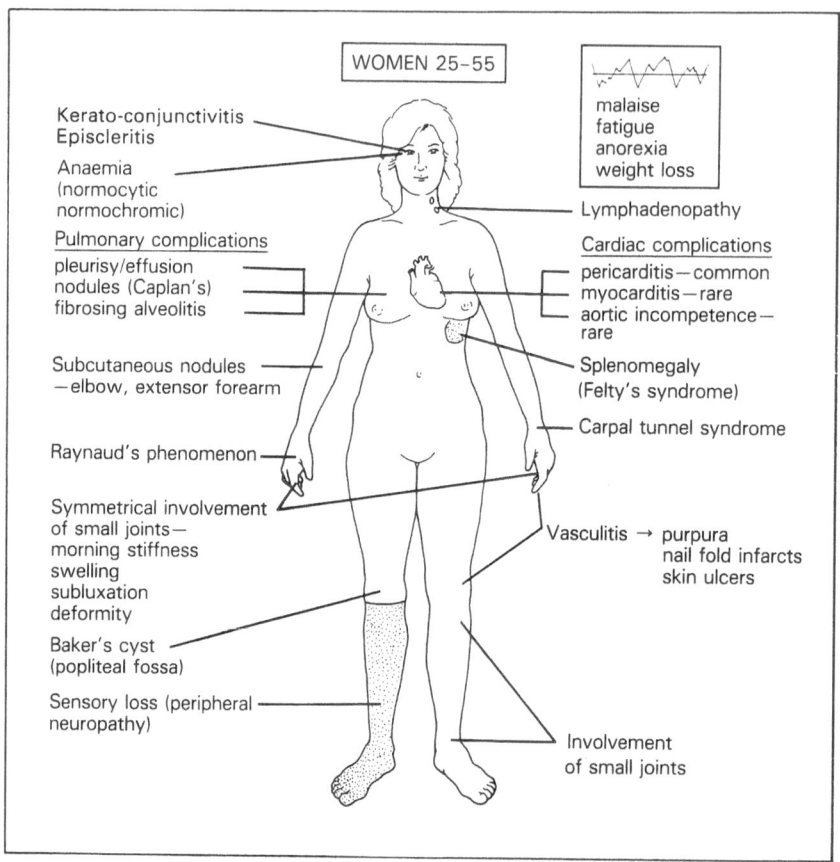

Fig. 4.4   *Clinical manifestations of rheumatoid arthritis*

- investigations: normocytic normochromic anaemia

ESR ↑

C-reactive protein ↑

plasma viscosity ↑

rheumatoid factor (80%)

X-rays

soft tissue swelling

juxta-articular osteoporosis

joint destruction

synovial fluid – reduced complement (CH50)

Osteoarthrosis (OA) (Fig. 4.5)

Causes

- developmental, e.g. Perthes' disease
- trauma, e.g. fractures involving joint
- occupational, e.g. pneumatic drill worker
- metabolic, e.g. haemachromatosis, Wilson's disease
- endocrine – acromegaly
- inflammatory – rheumatoid, gout
- neuropathic, e.g. tabes, diabetes
- Paget's disease

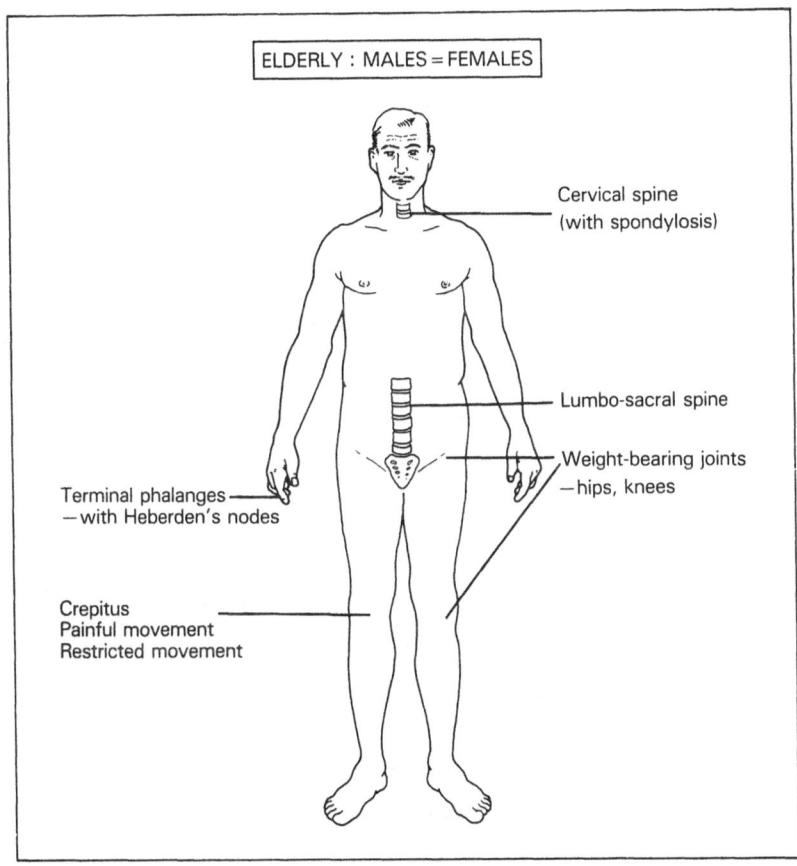

Fig. 4.5   *Clinical features of osteoarthrosis*

Features

- M = F
- sometimes polyarthritic (usually monoarthritic)
- slow onset – progressive
- synovial joints affected
  - knees
  - hips
  - distal i-p joints of hands
  - 1st metacarpo-phalangeal joint
  - Heberden's nodes
  - neck
  - lumbo-sacral
- degenerative 'joint failure'
- worse at end of day
- varies with weather, activities, and day to day
- exacerbations and remissions
- family history negative

Investigations

- only test of value is X-ray

Gout (Fig. 4.6)

- M > F
- onset earlier in men (40–50) than women (60+)
- FH+ in males
- *acute attack*
  - dramatic severe pain
  - most single joint – foot
    - knee
    - ankle
    - wrist
  - skin red, shiny and hot
  - exquisite tenderness
  - often recurs
  - may be precipitated by diuretics, alcohol
  - relief with NSAID, steroid, colchicine

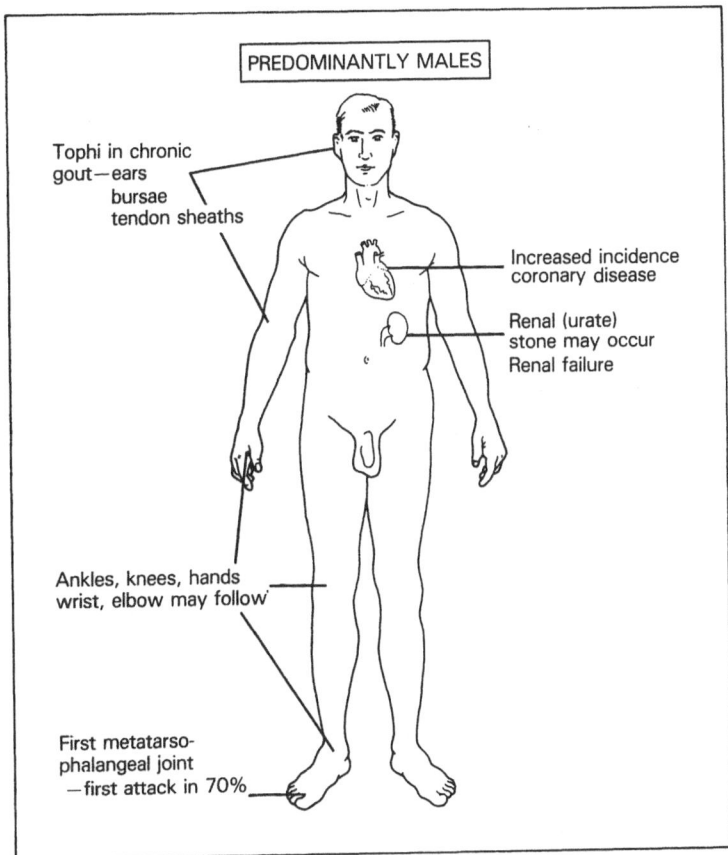

Fig. 4.6   *Common features of gout*

- *polyarthritic*

    slow onset

    tophi – ears, elbows, big toe, Achilles tendon

    destructive arthritis

- investigations

    serum uric acid level ↑

    X-rays – punched-out erosions at edge of joint margins

    renal: blood urea/creatinine may be ↑

             IVP – urate stones

    synovial fluid – urate crystals

- *other causes of hyperuricaemia*
    blood – leukaemia, polycythaemia
    renal failure
    hyperparathyroidism
    drugs – thiazides, salicylates, nicotinic acid
    lead poisoning
    psoriasis
    Down's syndrome

Psoriatic arthropathy (Fig. 4.7)

- M = F
- in 10% of psoriasis
- rash present (arthropathy may precede rash)
- acute or slow onset
- unrelated to severity of skin disease
- distal finger joints
- neck/spine may be affected
- 'sausage fingers or toes' – whole digit affected
- nails pitted

- investigations
    rheumatoid factor absent (sero-negative)
    X-rays
      terminal interphalangeal joint involvement and asymmetry distinguishes from rheumatoid arthritis
      spine – ankylosing spondylitis
      sacro-iliac joints – sacro-iliitis

Pseudogout (pyrophosphate arthropathy)

- M = F
- age related – increasing incidence after 70 years
- deposition of calcium pyrophosphate in articular cartilage
- knees, wrists, pubis, lumbar spine, shoulders

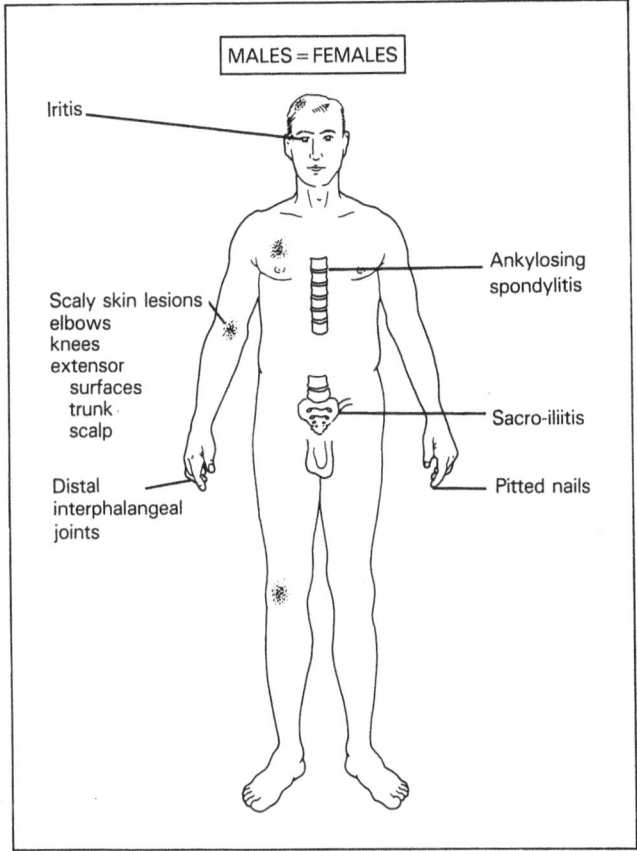

MALES = FEMALES

Iritis

Ankylosing
spondylitis

Scaly skin lesions
elbows
knees
extensor
 surfaces
  trunk
  scalp

Sacro-iliitis

Distal
interphalangeal
joints

Pitted nails

Fig. 4.7   *Clinical features of psoriatic arthropathy*

- acute attacks (commonest cause of acute arthritis in elderly)

- chronic progressive type causes destructive de-generative changes with bone cysts – knees, wrists, hips, shoulders

- investigations

  X-rays – crystals in articular cartilage

  synovial fluid – crystals of calcium pyrophos-phate

Reiter's syndrome (Fig. 4.8)
- M>F
- age 15–30
- polyarthritis follows non-specific urethritis (NSU) or diarrhoea
- knees, ankles, feet, hips
- asymmetrical
- plantar fasciitis and Achilles tendinitis
- acute onset 10 days after NSU or diarrhoea
- susceptible individuals (often HLA B27 positive)
- conjunctivitis/iritis
- urethritis
- mouth ulceration
- attack may last up to 6 months
- recurrence common

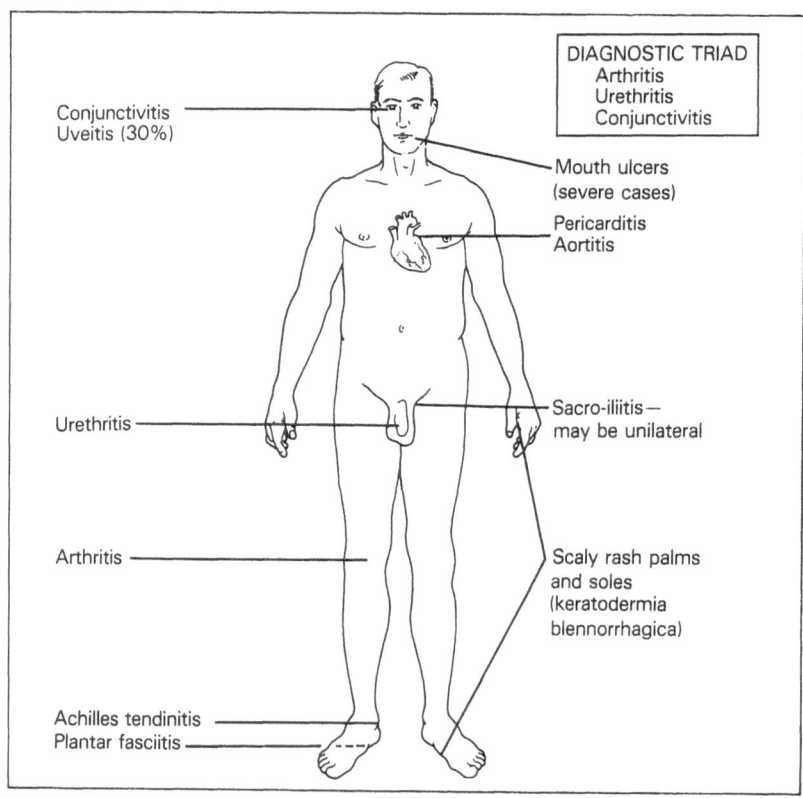

Fig. 4.8   *Clinical features of Reiter's disease*

Joint swellings

- investigations
- ESR – very high, persistent
- HLA B27 in >70%
- rheumatoid and antinuclear factors absent
- synovial fluid: high leucocyte count
                        macrophages
- X-rays –   periostitis – 'whiskering' in pelvis
                  calcaneal spur
                  knee erosions
                  periostitis – fingers

SLE (Fig. 4.9)

- F > M
- 15–30 years
- acute onset
- severely ill
- small joints: asymmetrical
- flitting pains
- butterfly rash (face)
- lymph glands +
- endocarditis/pericarditis
- lung/pleura involved
- renal: glomerulonephritis
             nephrotic syndrome
- peripheral neuritis

- investigations
  blood count – pancytopenia
  antinuclear antibodies >90%
  anti-DNA antibodies > 90%
  rheumatoid factor – 40%
  renal biopsy: focal change
                  membraneous nephritis
                  proliferative nephritis

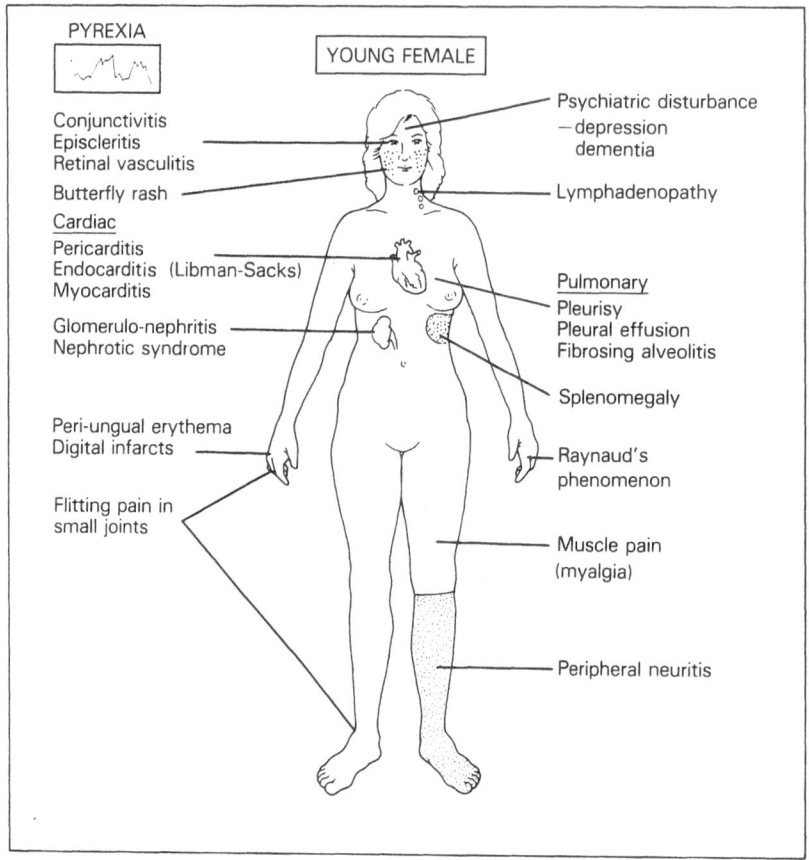

Fig. 4.9 *Common features of SLE*

Pitfalls in diagnosis

- 'Rheumatoid' type polyarthritis may be associated with systemic disease.
- In young – think of SLE.
- In elderly – think of neoplasm especially in men, e.g. bronchus.
- Always check other systems and examine the whole patient.
- Septic arthritis may be overlooked in a rheumatoid patient on steroids.
- Gout can be overlooked if a single large joint is affected.
- X-ray changes of osteoarthrosis are universal in elderly and may easily be blamed for joint pain which it is not in fact causing – this applies especially to the cervical spine.
- Underlying rheumatoid arthritis may easily be missed in a joint showing the secondary development of osteoarthrosis.

Useful practical points

- OA may be polyarthritic.
- ESR is a useful simple screening test.
- 'Cures' are unusual but much can be done to relieve and rehabilitate.
- 'Care' is often life long and has to be regularly supervised.
- The anaemia of rheumatoid arthritis is related to disease activity and doesn't respond to iron treatment.
- Loss of lateral flexion of the spine is the first physical sign of ankylosing spondylitis.
- Treat old people with arthritis at home if possible – they do not do well in hospital.

Case challenge

A 48-year-old woman with a long history of arthritis presented with acute pain in both knees worse on the right side. The arthritis had been present for at least 15 years and had initially affected her hands but had subsequently spread to involve her wrists, elbows, knees and ankles. For the past 5 years she had been treated with oral prednisolone 7.5 mg daily, and during a recent exacerbation the oral prednisolone was supplemented with local injections of hydrocortisone into both knees with some relief of the pain.

There was a past history of recent pleurisy since when she had been breathless on exertion and also had been left with an irritating dry cough.

The examination findings are shown in Fig. 4.10

Questions

What is your differential diagnosis?

What tests would you do?

What treatment would you recommend?

Possible diagnoses

- relapse of rheumatoid arthritis
- systemic lupus erythematosus
- ruptured Baker's cyst
- septic arthritis

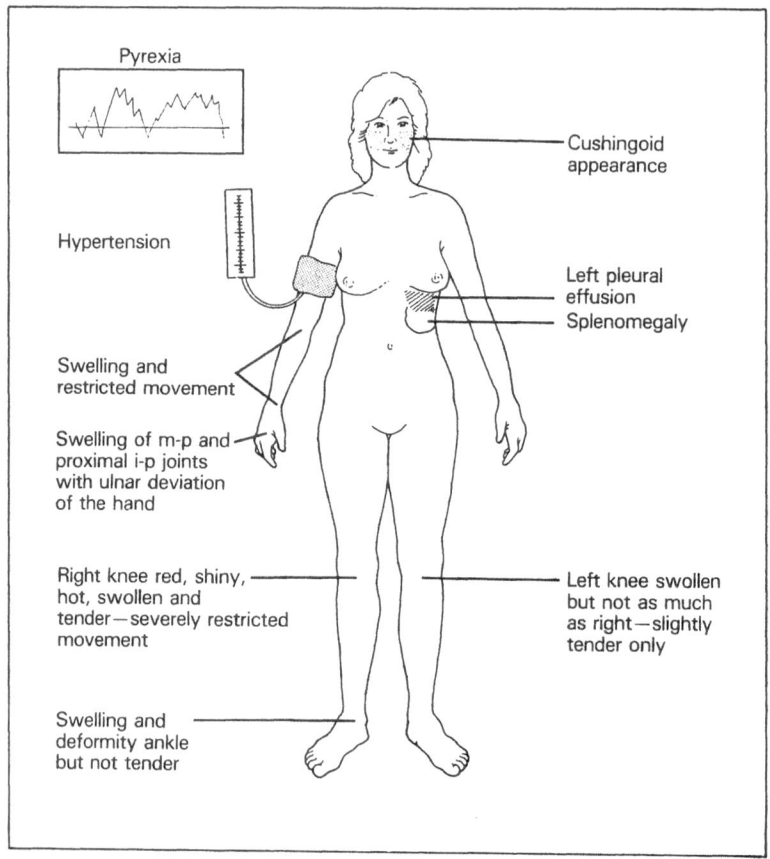

Fig. 4.10   *Findings on examination*

Relapse of rheumatoid arthritis

For	history	● long history of arthritis affecting small joints
		● acute exacerbations frequently occur
	exam	● changes typical of rheumatoid arthritis in the hands
		● pleural effusion – can occur in RA
		● splenomegaly – can occur in RA
Against	history	● joint involvement in acute exacerbations of rheumatoid arthritis tends to be symmetrical
	exam	● same point – asymmetrical involvement of the knees

96

Joint swellings

Tests		• synovial fluid analysis from joint aspiration is the best differentiating test between RA and septic arthritis
		• antinuclear antibodies – best test to distinguish RA from SLE – present in virtually all SLE but only 30% of patients with RA.

Systemic lupus erythematosus

For	history	• pleurisy – more frequent in SLE than RA
	exam	• pleural effusion
		• splenic enlargement
Against	history	• no permanent joint changes in SLE
	exam	• findings in knees very unusual in SLE – joints rarely show a severe acute inflammatory reaction
Tests		• antinuclear antibodies – 99% positive in SLE
		• anti-DNA antibodies – virtually all active SLE

Baker's cyst

For	history	• a ruptured Baker's cyst can produce severe pain in knee
		• common in association with rheumatoid arthritis
	exam	• nil
Against	history	• patient presented with acute pain in *both* knees
		• no pain in calf
	exam	• no calf tenderness or calf signs simulating venous thrombosis which is common with Baker's cyst
Tests		• best test is arthrogram

Septic arthritis

For	history	• steroid treatment in RA encourages infection
		• right knee more painful than left
	exam	• findings in right knee very compatible with acute infection
		• marked pyrexia

Against	history	• nil
	exam	• nil
Tests		• synovial fluid analysis
		• blood culture

	Septic arthritis	RA
Appearance	turbid green	less turbid yellow
WBC/mm^3	> 100 000	< 75 000
Neutrophils %	> 75%	< 75%
Organisms	+ film/culture	negative
Complement	normal	CH50

Actual diagnosis:

Septic arthritis right-knee

Penicillin-G sensitive *Staph. aureus* isolated

Diagnosis made on joint aspiration

Treatment

joint immobilized with a splint

IV penicillin – four megaunits 6 hourly for 2 weeks then oral amoxycillin 250mg eight hourly for a further month (if penicillinase-producing organisms resistant to penicillin G, use cloxacillin)

joint aspirated daily till no more fluid (surgical drainage may be necessary if joint aspiration blocked)

Outcome

rapid pain relief

control of infection within 48 hours

progressive improvement and full recovery in 6 weeks

5 Indigestion

Introduction

'*Indigestion*' is a patient's way of communicating a package of symptoms apparently referable to the gastrointestinal tract.

At the patient's level it implies:

consciousness of actions of process of digestion

abdominal discomfort

vagueness and imprecision of symptoms

common symptoms	
	• pain/ache
	• fullness/distension
	• wind/flatulence/flatus
	• heartburn/reflux
	• problems with swallowing
	• rumbling/'butterflies'
	• anorexia
	• nausea and vomiting

Causes of 'indigestion' (dyspepsia)

Oesophagus	
	• acid regurgitation
	• spasm
	• aerophagy
Stomach	• acute gastritis
	alcohol
	drugs
	• gastric ulcer

- gastric carcinoma
- hiatus hernia

Duodenum
- duodenal ulcer

Gall bladder disease

Pancreatic disease
- pancreatitis
- carcinoma

Small intestine disease
- malabsorption
- Crohn's disease
- mesenteric ischaemia

Large intestine disease
- irritable bowel syndrome
- diverticulitis
- carcinoma
- ulcerative colitis

Endocrine/metabolic
- diabetes
- uraemia

Chronic heart/lung disease

Psychogenic

Grades of severity

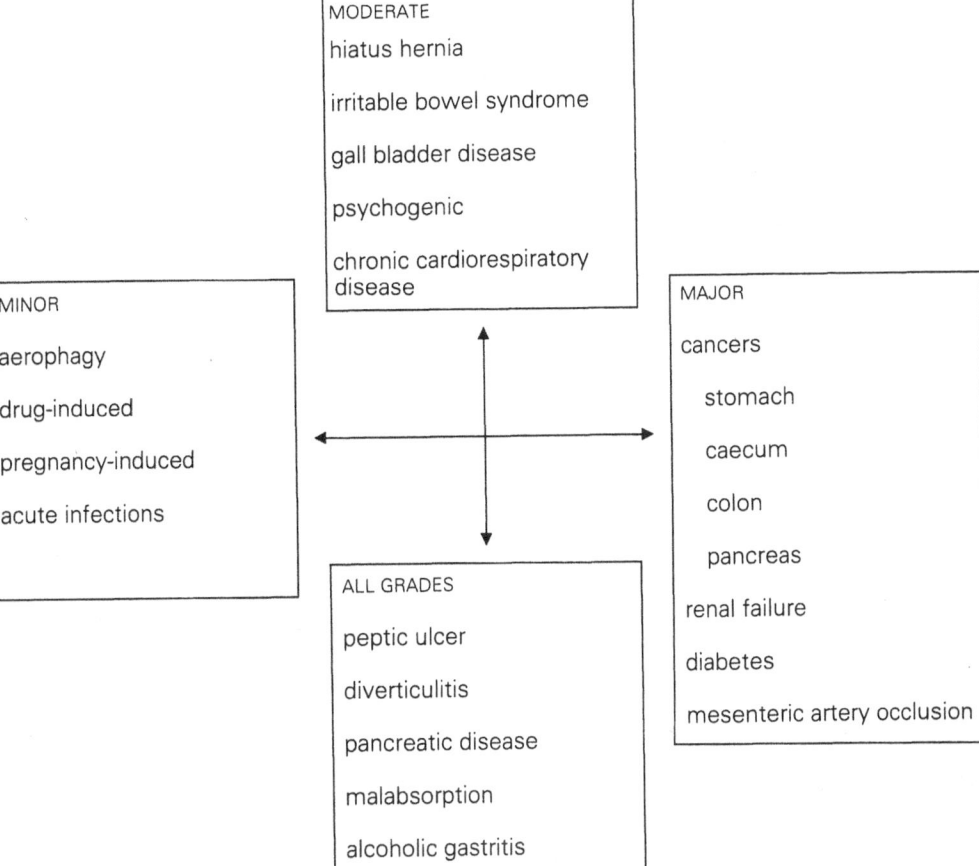

MODERATE

hiatus hernia

irritable bowel syndrome

gall bladder disease

psychogenic

chronic cardiorespiratory disease

MINOR

aerophagy

drug-induced

pregnancy-induced

acute infections

MAJOR

cancers

  stomach

  caecum

  colon

  pancreas

renal failure

diabetes

mesenteric artery occlusion

ALL GRADES

peptic ulcer

diverticulitis

pancreatic disease

malabsorption

alcoholic gastritis

Frequency

Annual prevalence of 'indigestion' *in a general practice of 2500 persons*	
Abdominal discomfort (fullness, distension, ache, pain) no specific cause	100
flatus, wind	20
flatulence, belching	10
heartburn – reflux	10
appetite disturbance	10
nausea	5
others	20

Age incidence

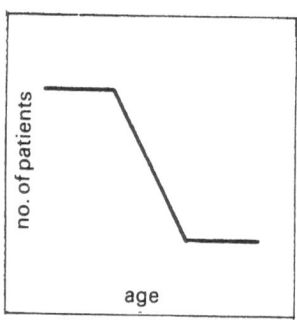

- abdominal pain (non-specific)
- acute infections
- appetite disturbances
- malabsorption

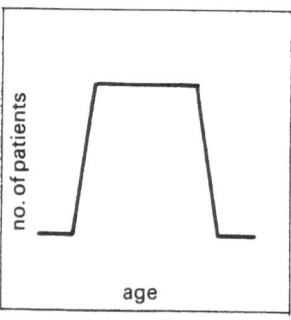

- flatulence
- heartburn
- loose stools (IBS)
- smoking +
- gastritis (alcoholic)
- psychogenic
- gall bladder disease

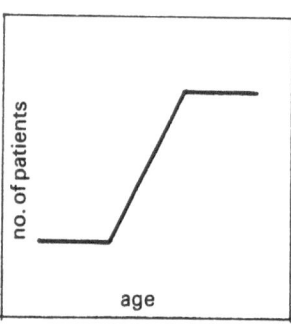

- constipation
- cancers GI tract
- diverticular disease
- mesenteric artery occlusion
- chronic cardio-respiratory disease

Diagnostic approach

History

Individual symptom and possible significance

Abdominal pain
Diagnosis depends on assessment of

- site of pain
- radiation of pain
- character of pain
- aggravating factors
- relieving factors
- associated symptoms

Site of pain

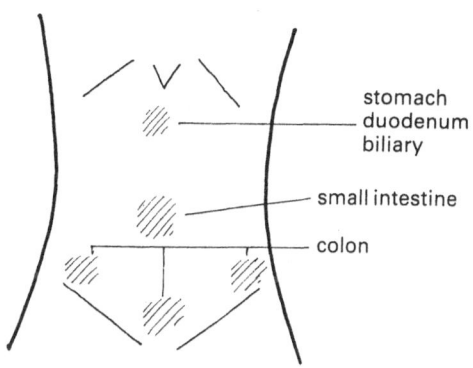

stomach
duodenum
biliary

small intestine

colon

Radiation of pain

- to interscapular area → gall bladder disease
- to tip of right shoulder → gall bladder disease
- to upper lumbar area → posterior duodenal ulcer, pancreatic disease
- to left shoulder and arm → oesophagitis

Character

- epigastric deep-seated gnawing pain → peptic ulcer
- retrosternal burning pain → gastro-oesophageal regurgitation
- deep-seated aching substernal pain → oesophageal spasm
- central abdominal colicky pain → small intestine

103

- cutting or burning pain → referred pain
- momentary 'stitch-like' pain → psychogenic

Aggravation
- food → gastric ulcer
- fried/fatty food → gall bladder disease
- bending → gastro-oesophageal regurgitation
- worse in evening/night → duodenal ulcer
- lying flat → pancreatitis
- movement, sneezing → peritonitis musculoskeletal pain
- deep breathing, coughing → referred from lungs
- anxiety, stress → psychogenic

Relief
- food → duodenal ulcer
- vomiting → gastric ulcer
- alkalis → gastric or duodenal ulcer
- better in morning → peptic ulcer
- passing flatus → colonic disease
- evacuation of bowels → colonic disease
- sitting up and crouching → pancreatic disease

Associated symptoms
- belching, flatulence, rumbling → irritable bowel syndrome
- acid regurgitation → oesophagitis
- waterbrash → duodenal ulcer
- anorexia, loss of weight → carcinoma of stomach
- symptoms of anaemia → carcinoma stomach or colon
- difficulty in swallowing → oesophagitis
- 'lump in throat' → psychogenic
- projectile vomiting → pyloric stenosis
- constipation/diarrhoea → irritable bowel syndrome
- diarrhoea 30 min after meal → mesenteric 'angina'

Anorexia

The causes are shown in Fig. 5.1.

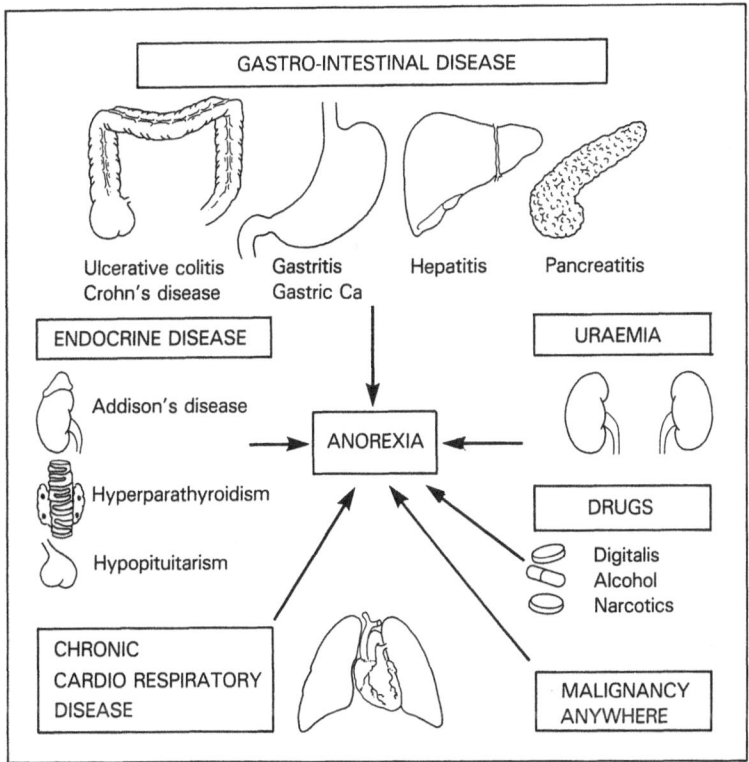

Fig. 5.1 *Causes of anorexia*

Nausea and vomiting

The causes are shown in Fig. 5.2.

Difficulty in swallowing
- solids only
  - pharyngeal/laryngeal infection
  - cricoid web
  - early carcinoma oesophagus
- nasal regurgitation
  - neuromuscular disease
- oesophageal regurgitation
  - pharyngeal pouch
  - achalasia of cardia

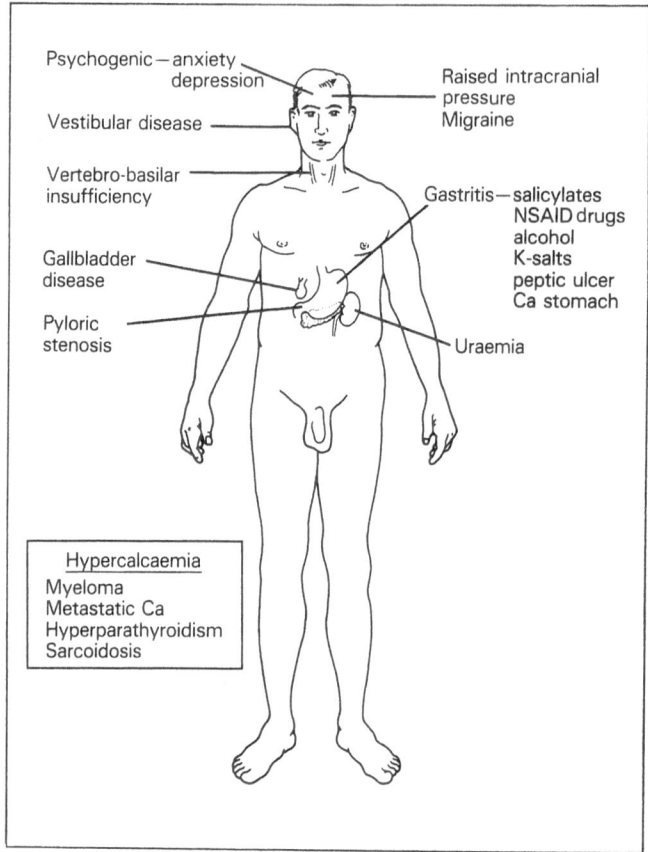

Fig. 5.2   *Causes of recurrent nausea/vomiting*

- reflux of acid
    oesophagitis
    scleroderma
- rapid weight loss
    carcinoma of oesophagus
- swallowing easier standing than sitting
    achalasia of cardia

Flatulent dyspepsia
    types

- belching
- abdominal distension
- bloating
- passing flatus per rectum
- rumbling/wind

Belching – this is usually functional and due to swallowing air which is caused by

- fear/anxiety
- hurried meals
- dry mouth (nervousness)
- excessive salivation

belching is rarely due to organic obstruction of gastric outlet caused by

- peptic ulcer
- cancer stomach

Abdominal distension – this is always intermittent and is usually due to excessive air in the bowel caused by

- aerophagy
- abnormal bacterial fermentation in the bowel

Bloating – this is a functional fluctuating abdominal swelling occurring more frequently in women and often accompanied by backache: it is thought to be due to contraction of the diaphragm and lumbar muscles

Excessive flatus per rectum – due to excessive fermentation by intestinal bacteria. It occurs with

- high fibre foods –beans, cabbage, broccoli
- malabsorption states

Rumbling/wind – this is due to excessive gut motility and is a distinctive symptom in irritable bowel syndrome. Although the symptom is usually functional it may occasionally be due to intestinal obstruction when other symptoms are present:

- colicky abdominal pain
- vomiting – faeculent eventually
- abdominal swelling
- increasing constipation

Heartburn – this is a retrosternal burning sensation radiating upwards from the epigastrium

it may radiate into
- the neck
- the shoulder
- arms

often accompanied by regurgitation of
- acid – hiatus hernia
- bile – duodenal ulcer, after gastric surgery

precipitated by
- heavy meal
- bending/stooping
- lying flat

causes
- pregnancy
- hiatus hernia
- obesity
- peptic ulcer
- gastritis
- gall bladder disease

differential diagnosis
- ischaemic heart disease
- pericarditis
- oesophageal spasm

Family history

peptic ulcer – strongest association, 3 × 'normal' population

inflammatory bowel disease – auto-immune disease
- rheumatoid arthritis
- collagen disease
- Hashimoto's thyroiditis
- pernicious anaemia
- hypoparathyroidism

gallstones – only in pigment stones due to hereditary haemolytic conditions
- congenital spherocytosis
- thalassaemia
- sickle cell disease

carcinoma stomach if due to pernicious anaemia

Indigestion

Smoking

Cigarettes may contribute to the development of

- peptic ulcer – more relevant in gastric ulcer than duodenal ulcer
- reflux oesophagitis – may be worse after cigarette
- gastritis – irritation of gastric mucosa
- oesophageal carcinoma
- mesenteric angina – due to atherosclerosis

Alcohol

may exacerbate

- gastritis
- reflux oesophagitis
- duodenal ulcer
- pancreatitis

Clinical examination

The findings which may help in deciding the cause of the 'indigestion' are shown in Fig. 5.3.

Investigation

the use of tests to investigate indigestion should be based on definite indications and with specific aims in mind either diagnostic or for management purposes.

the tests which may be of some value are:

- blood tests
- urine tests
- examination of faeces
- radiology
- endoscopy
- isotope studies

Blood tests

Hb – anaemia

- peptic ulcer
- hiatus hernia
- carcinoma
- haemolysis (gallstones)

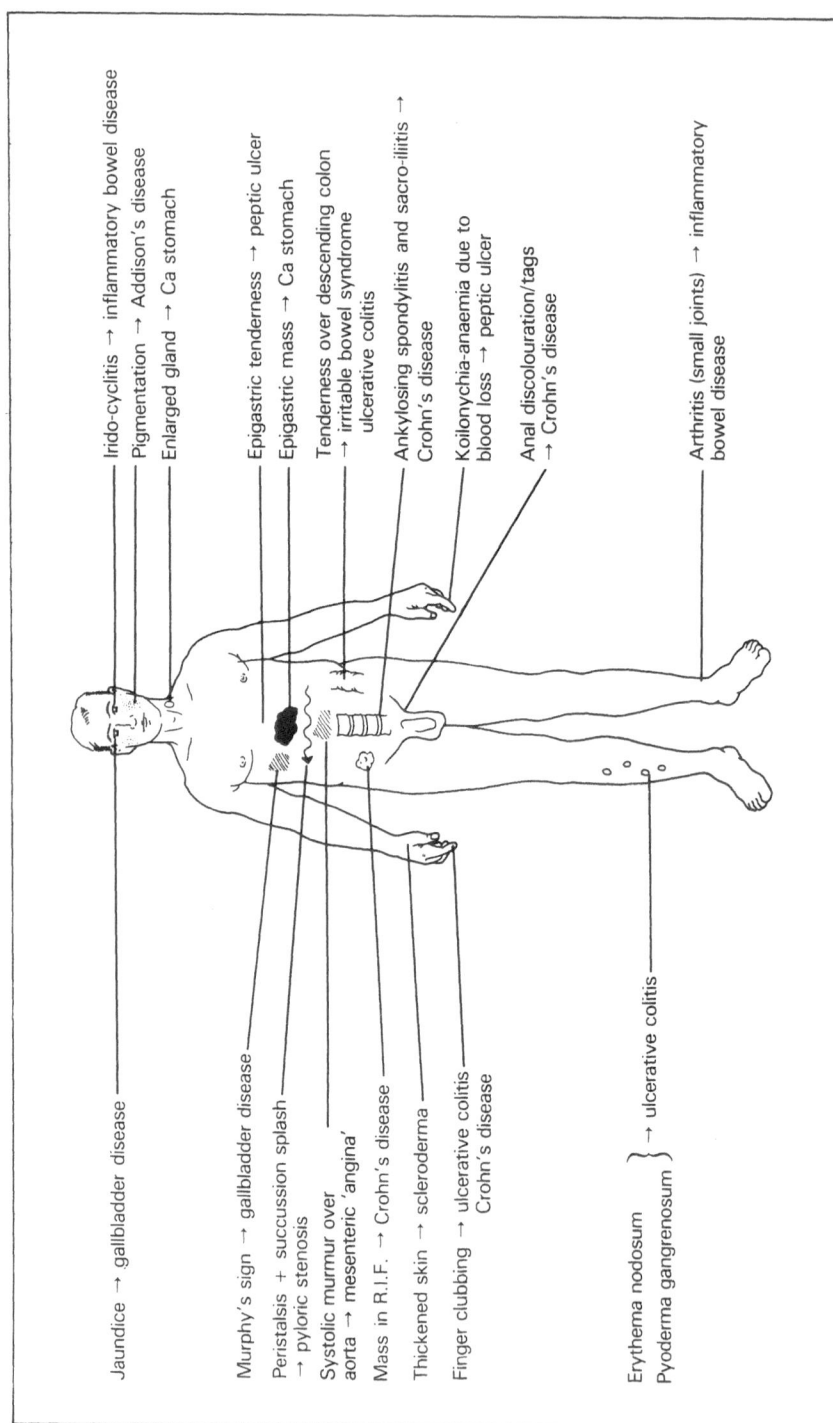

Fig. 5.3   *Clinical examination findings in 'indigestion'.*

blood film –
abnormal red cells

- thalassaemia
- sickle cell disease

ESR ↑

- inflammatory bowel disease
- malignancy
- collagen disease

serum amylase ↑

- acute pancreatitis

liver function

   bilirubin ↑
   alkaline phosphatase ↑ }   • gall bladder disease
   gamma-GT ↑

blood sugar ↑

- diabetes (gastric stasis)

serum calcium ↑

- hypercalcaemia (peptic ulcer)

Urine tests

- bilirubin   } → gall bladder disease
- urobilinogen ↑ }
- glycosuria   → diabetes
- protein   } → uraemia
- granular casts   }

Stools

- frank melaena → peptic ulcer
- occult blood present →

    peptic ulcer

    carcinoma

      stomach

      colon

- pale stools → gall bladder disease
- bulky, offensive, floating → pancreatic disease
- ribbon-like or pellets → irritable bowel
- loose with blood/slime →

    ulcerative colitis

    Crohn's disease

Radiology

  plain X-ray

    gall bladder disease

- radio-opaque gallstones (10–30%) (Fig. 5.4)
- hydrops of gall bladder
- empyema gall bladder
- 'limey' bile
- 'porcelain' gall bladder

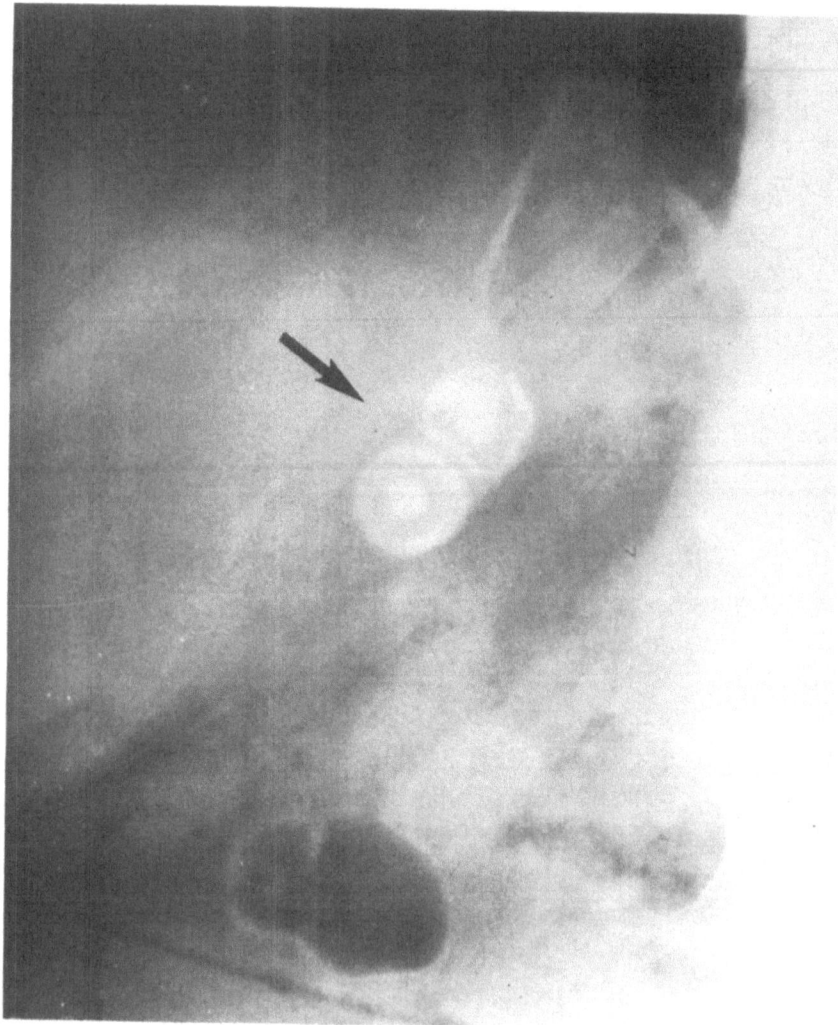

Fig. 5.4 *Plain X-ray of the abdomen showing radio-opaque multi-faceted gall-stones*

ulcerative colitis	• air in bowel may outline abnormal mucosal pattern
Crohn's disease	• mass in RIF
intestinal obstruction	• gas-distended loop
	• fluid levels in erect film
mesenteric ischaemia	• 'thumbprinting' due to sub-mucosal oedema in gas pattern

barium studies

gastric ulcer (Fig. 5.5a)	• niche of barium in stomach wall
	• sharply punched out margins
	• mucosal folds radiating to edge of crater

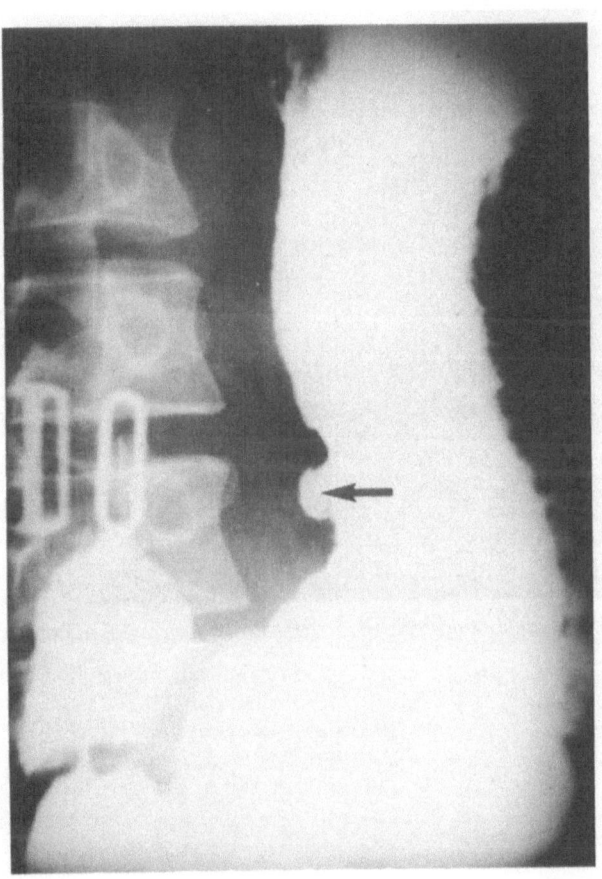

Fig. 5.5a   *Barium meal showing niche on lesser curve (arrowed) due to benign gastric ulcer*

duodenal ulcer

- tricorn deformity of duodenal cap (Fig. 5.5b)
- ulcer crater may be seen but difficult

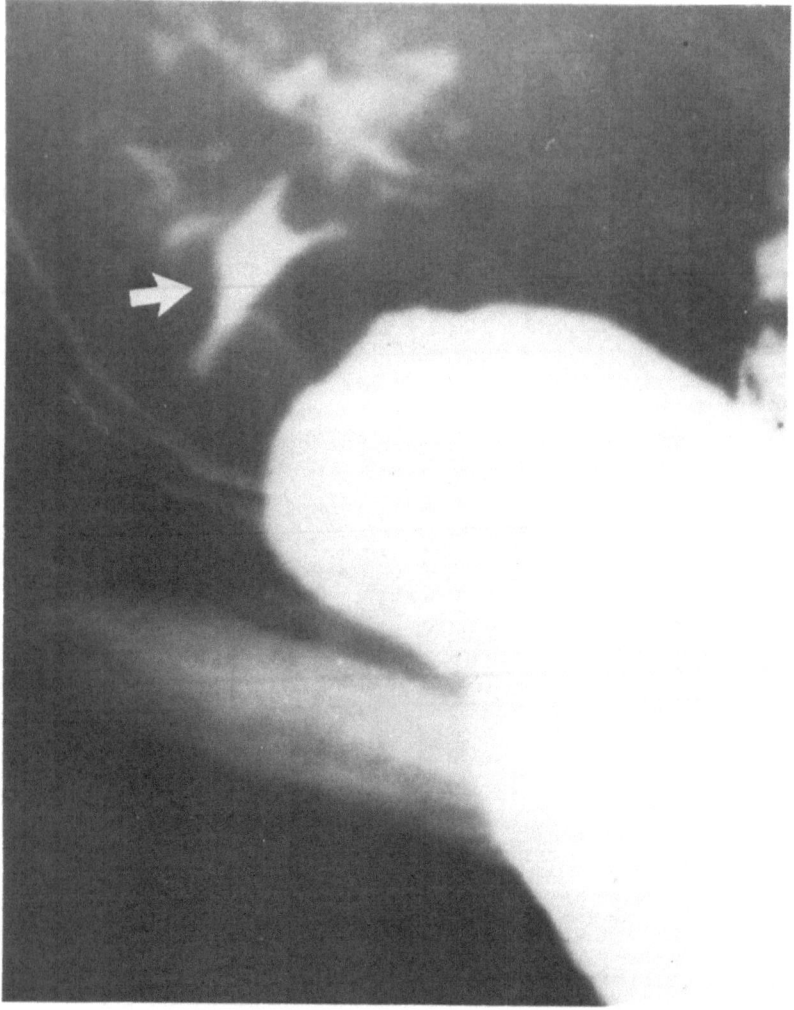

Fig. 5.5b *Barium meal showing the tricorn deformity (arrowed) of chronic duodenal ulcer*

carcinoma stomach

- filling defect antrum or body of stomach (Fig. 5.5c)
- ulcer on greater curve with irregular margin
- rigid tube in diffuse scirrhous cancer

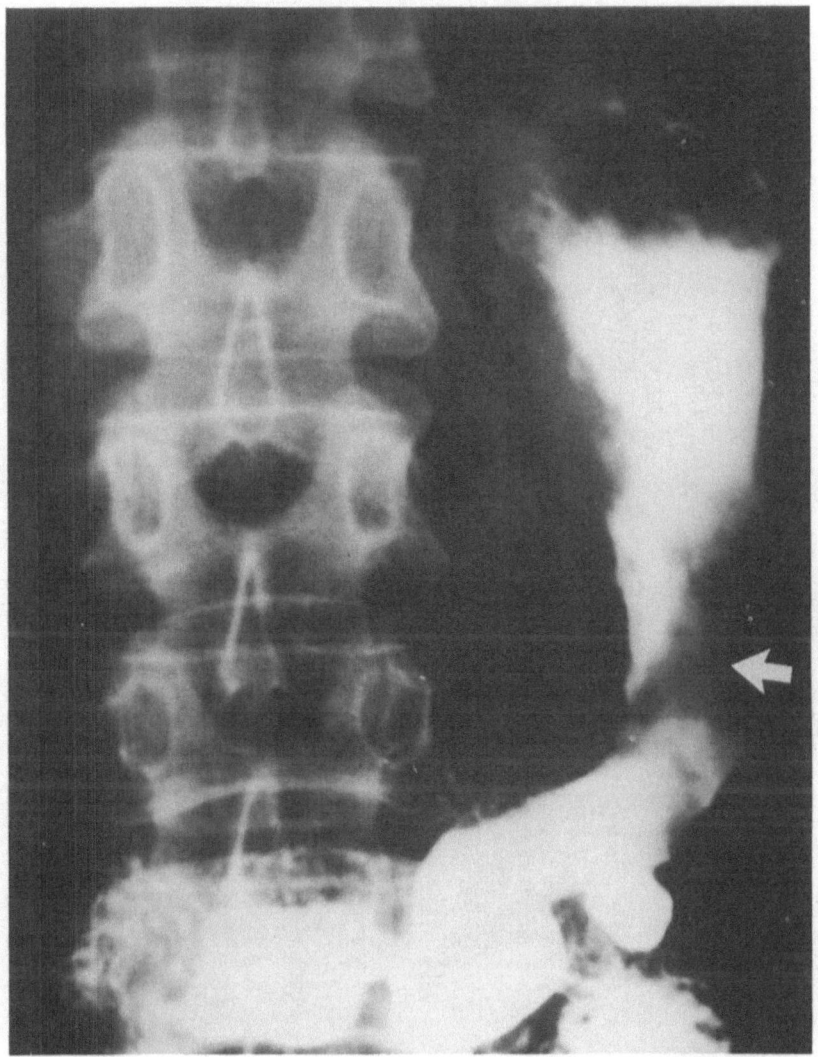

Fig. 5.5c *Barium meal showing filling defect due to carcinoma of the stomach*

Crohn's disease (small
intestine)
- terminal ileum narrow, irregular (Fig. 5.5d)
- segmental involvement
- cobblestone appearance
- deep transverse linear fissures
- strictures
- sinuses
- fistulae

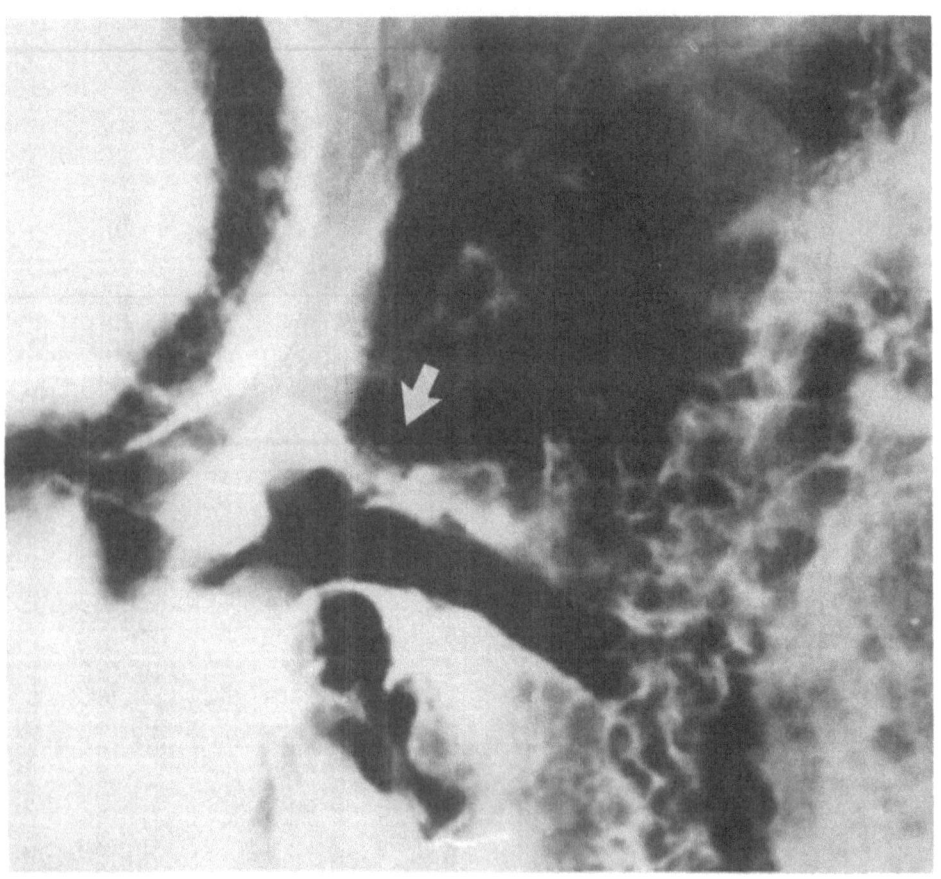

Fig. 5.5d *Small bowel enema showing narrowing and irregularity of the terminal ileum in Crohn's disease*

ulcerative colitis
(Fig. 5.5e)

- shallow ulceration
- loss of haustral pattern
- uniform constriction and shortening
- pseudo-polyps

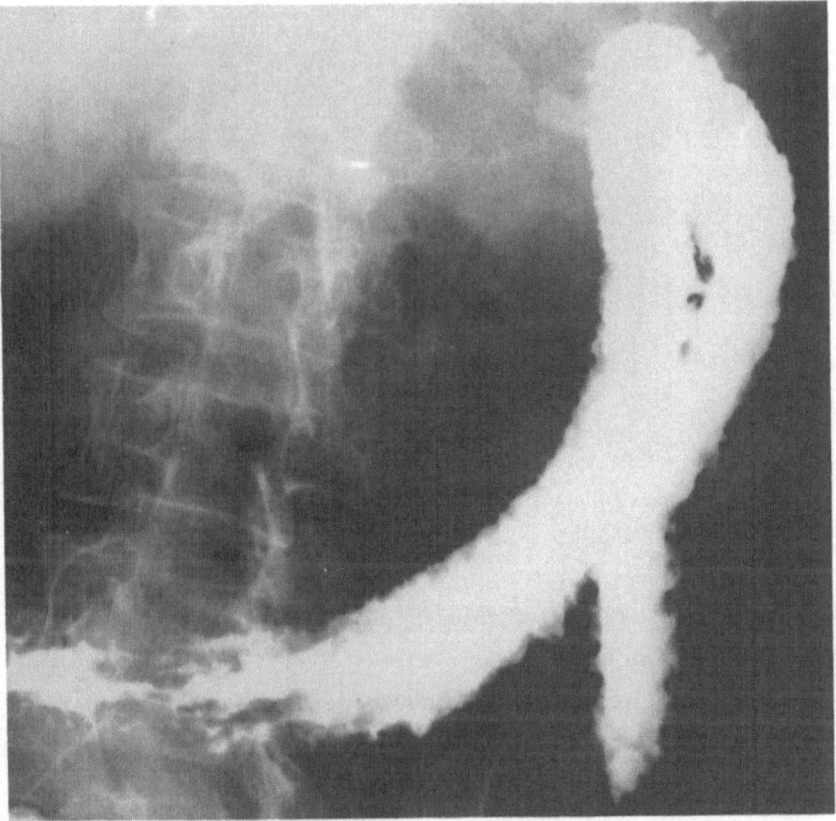

Fig. 5.5e   *Barium enema showing ulcerative colitis with a ragged mucosa and loss of haustration*

colonic carcinoma

- stricture (usually descending colon)
- filling defect (**Fig. 5.5f**) (usually ascending colon)

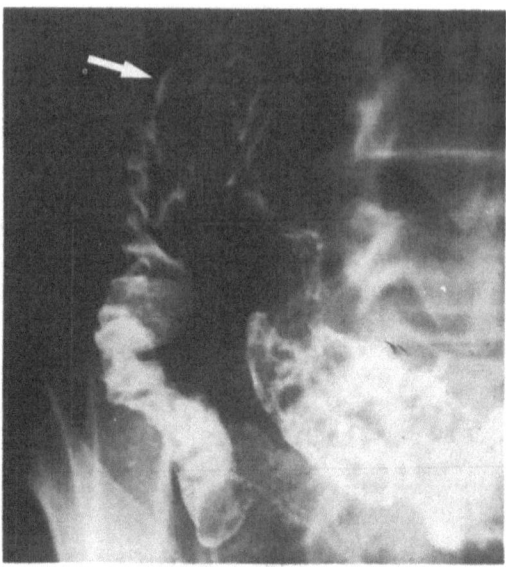

Fig. 5.5f *Barium enema showing filling defect in hepatic flexure of colon due to carcinoma (arrowed)*

cholecystogram – gall bladder disease (Fig. 5.5g)

identifies 70% of stones

10% of non-visualized gall bladders may be seen on second examination

'poorly-functional' gall bladder is not significant – 50% turn out to be normal

Intravenous cholangiography

indications

- previous cholecystectomy
- for confirmation of non-visualized gall bladder on oral cholecystography
- differential diagnosis of acute abdomen to exclude gallstones
- oral cholecystogram not possible because of gastro-duodenal disease
- stones suspected in common bile duct (CBD)

(liver function tests must be normal)

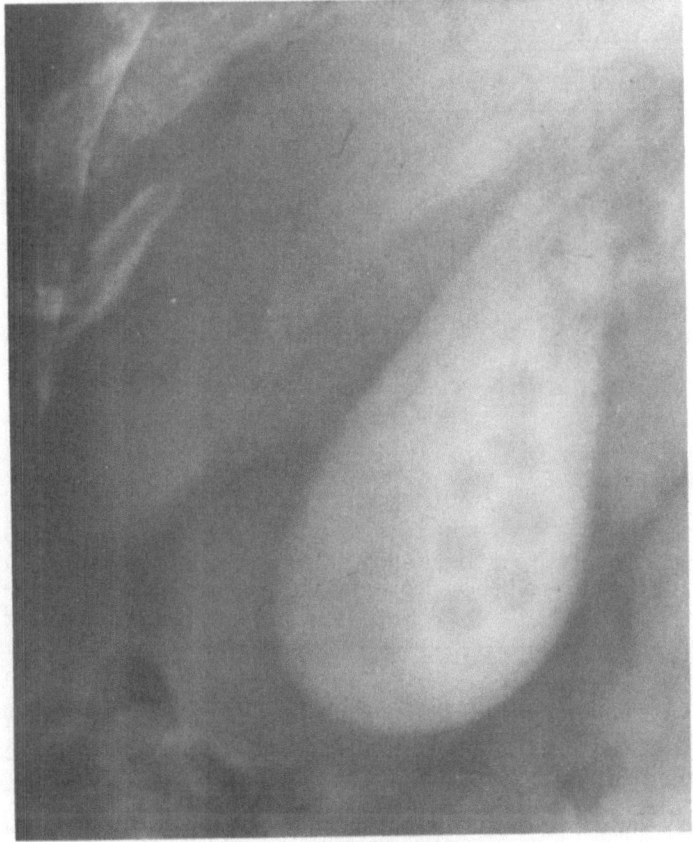

Fig. 5.5g *Cholecystogram showing radiotranslucent (cholesterol) gallstones*

ERCP (endoscopic retrograde cholangio-pancreatography)

provides diagnosis in 85% of jaundiced patients

indications
- to show bile ducts not seen on cholecystogram
- to distinguish stricture from overlooked stones after biliary surgery
- to distinguish gall bladder disease from pancreatic or gastroduodenal disease
- to remove small stones through sphincterotomy

Endoscopy

this is superior to barium meal examination in the investigation of upper gastrointestinal disease

a comparison of the two procedures is shown in Table 5.1.

Table 5.1

	Barium meal	Endoscopy
Advantages	simple	accurate
	inexpensive	reliable
	widely available	distinguishes benign and malignant ulcers
	little discomfort	biopsy possible
		can assess healing
		can control bleeding
Disadvantages	may miss ulcer (10–30%)	not readily available
	unreliable differentiation between benign and malignant ulcer	complications possible perforated oesophagus bursting of recent perforation bursting of recently healed ulcer

endoscopy can show active ulceration in 50% of patients with indigestion in whom barium examination has been non-specific and in 30% of those with a completely normal barium meal

endoscopy changes diagnoses and managements in 30–35% of patients who have had a previous barium meal examination

endoscopy of the lower bowel (colonoscopy) may be of value:

when doubt exists about the differential diagnosis of ulcerative colitis and Crohn's disease

to exclude carcinoma in long-standing ulcerative colitis

Ultrasound

Indications

abdominal masses
- cysts
- tumours

gall bladder
- to detect gallstones in non-functioning gall bladder on cholecystography
- to pick up very small stones – down to 3 mm diameter
- differential diagnosis of jaundice
- good demonstration of intrahepatic ducts
- preferable to radiology in pregnant women and in children

detection of hepatic metastases/hepatoma

pancreatitis – diffuse enlargement

ascites easily detectable

Computed tomography

extremely expensive equipment and not widely available

can detect
- cysts
- solid abdominal masses
- abscesses
- hepatic metastases
- lymphadenopathy
- gall bladder disease/dilated bile ducts

Manometric studies

measurement of pressure changes inside the oesophagus or colon may help in the diagnosis of oesophageal spasm or stasis, and irritable bowel syndrome

these tests are usually confined to research units and are not widely available in practice

Specific Conditions

Hiatus hernia/reflux oesophagitis
- F>M
- predisposing factors
  - obesity
  - pregnancy
  - ascites
- cardinal symptom – heartburn

- aggravated by

    bending or stooping

    lying flat in bed

    lifting or straining

    big meal

- substernal discomfort may radiate to left arm mimicking angina pectoris – distinguish by relationship to meals/posture and not exercise

- associated often with regurgitation of acid into mouth

- complications

    chronic blood loss → anaemia

    severe acute blood loss → haematemesis

    oesophageal stricture → dysphagia

- tests

    barium meal

        regurgitation of barium

        hiatus hernia (rolling/sliding)

        stricture

    oesophagoscopy

        oesophagitis

        oesophageal ulcer

        stricture

        site of bleeding

Peptic ulcer

- types of peptic ulcer

    gastric ulcer

    duodenal ulcer

    lower oesophagal ulcer

    stomal after gastric surgery

    rarely in Meckel's diverticulum

- affects 10% of all adult males in West

- male : female – duodenal ulcer 4 : 1

    gastric ulcer 2 : 1

Indigestion

- aetiology

    heredity, especially duodenal ulcer

    smoking, especially gastric ulcer

    commoner in blood group O

    social class – commoner in poor

    gastric acidity high in DU

    stress – probably minimal contribution

- presentation

    episodic epigastric pain related to meals

    waterbrash – especially DU

    vomiting

    GU – relieves pain

    outlet obstruction → large vomit containing food

    acute gastrointestinal bleed → haematemesis and melaena

    chronic iron deficiency anemia

- clinical examination

    most frequent – epigastric tenderness

    pyloric stenosis – succussion splash, peristalsis L → R

- investigations

    barium meal

    GU – punched-out ulcer niche

    DU – tricorn deformity

    ulcer crater difficult to see

    endoscopy – more accurate than barium meal (for comparison see Table 5.1)

- complications

    perforation – X-ray → air under diaphragm

    bleeding → haematemesis and melaena

    pyloric stenosis

    chronic hypochromic anaemia

    development of carcinoma from GU

Carcinoma of stomach

- male : female   3 : 1
- suspicious symptoms

    new onset indigestion in middle age

    changing indigestion in gastric ulcer

    failure of indigestion to improve with treatment

    persistent vomiting

    anorexia

    loss of weight

    abdominal symptoms or loss of weight in pernicious anaemia

    unexplained iron-deficiency anaemia in older patients

- clinical examination – see Fig. 5.6

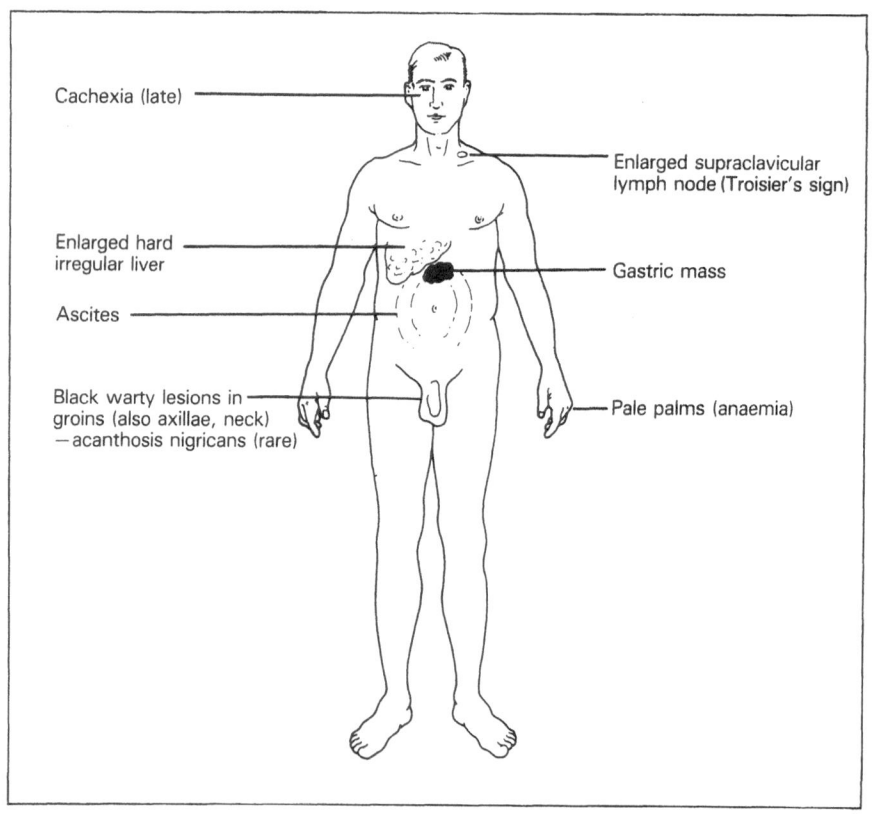

Cachexia (late)

Enlarged supraclavicular lymph node (Troisier's sign)

Enlarged hard irregular liver

Gastric mass

Ascites

Black warty lesions in groins (also axillae, neck) — acanthosis nigricans (rare)

Pale palms (anaemia)

Fig. 5.6 *Signs of gastric carcinoma (late)*

124

Indigestion

- investigation

  barium meal may easily miss

  best test is endoscopy and biopsy

  a positive barium meal may show a filling defect in body or antrum of the stomach, or rarely a rigid tube due to infiltrating scirrhous cancer

  exfoliative cytology from gastric washings may help

- all gastric ulcers should be followed up, endo-scopically if possible, to confirm healing because of their potential to become malignant

Gall bladder disease

Gallstones

- types of stones

  pigment (bilirubin)

  cholesterol

  mixed

- predisposing factors

  cholesterol

      female

      fair

      fat

      forty

      fertile

  (*also* oral contraceptives)

  pigment – haemolytic conditions:

      congenital spherocytosis

      thalassaemia

      sickle cell disease

- presentation

  symptomless if free in gall bladder – discovered incidentally

  biliary colic (cystic duct)

  jaundice (common bile duct)

  cholecystitis

  hydrops of gall bladder → slow distension

- diagnosis

    plain abdominal X-ray – 10–30% opaque

    cholecystogram – positive in 70%

    intravenous cholangiography – for indications see page 118.

    ultrasound – if non-functioning gall bladder (see page 120)

    ERCP – see page 119

    urine test – bile present

    liver function – increase in bilirubin and alkaline phosphatase

Cholecystitis

acute

- usually follows gallstone impaction
- 80% subside spontaneously
- diagnosis

    pain in right hypochondrium – may be referred to right shoulder or scapula

    fever

    local tenderness (Murphy's sign)

- complications

    gangrene of gall bladder with perforation

    empyema of gall bladder

    ascending cholangitis

- investigation

    gallstones on plain X-ray (10–30%)

    leucocytosis

    bile in urine

    abnormal liver function

chronic

- due to recurrent attacks acute cholecystitis
- flatulent dyspepsia occurs as frequently in patients without chronic gall bladder disease as with it
- may get recurrent bouts of pain in right hypochondrium

126

Indigestion

- complications
    - acute exacerbations
    - pancreatitis
    - fistula formation
    - carcinoma (rare)
- diagnosis
    - cholecystogram – no function
    - intravenous cholangiogram
    - ultrasound
    - ERCP

Irritable bowel syndrome

- the cardinal symptoms are
    - abdominal pain
    - disturbance of the bowels
- forms 70% of all patients with chronic digestive complaints
- male : female   2 : 1
- aetiology unknown – possible factors are
    - psychological disturbance
    - post-infective – may follow episode of infective enteritis
    - inadequate bulk in diet (fibre)
    - purgative abuse
    - lactose intolerance – rare
- pain variable in all aspects
    - severity – mild to intense
    - site – commonest lower abdominal and LIF but can be anywhere
    - character
        - dull ache
        - colicky
        - stabbing
        - burning
    - may be worse after food (30%)
    - relieved by defaecation (30%)

- bowel disturbance

    painless watery diarrhoea 10%

    diarrhoea with severe colic

    constipation may occur alone or may alternate with diarrhoea

    tenesmus may be present

- stool

    ribbon or pencil-like

    small hard pellets

- associated symptoms

    abdominal distension

    flatulence and belching

    heartburn

    nausea, anorexia

    anxiety

        excessive fatigue

        palpitations

        hyperventilation

- examination

    may have scars of previous operations

    may feel tender descending colon in LIF

    may feel fluctuant gas-filled caecum in RIF

- sigmoidoscopy

    often normal

    may show slight hyperaemia, excess of mucus

    spasm or hypermotility

- barium studies from both ends of the GI tract are desirable to

    exclude organic disease

    reassure the patient

Diverticular disease

- usually middle-aged or elderly – M = F
- 'diverticulitis' is inflammation in diverticulosis

Indigestion

- diverticulae found mainly in colon (left and sigmoid)
- probably due to inadequate bulk (fibre) in the diet
- presentation

    pain and tenderness in LIF

    alteration of bowels → usually increasing constipation

    subacute obstruction may occur

        abdominal distension

        colicky pain

        borborygmi

    may spread to bladder → frequency dysuria

    occasionally fistulates into bladder → air in the urine

- investigation

    sigmoidoscopy – to exclude cancer

    barium enema – diverticulae

    colonoscopy

Mesenteric ischaemia

- due to atherosclerotic narrowing of superior mesenteric artery
- presentation

    post-prandial colicky peri-umbilical pain with diarrhoea 15–30 min after meals (abdominal 'angina')

    weight loss

- clinical examination – signs of atherosclerosis (Fig. 5.7)
- investigation

    plain X-ray abdomen – 'thumbprinting' due to patches of mucosal oedema imprinted on gas in bowel

    aortic calcification may be seen on plain X-ray abdomen

    mesenteric arteriography is the definitive test to show atherosclerotic obstruction

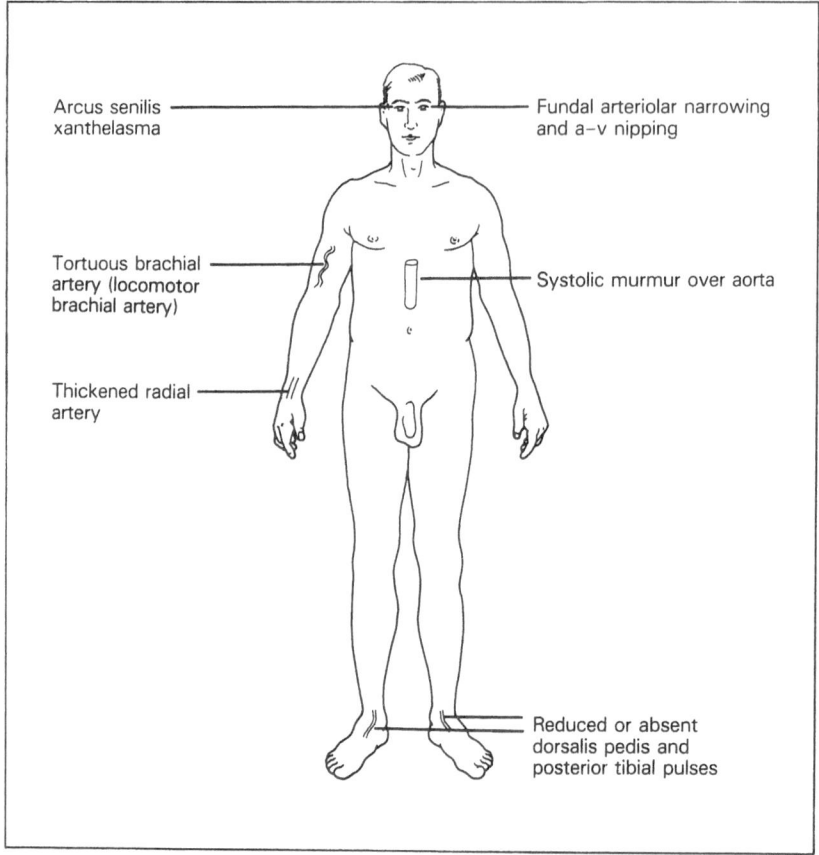

Arcus senilis
xanthelasma

Fundal arteriolar narrowing
and a–v nipping

Tortuous brachial
artery (locomotor
brachial artery)

Systolic murmur over aorta

Thickened radial
artery

Reduced or absent
dorsalis pedis and
posterior tibial pulses

Fig. 5.7 *Signs of arteriosclerosis in abdominal 'angina'*

Pitfalls in diagnosis

- Peptic ulcer and reflux oesophagitis can mimic angina pectoris and myocardial infarction.
- Night pain and the relationship of the pain to meals does not reliably distinguish gastric and duodenal ulcer.
- The pain of gastric carcinoma may improve temporarily with rest, alkalis or an H_2-blocker.
- The association between gastric carcinoma and pernicious anaemia may be overlooked.
- Peptic ulcer and chronic gall bladder disease may co-exist – if gallstones are seen on a plain X-ray of the abdomen the peptic ulcer may easily be overlooked.
- Central abdominal pain and diarrhoea may easily be attributed to irritable bowel syndrome and the possibility of chronic mesenteric ischaemia overlooked.

Useful practical points

- Flatulent dyspepsia is not indicative of chronic gall bladder disease.

- Always confirm objectively that a gastric ulcer has healed with treatment because of its potential to become malignant.

- If there is evidence of extensive arteriosclerosis always consider chronic mesenteric ischaemia as a possible cause of abdominal pain, especially if associated with diarrhoea.

- Biliary colic with an increase in serum bilirubin or alkaline phosphatase is highly suggestive of gallstones.

- Dissolving cholesterol gallstones with chenodeoxycholic acid is prolonged and rarely permanent – 70% recur in 5 years.

- Endoscopy is the investigation of choice in peptic ulcer because of its high accuracy, biopsy opportunity and potential for arresting bleeding.

Case challenge

A 73-year-old lady presented with a 6 month history of epigastric discomfort sometimes half-an-hour after meals and at other times unrelated to meals. She had a past history of gastric ulcer first diagnosed when she was 50 years old and which had recurred several times since, the last time being eighteen months ago for which she had a 3 month course of cimetidine. She was losing weight but attributed this to being afraid to eat because of the pain. She also admitted to increasing constipation but had not noticed any colour change or seen any blood in her stools. Other symptoms included breathlessness on exertion, dizziness, palpitations and swelling of the ankles but she thought these symptoms had been coming on slowly over the past 2 or 3 years.

There was a past history of arthritis for which she has been taking ibuprofen (Brufen) intermittently for years. She had also had gallstones in the past but had refused to have an operation and was subject to a lot of wind and abdominal rumbling particularly after she had a fatty or fried meal.

The findings on examination are shown in Fig. 5.8.

Questions   What diagnoses would you consider?

           What tests would you do?

           What treatment would you suggest?

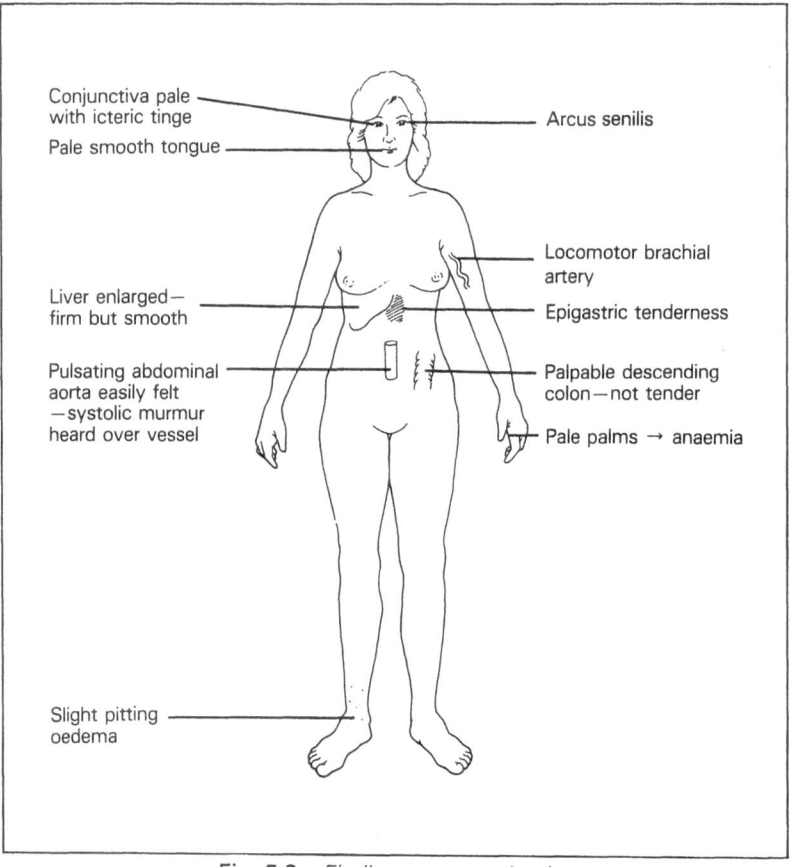

Conjunctiva pale with icteric tinge

Pale smooth tongue

Arcus senilis

Liver enlarged— firm but smooth

Locomotor brachial artery

Epigastric tenderness

Pulsating abdominal aorta easily felt —systolic murmur heard over vessel

Palpable descending colon—not tender

Pale palms → anaemia

Slight pitting oedema

Fig. 5.8   *Findings on examination*

Possible diagnoses	
	• reactivation of old gastric ulcer
	• gall bladder disease
	• irritable bowel syndrome
	• chronic mesenteric ischaemia
	• carcinoma of stomach

Gastric ulcer

For   history   • previous history
        • chronic relapsing condition
        • pain sometimes related to meals
        • indomethacin treatment might activate GU

        exam   • epigastric tenderness

Indigestion

Against	history	• pain sometimes not related to meals
		• age – malignancy commoner in elderly
		• marked loss of weight
	exam	• enlarged liver
Tests		• gastroscopy, biopsy
		• barium meal – less diagnostic

Gall bladder disease

For	history	• past history of gallstones
		• flatulent dyspepsia after fatty meal
	exam	• slight jaundice
Against	history	• no pain in right hypochondrium
		• pain not referred to R shoulder or scapula
		• no pale stools to suggest obstructive jaundice
	exam	• no tenderness in right hypochondrium
Tests		• oral cholecystogram
		• plain abdominal X-ray for stones
		• ultrasound for duct dilatation
		• oral cholecystogram for stones or lack of function
		• intravenous cholangiography for duct dilatation

Irritable bowel

For	history	• wind and abdominal rumbling after meals
		• constipation
	exam	• palpable descending colon
Against	history	• pain localized to epigastrium
		• no diarrhoea alternating with constipation
	exam	• colon not tender
		• enlarged liver
Tests		• sigmoidoscopy may show
		hyperaemia
		mucus +
		• barium studies primarily to exclude organic disease

Mesenteric ischaemia

For   history   • loss of weight

       exam   • elderly atherosclerotic lady

               • murmur over diseased aorta

Against   history   • epigastric not peri-umbilical pain

               • not consistently 20–30 min after meals

               • no associated diarrhoea

       exam   • nil

Tests   • plain X-ray abdomen for 'thumbprinting'

           • mesenteric arteriogram ?justified in this elderly patient

Gastric carcinoma

For   history   • elderly

               • pain not consistently related to meals

               • loss of weight

       exam   • possibility of pernicious anaemia

                   symptoms of anaemia

                   atrophic glossitis

                   anaemia-palms

                   slight jaundice

               • enlarged liver

Against   • nil

Tests   • gastroscopy and biopsy

           • barium meal – less reliable

           • blood count and film for macrocytic anaemia

           • serum vitamin B12 level to confirm pernicious anaemia

---

Actual diagnosis:
Malignant gastric ulcer
Hepatic metastases found by ultrasound

Treatment and outcome

no curative treatment was possible

the patient deteriorated rapidly and died within 7 weeks.

a palliative bypass operation may be worthwhile if pyloric obstruction severe

only 20% survival in 5 years

6   Acute Abdominal Pain

Introduction

The 'acute abdomen' is a life–death situation in clinical practice.

Its rather wide title is intentional because its range of possible conditions also is wide and with various symptoms and signs.

The acute abdomen crosses all specialist boundaries presenting in surgical, medical, gynaecological, paediatric, geriatric, psychiatric and other specialist units as well as in general practice.

Probably, it is in general practice that the greatest difficulties occur since the earliest features are so difficult to unravel.

The acute abdomen poses challenges to personal clinical acumen.

Causes of acute abdomen

Intra-abdominal
- inflammatory (Fig. 6.1)
- perforation (Fig. 6.2)
- obstruction (Fig. 6.3)
- haemorrhage (Fig. 6.4)
- torsion (Fig. 6.5)
- vascular (Fig. 6.6)

Extra-abdominal (Fig. 6.7)

respiratory
- pneumonia/pleurisy
- oesophageal – hiatus hernia, ruptured oesophagus

CVS
- myocardial infarction
- ruptured aneurysm of abdominal aorta
- dissecting aneurysm

skin
- herpes zoster

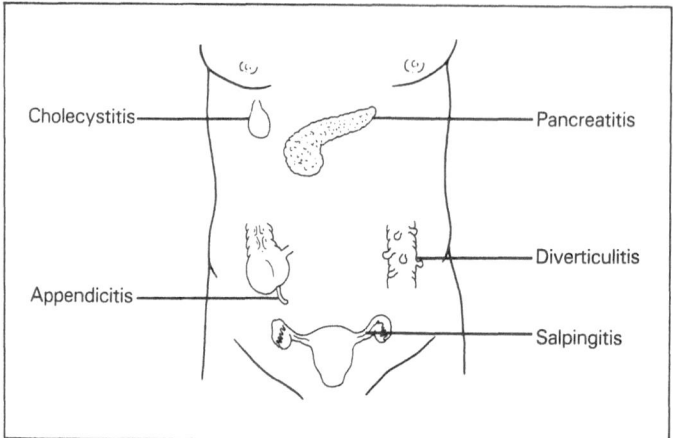

Fig. 6.1   *Inflammation*

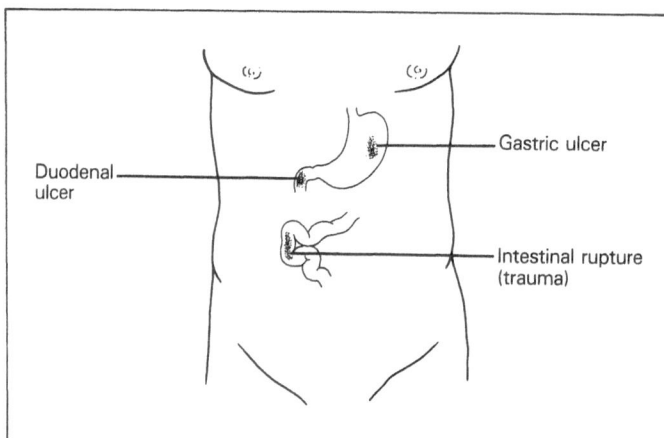

Fig. 6.2   *Perforation*

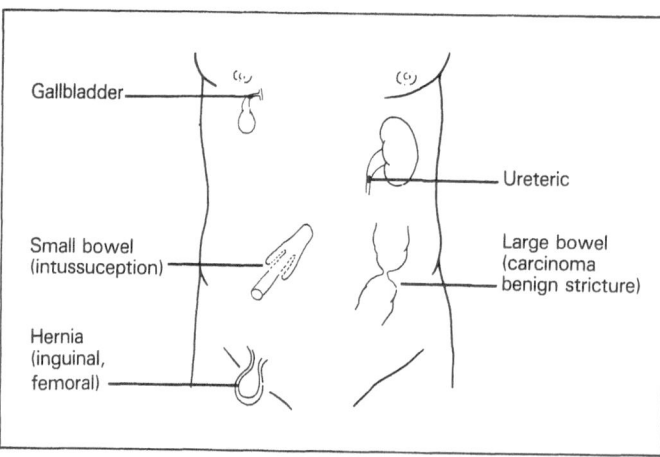

Fig. 6.3   *Obstruction*

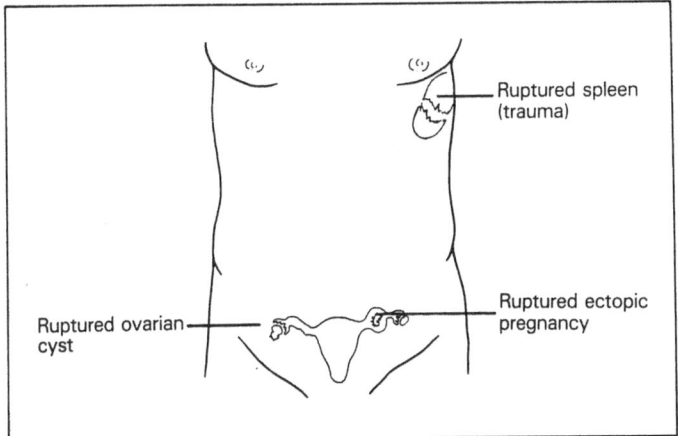

Fig. 6.4   *Haemorrhage*

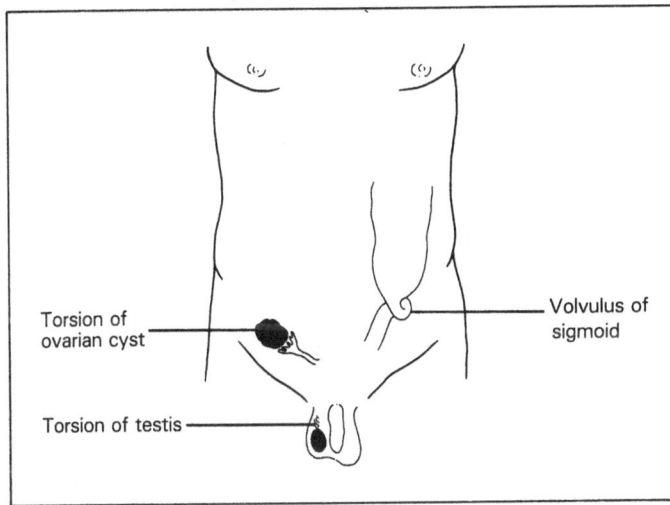

Fig. 6.5   *Torsion*

metabolic	• porphyria
CNS	• nerve root irritation
	• tabes dorsalis
endocrine	• diabetes
	• Addison's disease
others	• Henoch–Schönlein

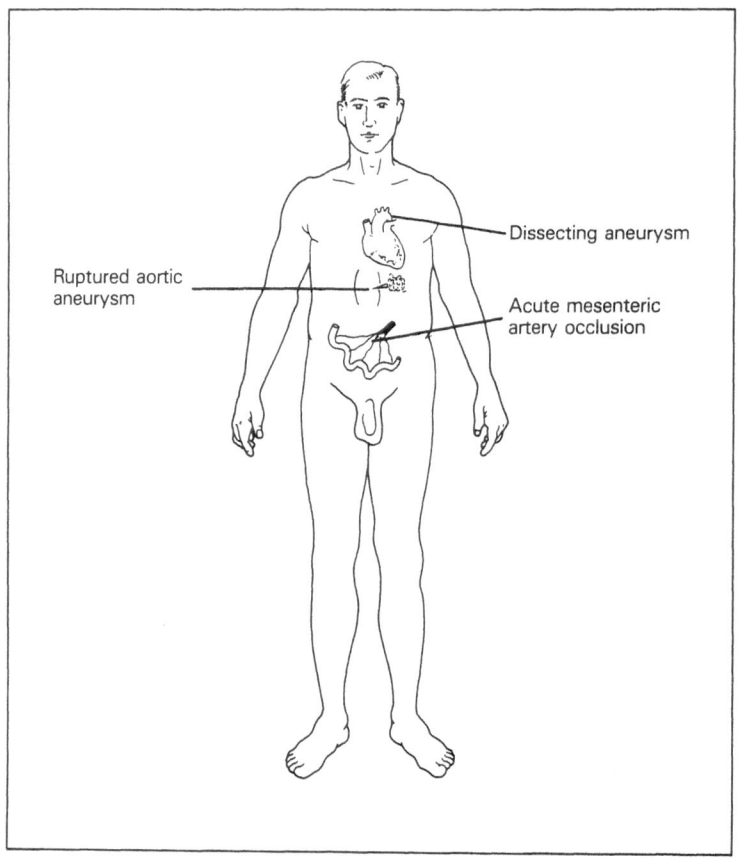

Fig. 6.6 *Vascular*

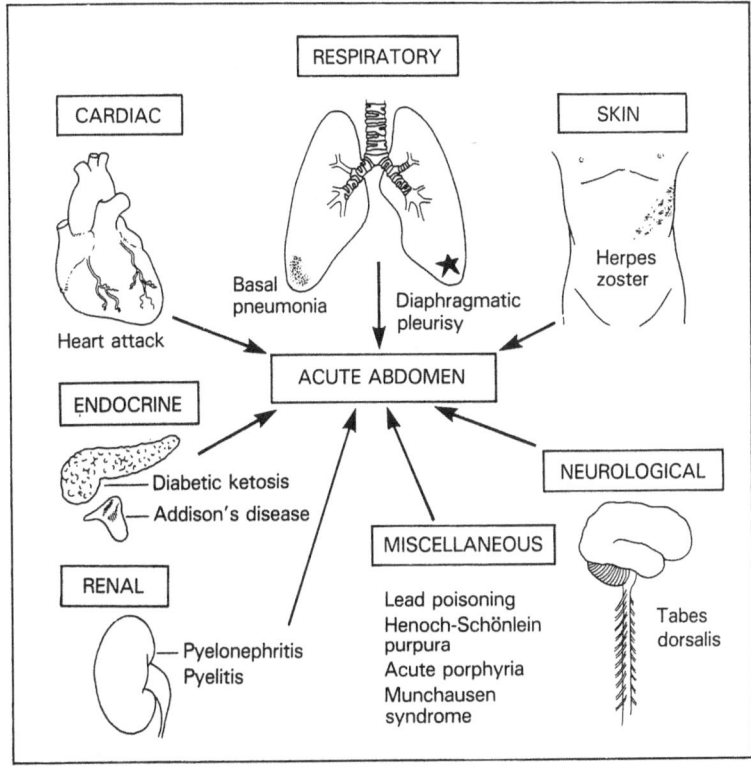

RESPIRATORY

CARDIAC

SKIN

Basal
pneumonia

Diaphragmatic
pleurisy

Herpes
zoster

Heart attack

ACUTE ABDOMEN

ENDOCRINE

NEUROLOGICAL

— Diabetic ketosis
— Addison's disease

MISCELLANEOUS

RENAL

Lead poisoning
Henoch-Schönlein
purpura
Acute porphyria
Munchausen
syndrome

Tabes
dorsalis

— Pyelonephritis
Pyelitis

Fig. 6.7   *Medical (extra-abdominal) causes of an 'acute abdomen'*

Grades of severity

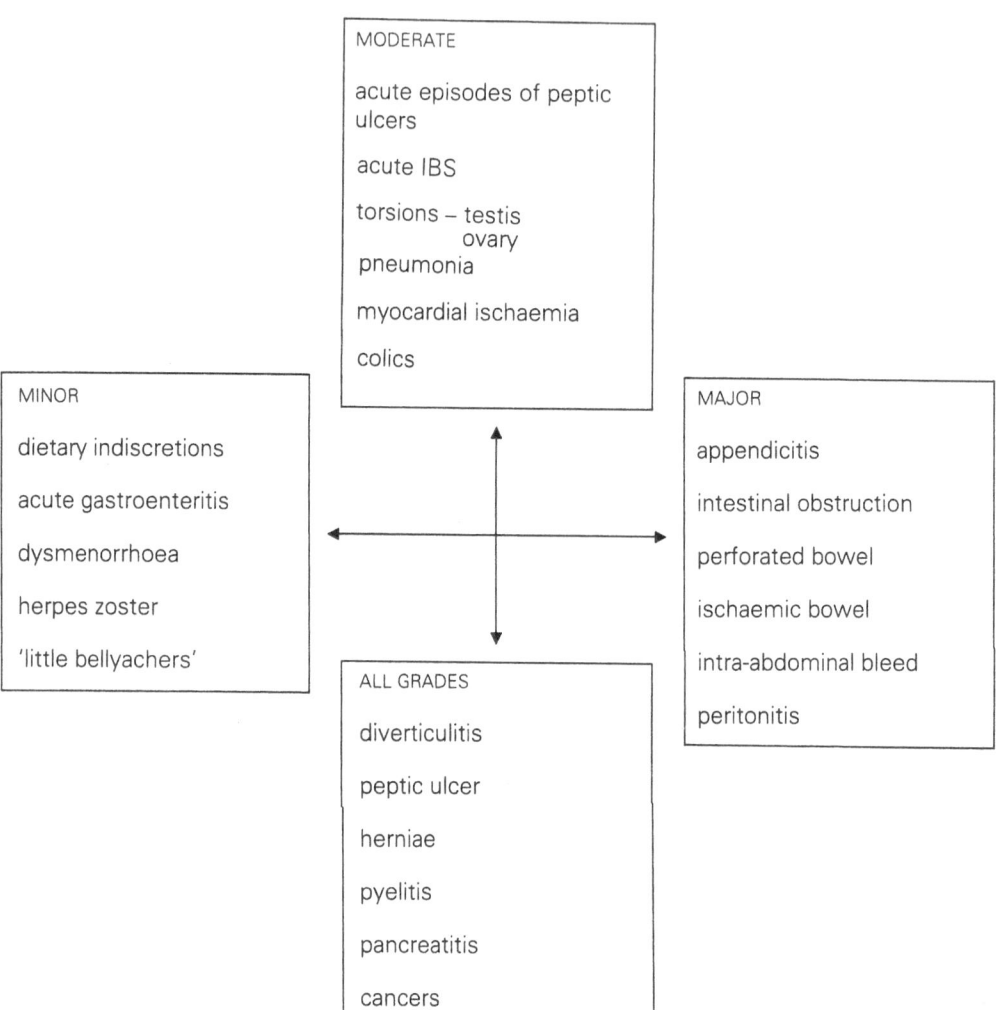

MODERATE

acute episodes of peptic ulcers

acute IBS

torsions – testis
            ovary
pneumonia

myocardial ischaemia

colics

MINOR

dietary indiscretions

acute gastroenteritis

dysmenorrhoea

herpes zoster

'little bellyachers'

MAJOR

appendicitis

intestinal obstruction

perforated bowel

ischaemic bowel

intra-abdominal bleed

peritonitis

ALL GRADES

diverticulitis

peptic ulcer

herniae

pyelitis

pancreatitis

cancers

Frequency

Annual prevalence of acute abdomen (major) in a general practice of 2500 persons	
Acute appendicitis	3
Renal colic	3
Intestinal obstruction	1
Peptic ulcer (bleed or perforation)	1
Others	<1

Thus the major acute abdomen is not that frequent in general practice.

However since there are approximately 100 GPs to a district general hospital the annual number of cases likely to be seen at the hospital must be multiplied by 100, i.e. 300 acute appendicitis per year.

The order of frequency by percentages of cases of acute abdomen in general practice are (Fry, 1985):

acute appendicitis	31%
colics (renal 21, biliary 8)	29%
intestinal obstruction	11%
peptic ulcers (bleed 6, perforation 3)	9%
gynaecological (torsions, ectopics)	5%
strangulated herniae	5%
acute pancreatitis	3%
mesenteric artery occlusion	2%
others	5%
	100%

In addition to such 'surgical' 9 acute abdomens a GP may expect to see and assess another 30 'non-surgical' cases.

Age incidence

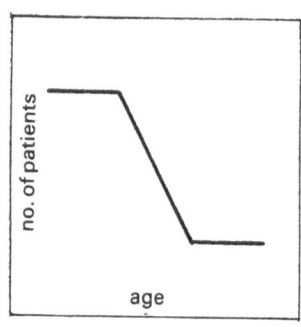

- appendicitis
- intussusception
- torsion of testis
- congenital abnormalities
- bellyachers
- Henoch–Schönlein
- pyelitis

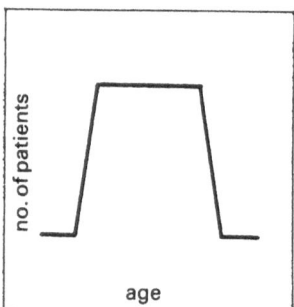

- renal/biliary colic
- peptic ulcers
- gynaecological

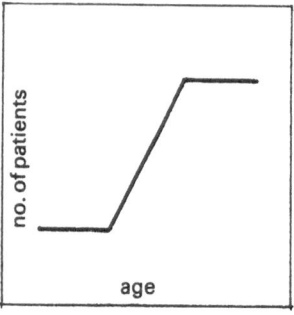

- intestinal obstruction (NG)
- mesenteric artery occlusion
- strangulated hernia
- diverticulitis

Significance

the dangers to life of an acute abdomen may be –

- shock
- sepsis
- bleeding
- body fluid disturbances

time is a major factor
- dangers increase with each hour
- any abdominal pain that persists for more than hours is a possible acute abdomen

dangers of misdiagnosis
- gangrenous appendix → peritonitis
- perforated ulcer → peritonitis
- obstructed bowel → gangrene
- hazardous laparotomy in acute pancreatitis

premature treatment with analgesics in response to patient's appeals for relief of pain may mask diagnosis

special diagnostic difficulties

infants
- history and examination difficult
- rapid deterioration occurs

elderly
- history difficult
- presentation unusual
- high pain threshold

steroid treatment
- masks symptoms

immediate post-operative period
- heavily sedated
- residual pain
- post-operative ileus may be present

previous gastric surgery
- perforated stomal ulcer presents differently to perforated gastric/duodenal ulcer

Diagnostic approach

General

The *general practitioner's roles* are *not* necessarily to make a specific pathological diagnosis, rather to decide
- does it require immediate hospital admission?
- if not, should the patient be reassessed, and if so when?

145

- if not, what instructions should be given to the patient to report any problems?

The *hospital doctor's roles* are to decide

- is it surgical or medical?
- if surgical when should surgery be undertaken?

History

Age – the age incidence of the acute abdomen is shown on page 144

Sex

females	• cholecystitis
	• cancer of colon (except rectum)
	• gynaecological crises
males	• perforated peptic ulcer
	• carcinoma rectum
	• mesenteric occlusion
	• torsion of testes

Mode of onset

sudden	• perforated peptic ulcer
	• haemorrhage
	ruptured ectopic
	ruptured aneurysm
	• mesenteric arterial occlusion
	• biliary colic
	• renal colic
	• volvulus sigmoid/caecum
	• torsion of the testis/ovarian cyst
gradual	• appendicitis
	• cholecystitis
	• diverticulitis
	• pancreatitis
	• intestinal obstruction
	• salpingitis

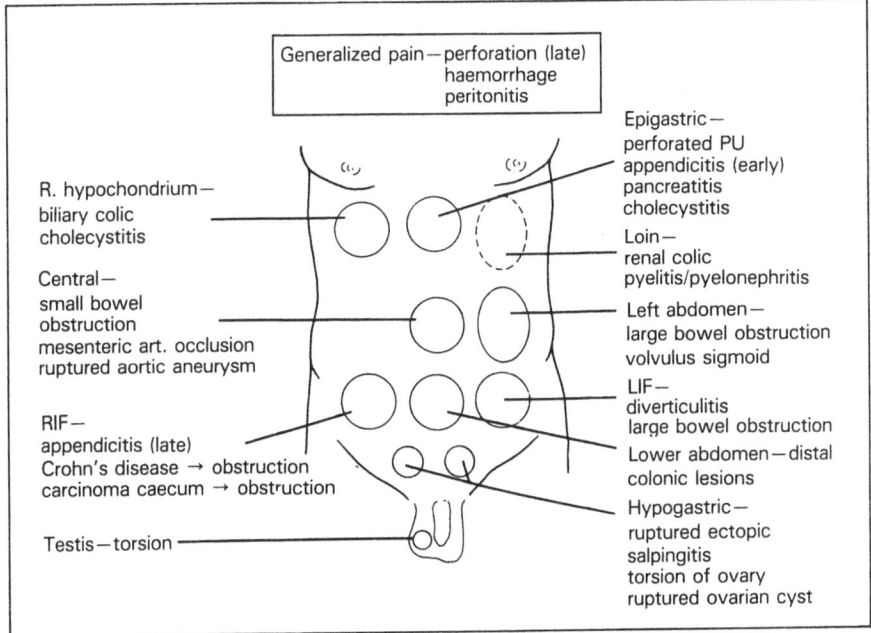

Generalized pain—perforation (late)
haemorrhage
peritonitis

Epigastric—
perforated PU
appendicitis (early)
pancreatitis
cholecystitis

Loin—
renal colic
pyelitis/pyelonephritis

R. hypochondrium—
biliary colic
cholecystitis

Central—
small bowel
obstruction
mesenteric art. occlusion
ruptured aortic aneurysm

Left abdomen—
large bowel obstruction
volvulus sigmoid

LIF—
diverticulitis
large bowel obstruction

RIF—
appendicitis (late)
Crohn's disease → obstruction
carcinoma caecum → obstruction

Lower abdomen—distal
colonic lesions

Hypogastric—
ruptured ectopic
salpingitis
torsion of ovary
ruptured ovarian cyst

Testis—torsion

Fig. 6.8 *Sites of abdominal pain in 'acute abdomen'*

Site of the pain

This is shown in Fig. 6.8

Character

The main feature of diagnostic help in relation to the character of the pain is whether it is *colicky* or *constant*

colic occurs in
- renal/ureteric stone
- small intestinal obstruction
- lead poisoning (but may be constant)
- colonic pain

NB biliary pain is usually constant, not colicky

Radiation
- perforated PU epigastric → all over abdomen and shoulder tips
- biliary 'colic' R. hypochondrium → interscapular
  R. shoulder tip
  lower sternum

- pancreatitis epigastric → straight through to back
- appendicitis epigastric → RIF
  pelvic pain (pelvic appendix)
  pain in R loin (retrocaecal appendix)
- renal colic loin → anteriorly to hypochondrium
  lateral side of abdomen
  testis/labia
  thigh

Aggravating/relieving factors
- perforated PU – worse with movement
- biliary colic – can't lie still
- renal colic – can't lie still
- pancreatitis – better sitting up
- pneumonia/pleurisy (referred pain) – worse deep breathing and coughing
- appendicitis – worse on coughing

Associated symptoms

constipation →
- intestinal obstruction
- diverticulitis
- peritonitis with ileus

diarrhoea →
- pelvic appendicitis
- appendicitis in infants

bleeding from bowel →
- carcinoma bowel
- intussusception ('redcurrant jelly')
- Crohn's disease
- mesenteric artery occlusion
- Henoch–Schönlein purpura

dysuria/frequency →
- pyelitis
- secondary infection after renal stone
- salpingitis

related to menses →
- salpingitis

cough →
- referred from the lung

breathlessness →
- referred from lung (infection)
- referred from the heart (heart attack)

thirst/polyuria weight loss → • diabetic ketosis

'lightning pains' →   • tabes dorsalis (gastric crisis)

Past history

indigestion →   • perforated peptic ulcer

jaundice →   • biliary colic/acute cholecystitis

grumbling left-sided abdominal pain and constipation

→ • acute diverticulitis

progressive constipation → • intestinal obstruction (colon)

progressive weight loss → • carcinoma colon

bloody diarrhoea →   • carcinoma colon/Crohn's disease

central colicky pain and diarrhoea after meals

→ • mesenteric artery occlusion

alcoholism →   • acute pancreatitis

missed period →   • ruptured ectopic

recent pregnancy or abortion →

• salpingitis

infant weaning →   • intussusception

Examination

General

shock →   • perforated peptic ulcer

• acute pancreatitis

• massive intra-abdominal bleed

• small bowel obstruction

• mesenteric artery occlusion

absolutely still →   • perforated peptic ulcer

• peritonitis

very restless →   • renal colic

• biliary 'colic'

jaundice →   • cholecystitis

• gallstones

Temperature (fever)

above normal →
- appendicitis (only slight, 1°C)
- cholecystitis
- diverticulitis
- salpingitis
- pyelitis
- peritonitis

below normal →
- perforated peptic ulcer
- acute pancreatitis
- ruptured ectopic
- ruptured aneurysm
- mesenteric occlusion

Respiration

increased →
- respiratory infection
- heart attack
- diabetic ketosis

depressed →
- perforated peptic ulcer
- peritonitis
- painful pleurisy

Abdominal findings

Look for

distension →
- intestinal obstruction
  central → small bowel
  flanks → large bowel
- peritonitis
- paralytic ileus
- volvulus of sigmoid

movement →
- absent in peritonitis
- reduced in perforation

masses →
- carcinoma colon
  RIF, LIF
  along colon
- Crohn's disease – RIF

Acute abdominal pain

- diverticulitis – LIF
- pulsating epigastric → aortic aneurysm
- irregular liver → metastases

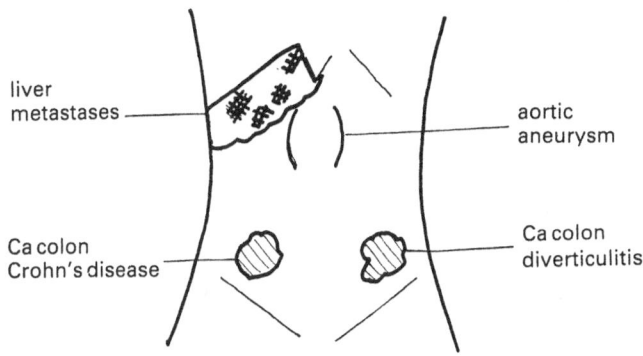

liver metastases

aortic aneurysm

Ca colon
Crohn's disease

Ca colon
diverticulitis

discolouration →	• in pancreatitis blue discolouration around umbilicus (Cullen's sign) or flanks (Grey–Turner's sign)
rash →	• herpes zoster → root distribution
	• purpuric → Henoch–Schönlein
	• photosensitivity → acute porphyria
hernia →	• a strangulated hernia is a common cause of an acute abdomen
	• a femoral hernia may be difficult to see
previous scars →	• adhesions
	• unrecognized porphyria
	• Munchausen syndrome
peristalis →	• important sign of intestinal obstruction
	• irregular in small bowel obstruction ('bag of worms')
	• less common in large bowel obstruction – runs from R to L

Feel for

local tenderness →	• inflammatory lesion
Rovsing's sign →	• pressure LIF → pain RIF → appendicitis
voluntary guarding →	• organ inflammation
reflex rigidity →	• local → local peritonitis

- general → peritonitis widespread

rebound tenderness →
- peritonitis

inflammatory masses →
- appendix abscess
- diverticulitis
- Crohn's disease
- cholecystitis
- intussusception

emptiness in RIF →
- intussusception

pancreatic pseudo-cyst →
- epigastric mass (pancreatitis)

liver
- tenderness → cholangitis (cholecystitis)
  pylephlebitis (appendicitis, diverticulitis)
- enlargement → smooth → stone in CBD
  hard/irregular → carcinoma
  metastases

spleen →
- very tender in traumatic tear

kidney →
- loin tenderness in pyelonephritis

hernial orifices →
- inguinal – direct
  indirect
- femoral
- epigastric
- incisional
- umbilical (infants)

Percuss for

hyper-resonance →
- intestinal obstruction
- gas-filled bowel abscess

shifting dullness (fluid) →
- intra-abdominal bleed

Listen for

bowel sounds
- absent → peritonitis
  paralytic ileus
- excessive → intestinal obstruction (tinkling sound)

systolic murmurs
- aortic aneurysm
- mesenteric atheroma

Acute abdominal pain

Rectal examination
(never omit)

- appendicitis → pelvic abscess
- diverticulitis → tender mass in rectum
- ruptured ectopic → tender mass pelvis
- salpingitis → tender mass pelvis
- peritonitis → exquisite tenderness pelvic peritoneum
- carcinoma rectum → proliferating tumour, craggy ulcer
- apex of intussusception (infants)
- perforated PU → tender recto-vesical pouch

Vaginal examination
(never omit)

- ruptured ectopic
    bleeding ('prune-juice')
    soft cervix
    moving cervix very painful
    fornices tender
- salpingitis
    fixed uterus
    soft cervix if post-pregnancy or abortion
    thickened tubal mass – unilateral or bilateral
- twisted ovarian cyst – tender lump in pelvis

Extra-abdominal examination

chest

- pleurisy → pleural rub
- pneumonia → dullness, crepitations
- pneumothorax → hyper-resonant chest
                    no breath sounds

CVS

- heart attack
    tachycardia
    low blood pressure
    muffled heart sounds
    gallop rhythm
    systolic murmur
    basal crepitations

153

- dissecting aneurysm

    shock

    BP lower left arm than R

    reduced or absent femoral pulses

- nervous sytem

    tabes dorsalis (see Fig. 6.9)

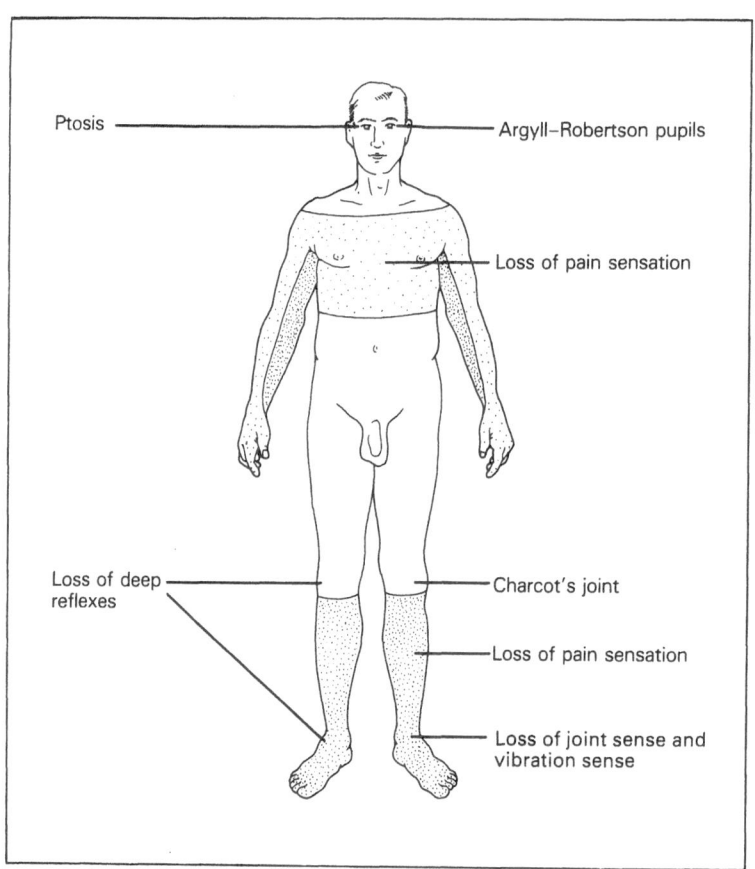

Fig. 6.9   *Signs of tabes dorsalis*

Investigation

Urine	blood	• renal colic (stone, blood clot)
		• pyelonephritis/pyelitis
	bile	• gallstone colic
	pus	• pyelonephritis/pyelitis
		• appendicitis –
		pelvic → bladder involvement
		retrocaecal → ureteric involvement
	sugar	• diabetes
		• acute pancreatitis
	ketones	• diabetic ketosis
	air (pneumaturia)	
		• diverticulitis, other pelvic infections
	uroporphobilinogen	• acute porphyria
Faeces	blood	• carcinoma colon
		• Crohn's disease (obstruction)
		• mesenteric infarction
		• intussusception ('redcurrant jelly')
	diarrhoea	• diverticulitis (sometimes)
		• pelvic appendicitis
		• infantile appendicitis
		• Crohn's disease

Blood tests

leucocytosis
- acute pancreatitis (↑ to $30\,000/mm^3$)
- appendicitis (75%) – can be normal
- mesenteric adenitis – first day only
- cholecystitis – especially with empyema
- kidney infections
- strangulated intestinal obstruction

serum amylase ↑
- acute pancreatitis (> 1000 units)
- perforated peptic ulcer.
- ruptured empyema of gall bladder
- ruptured aortic aneurysm

	• ruptured ectopic
serum bilirubin ↑	• biliary colic
	• cholecystitis
	• pancreatitis (even in absence of jaundice)
sugar ↑	• diabetic ketosis
electrolytes – Na ↓ K ↓	• intestinal obstruction
	• severe vomiting from any acute condition
calcium ↑	• renal stone (hyperparathyroidism)
calcium ↓	• acute pancreatitis
plasma fibrinogen ↑	• acute pancreatitis
methaemalbumin	• haemorrhagic pancreatitis – bad prognosis

Radiology

plain X-ray abdomen	• renal stones – 70% opaque
	• biliary stones – only 10–30% opaque
	• air under diaphragm → perforation (75% positive)
	• distended bowel with fluid levels → intestinal obstruction
	• gross distension of sigmoid → volvulus
	• blood in peritoneal cavity → haemorrhage
	• calcified aneurysm → ruptured aneurysm
	• blurred R psoas shadow → appendicitis
barium enema	• large bowel obstruction
IVP	• renal stone
chest X-ray	• pneumonia (basal → referred pain)
	• pneumothorax
	• fractured ribs L base → splenic tear

Some typical X-rays are shown (Figs. 6.10 a–c)

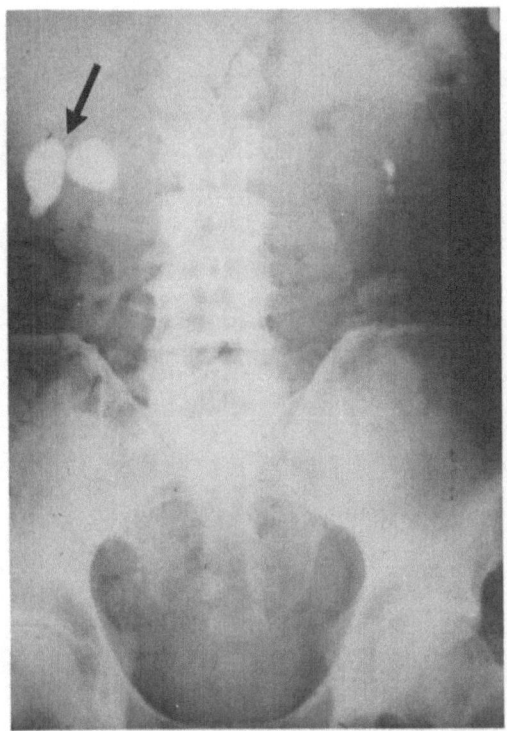

Fig. 6.10a   *Plain X-ray of the abdomen showing a radio-opaque renal stone (arrowed)*

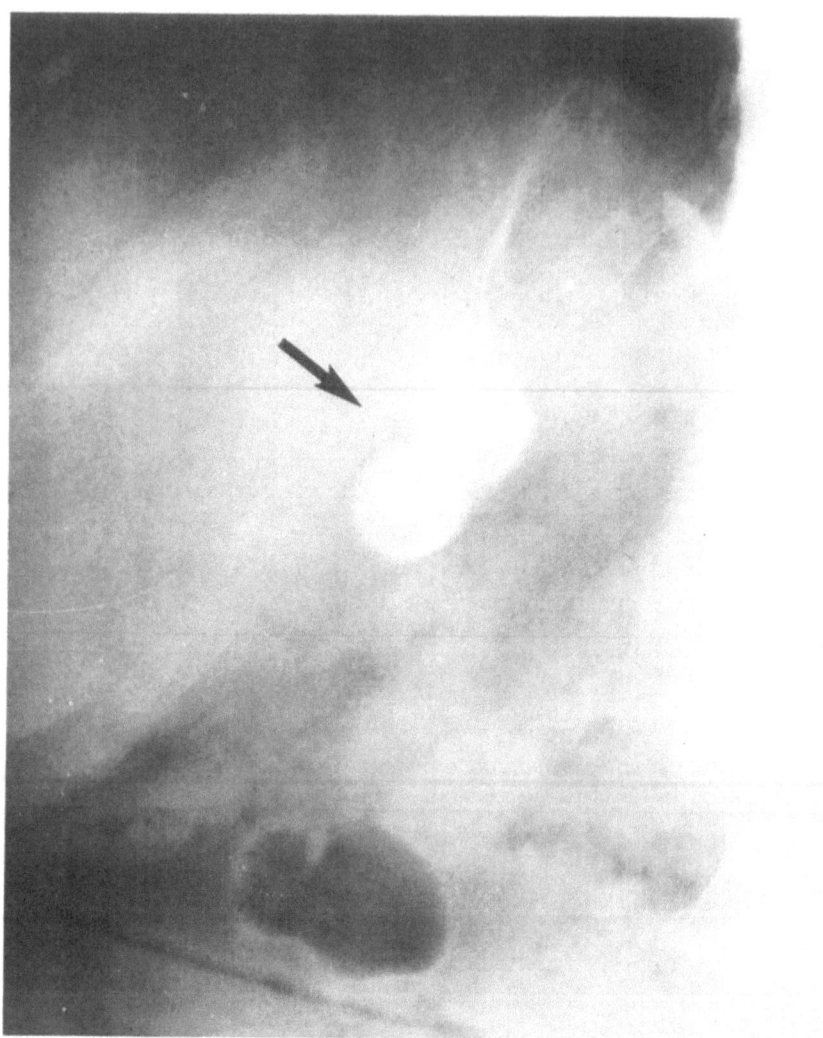

Fig. 6.10b *Plain X-ray of the abdomen showing radio-opaque multi-faceted gallstones*

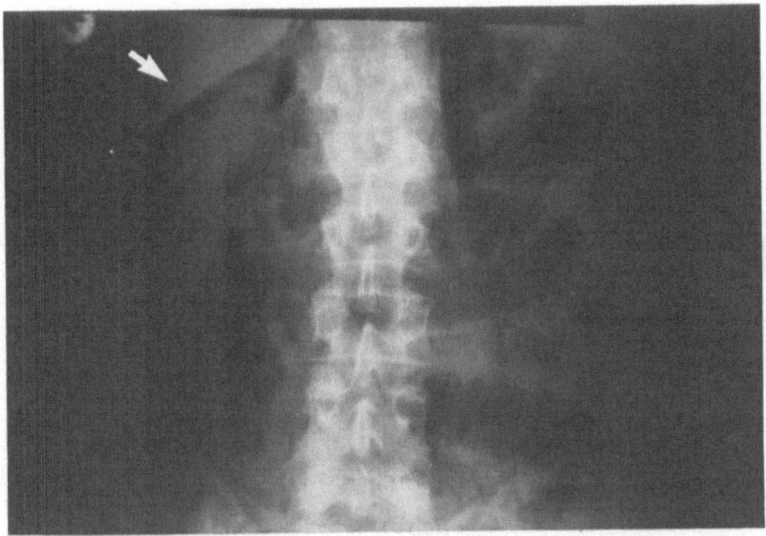

Fig. 6.10c   *Plain X-ray of the abdomen showing intraperitoneal gas due to perforation*

Laparoscopy (peritoneoscopy)

in experienced hands this is a useful diagnostic approach for the undiagnosed 'acute abdomen' and may remove the need for the more traumatic laparotomy

especially useful in young females with acute pain in RIF and pelvis

also useful for traumatic injuries to abdomen

contraindications
- generalized peritonitis
- ileus
- abdominal wall sepsis
- multiple previous operations

ECG

To diagnose myocardial infarction with referred pain to abdomen

Specific conditions

Acute appendicitis
- maximum incidence 20–30 years but occurs at all ages
- starts with central abdominal pain → RIF after 6 hours
- vomiting infrequent and of short duration
- slight pyrexia, slight tachycardia

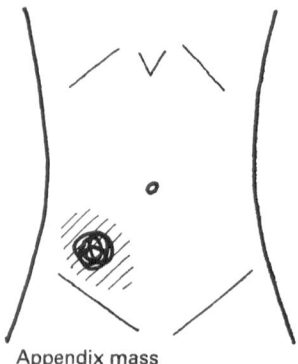

Appendix mass

- tenderness, guarding, rigidity, rebound tenderness RIF
- rectal examination – tender if
    pelvic appendix
    pelvic peritonitis
- appendix mass may develop in 4–5 days
- special cases
    retrocaecal
        little tenderness RIF
        rigidity absent
        loin tenderness
        R hip flexed
    pelvic
        no tenderness or rigidity RIF
        possible frequency
        possible diarrhoea
    infants
        inadequate history
        only 50% survive
        perforation and peritonitis common
        may be misdiagnosed as enteritis
    elderly
        rigidity slight or absent
        gangrene and peritonitis frequent
        may simulate obstruction → enema causes peritonitis
    pregnancy
        pain higher, more lateral
        peritonitis more common
        20% mortality in last trimester
        premature labour 30–50%

Acute abdominal pain

- tests – very few of value

  leucocytosis (75%)

  X-ray abdomen

    soft tissue shadow RIF

    fluid level caecum

    blurred psoas shadow

Renal colic (stone)

- M > F
- maximum incidence 30–50 years
- types of stone

    oxalate (mulberry stone) – radio-opaque

    phosphate (staghorn) – radio-opaque

    urate (multiple faceted) – radiolucent

    cystine – rare, young girls – radio-opaque

- stones may be symptomless → renal damage → uraemia
- ureteric colic

    agonizing pain from loin to groin

    lasts < 8 hours

    abdominal examination

      tender kidney

      tenderness, rigidity over ureter

- haematuria – smoky urine
- tests

    urine – blood and often pus

    plain X-ray – radio-opaque stone (70% cases)

    IVP –

      confirms opacity intrarenal

      shows function of opposite kidney

    cystoscopy

      may show urethral stricture or prostatic obstruction – encourages stone

      no urine from blocked ureter

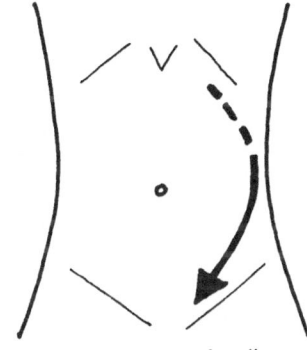

Radiation in ureteric colic

Biliary colic (gallstones)

- types of stone
  - pigment
  - cholesterol
  - mixed
- predisposing factors – 'five f's'
  - female
  - fair
  - fat
  - forty
  - fertile
- others
  - obesity
  - oestrogens
    - contraceptive pill
    - menopausal treatment
  - clofibrate (Atromid S) treatment
- presentations
  - gallstones – silent in 50%
  - biliary colic
    - epigastric or R hypochondriac (Fig. 6.11)
    - constant – not colicky
    - radiation → tip R shoulder, interscapular area
  - lasts 10 minutes–6 hours

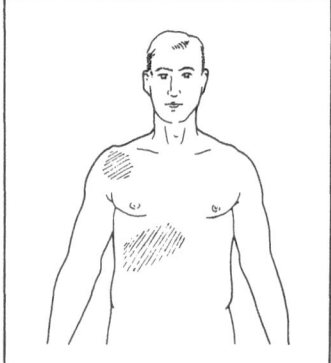

Fig. 6.11 *Sites of pain in biliary colic (gallstone)*

acute cholecystitis if stone remains impacted

passage into common bile duct →

    biliary colic

    obstructive jaundice

    cholangitis

- complications of gallstones

    recurrent cholecystitis

    hydrops of gall bladder

    empyema of gall bladder

    fistula formation into:

        colon

        duodenum

        stomach

    gallstone ileus following fistula into colon

    biliary cirrhosis → chronic obstruction

    carcinoma gall bladder – rare $< 0.5\%$

    acute pancreatitis

- tests

    straight X-ray abdomen – radio-opaque stones only in 10–30%

    ultrasound

    oral cholecystogram – identifies 70% of stones

    intravenous cholangiography if previous cholecystectomy

    liver function tests

        raised bilirubin

        raised alkaline phosphatase

Perforated peptic ulcer

- maximum incidence 45–55 years: DU > GU
- M : F = 20 : 1
- past history of indigestion in 80%
- sudden onset agonizing upper abdominal pain → generalized as peritonitis sets in after 6 hours
- shock but not for 3–4 hours
- abdominal board-like rigidity
- rectal examination – pelvic tenderness
- low-grade fever as peritonitis develops
- ileus develops (silent abdominal distension) following peritonitis
- pulse rate rises progressively with increasing deterioration
- special problems

   pain may ease as peritoneal fluid accumulates → false security

   elderly patient – may have little pain

   on steroids – painless perforation
- tests

   X-ray abdomen (erect)

      air under diaphragm – 70% cases (see Fig. 6.10c)

      later fluid levels due to paralytic ileus
- do not give morphine (or other potent analgesic) until diagnosis confirmed
- complications

   subphrenic or pelvic abscess →

      paralytic ileus

      adhesions → obstruction
- perforated GU confused with:

   diaphragmatic pleurisy

   heart attack

   ruptured aortic aneurysm

- perforated DU confused with appendicitis because of fluid tracking down R paracolic gutter – Rovsing's sign may help (pressure over left iliac fossa → pain in right iliac fossa)

Acute intestinal obstruction
- causes
    small bowel
        strangulated hernia
        adhesions
        regional ileitis
        intussusception
        volvulus – rare
    large bowel
        carcinoma (30%)
        diverticulitis
- cardinal features
    pain – colicky
    vomiting – more in small bowel obstruction, more in children
    absolute constipation – no faeces or flatus
    abdominal distension
    visible peristalis
    loud borborygmi
- always check hernial orifices for strangulated hernia
- dehydration rapidly ensues, especially in children
- a mass may be felt:
    carcinoma colon
    diverticulitis
    intussusception
    abscess
- rectal examination may show:
    empty rectum

carcinoma

apex of intussusception (rare)

- tests

    X-ray abdomen

        fluid levels in erect film

        sigmoid volvulus → distended U loop

        gallstone ileus

    marked leucocytosis → strangulated hernia

    electrolytes low → dehydration

    barium enema

        carcinoma

        diverticulitis

- if in doubt of diagnosis of intestinal obstruction an enema may help

Superior mesenteric artery occlusion

- M > F
- elderly
- sudden onset of colicky pain
- profuse vomiting
- shock develops early
- watery diarrhoea – blood in 1/3
- local tenderness, rigidity and rebound over infarcted bowel
- other clinical findings (Fig. 6.12)
- tests

    plain X-ray abdomen – 'thumbprinting' due to mucosal oedema superimposed on gas-filled bowel

    mesenteric arteriography

- early diagnosis (within a few hours) is essential otherwise gangrene, peritonitis and death are likely to ensue
- inferior mesenteric artery occlusion is less severe and survival is more likely

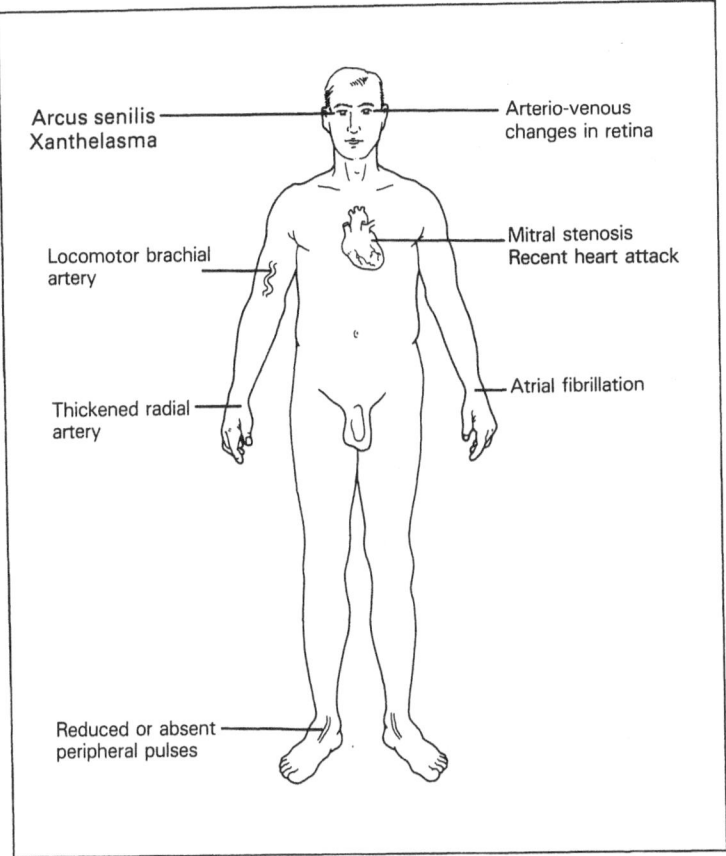

Fig. 6.12 *General signs in superior mesenteric artery occlusion*

Acute diverticulitis	• F > M
	• > 40 years of age
	• often long-standing grumbling left-sided abdominal pain and constipation
	• occurs in < 10% of patients with diverticulosis
	• acute onset pain in LIF
	• tenderness and guarding LIF
	• high fever
	• inflammatory mass may develop in LIF
	• constipation

167

- tests

  polymorph leucocytosis ⎫ distinguishes acute
  high ESR ⎬ diverticulitis from
  pus and blood in stools ⎭ painful diverticular
        disease

- complications

  perforation – mortality 40%

  abscess

  peritonitis

  fistula into:

       bladder → pneumaturia

       vagina

       small bowel

       renal tract

  excessive bleeding especially in elderly

  intestinal obstruction

  portal pyaemia – rare

Acute gastro-enteritis

- all ages
- pathogens

  bacterial

       Shigella

       Salmonella

       Staphylococcus aureus

       Clostridium welchii

  virus

  protozoa

       Entamoeba histtolytica

       Giardia lamblia

- mainly in communities – direct spread by touch
- most frequent < 10 years
- incubation 1–3 days
- diarrhoea – green, watery, mucus
- excessive offensive flatus

Acute abdominal pain

- vomiting – especially babies
- colicky abdominal pain < 50% – relieved by passing motion or flatus
- fever (30%)
- tender over descending colon or RIF – simulates appendicitis
- tests

    stool examination and culture rarely helpful

    serum electrolytes for dehydration
- complications

    severe dehydration especially babies

    recurrences common

    chronic carrier state may be established

Acute intermittent porphyria
- hereditary disorder of breakdown of haemoglobin
- abdominal crises mimic a surgical 'acute abdomen'
- may be precipitated by drugs e.g. phenobarbitone
- the clinical features are shown in Fig. 6.13
- skin photosensitivity may be present
- anaemia often present (haemolytic)
- tests

    urine – normal appearance on passing, change to 'port-wine' on standing

    X-ray abdomen – may show segments of intestinal spasm with dilated gas-filled bowel between

    serum sodium may be very low

    lab test for urinary porphobilinogen

Ruptured ectopic gestation
- commonest cause of intraperitoneal haemorrhage
- history of missed period
- may be past history of pelvic infection preventing normal implantation of the fertilized ovum
- intermittent abdominal pain – suprapubic or iliac fossa

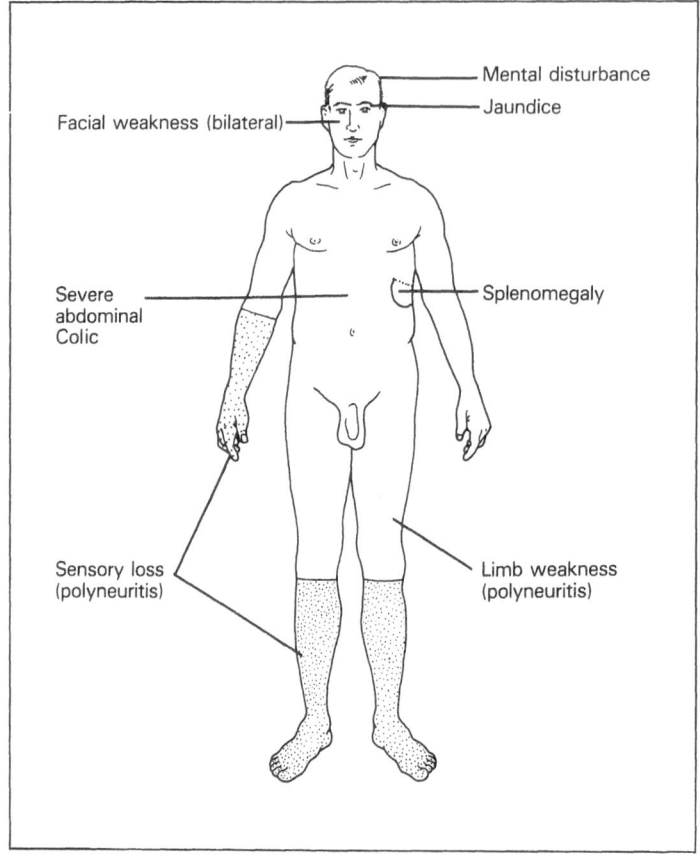

Fig. 6.13 *Acute intermittent porphyria*

- pain may radiate to:
    - rectum (lavatory sign)
    - vagina
    - leg
- brown vaginal discharge
- dysuria and frequency may occur
- abdomen
    - slight distension
    - deep tenderness in iliac fossa
    - rebound tenderness may be present
    - shifting dullness if enough blood

Acute abdominal pain

- vaginal examination

    dark thick blood ('prune-juice')

    soft cervix

    moving cervix → severe pain

    fornices tender

- temperature and pulse normal in early stages

Pitfalls in diagnosis

- Misdiagnosis of abdominal pain and diarrhoea due to appendicitis in children as gastro-enteritis – localized tenderness in RIF or on rectal examination will help.
- False reassurance when pain eases in perforated ulcer – may be due to the development of peritonitis.
- Misdiagnosing abdominal pain, frequency and dysuria as urinary tract infection in pelvic appendicitis, diverticulitis, salpingitis, ruptured ectopic.
- Missing a perforation in elderly or in patients on steroids because of lack of pain.
- Forgetting to examine hernial orifices in a patient with intestinal obstruction.
- Mistaking the brown vaginal discharge in ectopic gestation for a normal period thereby excluding the possibility of rupture.
- Forgetting the possibility of superior mesenteric artery obstruction in an elderly arteriosclerotic patient with colicky central abdominal pain.

Useful practical points

- Right sided abdominal pain and a *high* fever is unlikely to be appendicitis – pyelitis more likely.
- The urine may show pus and red cells in appendicitis when:

  pelvic – affects bladder

  retrocaecal – affects ureter
- Always think of referred respiratory pain where there is severe upper abdominal pain without tenderness or guarding – a chest X-ray will decide.
- Local tenderness in RIF and Rovsing's sign help to distinguish appendicitis from gastro-enteritis in childhood.
- Always think of uraemia when hiccups are present in a patient with abdominal distension and vomiting thought initially to be intestinal obstruction.
- Suspect a mesenteric artery embolism in a patient with mitral stenosis and atrial fibrillation who develops sudden abdominal pain mimicking an 'acute abdomen'.
- Don't forget herpes zoster in an elderly patient with excruciating unilateral abdominal pain especially if it follows a particular dermatome.
- Deep sighing respiration in a patient with abdominal pain, vomiting, tenderness and rigidity should suggest diabetic keto-acidosis – always test the urine for sugar in all patients with an 'acute abdomen'.

Case challenge

A 42-year-old male patient was admitted to hospital with acute abdominal pain which had been gradually getting worse over the previous 24 hours. The pain had started in the epigastrium and had spread to involve the whole of the abdomen and was associated with repeated vomiting. He had a long history of indigestion which had never been investigated by a barium meal; he attributed the indigestion to alcohol since he admitted to being a fairly heavy drinker, 4–5 pints of beer most days, for at least 20 years. He had a previous attack of abdominal pain and jaundice several years ago which had lasted for about a week but this had been treated at home by his family doctor and he had no special tests.

The examination findings are shown in Fig. 6.14.

Questions

What is the differential diagnosis?

What tests would help the decision on diagnosis?

Acute abdominal pain

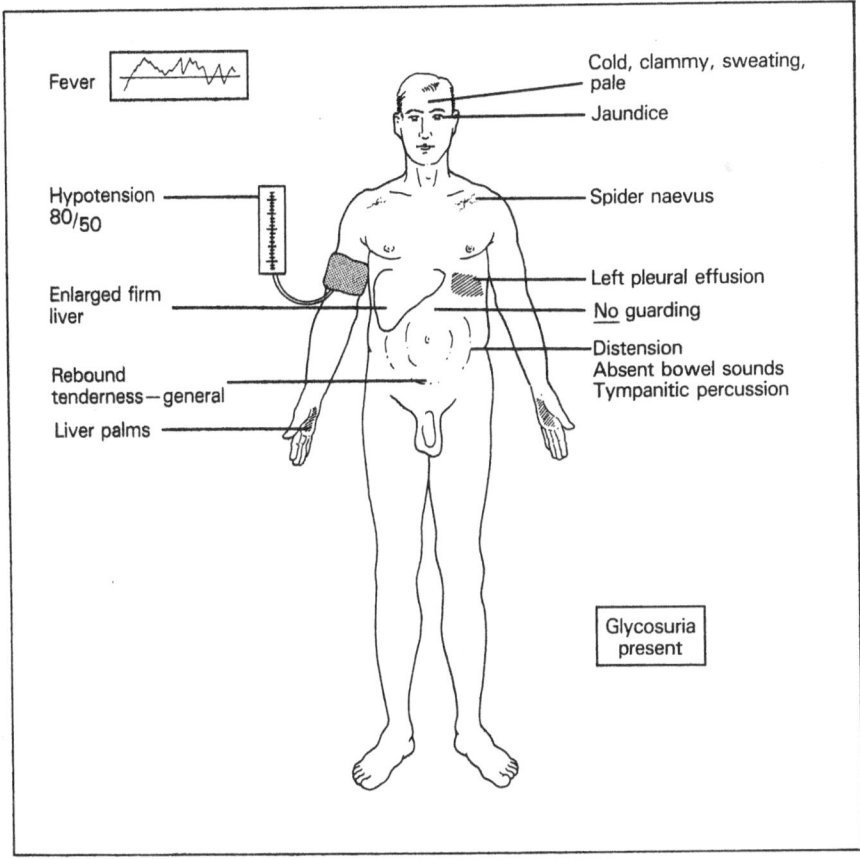

Fig. 6.14 *Examination findings in case challenge*

Differential diagnosis

- perforated peptic ulcer
- biliary disease
  gallstones
  acute cholecystitis
- acute pancreatitis
- acute mesenteric artery occlusion
- diabetic keto-acidosis

Perforated peptic ulcer

For	history	• long history of indigestion
Against	exam	• no board-like rigidity in epigastrium
Tests		• plain X-ray abdomen – air under diaphragm

Biliary disease

For	history	• previous attack of abdominal pain and jaundice
	exam	• jaundice
		• evidence of liver disease
Against	history	• no history of biliary colic
	exam	• no local tenderness over gall bladder
Tests		• plain X-ray abdomen – gallstones (opaque 10–30%)
		• ultrasound
		for gall bladder distension
		for bile duct dilatation
		• intravenous cholangiography
		• blood test
		bilirubin ↑
		alkaline phosphatase ↑

Acute pancreatitis

For	history	• past history of alcoholism
		• possible previous attack of pancreatitis
		• build up of pain over 24 hours
		• profuse vomiting
	exam	• shock
		• jaundice
		• lack of guarding or rigidity
		• evidence of peritonitis with paralytic ileus
		• evidence of cirrhosis (probably alcoholic)
		• left pleural effusion (10% of cases)
		• glycosuria

Acute abdominal pain

Tests

- serum amylase ↑ – over 1000 units but increased also in:

  perforated peptic ulcer

  gallstones

  mesenteric infarction

  (salivary disease)

- other blood tests

  WBC ↑

  serum calcium ↓

  serum albumin ↓

  bilirubin ↑

  blood sugar ↑

NB methaemalbuminaemia indicates severe hae-morrhagic necrosis of pancreas

- plain X-ray abdomen

  general distension with air – paralytic ileus

  may get segmented distension jejunum or transverse colon in ileus

  calcification in pancreas

Acute mesenteric artery occlusion

For	history	• nil
	exam	• lack of guarding on examination
		• evidence of paralytic ileus
Against	history	• no prior history of mesenteric angina
		• central colicky abdominal pain with diarrhoea 20–30 minutes after meals
	exam	• no obvious source of embolus
		• no evidence of arteriosclerosis
Tests		• plain X-ray abdomen – 'thumbprinting' due to patchy mucosal oedema superimposed on gas-filled bowel
		• mesenteric arteriography

Diabetic ketosis

For	history	• acute abdominal pain
	exam	• no local guarding in abdomen
		• circulatory collapse
		• glycosuria
Against	history	• no previous history of:
		thirst
		polyuria
		loss of weight
	exam	• no acidotic breathing
		• no reason for peritonitis and paralytic ileus
Tests		• blood sugar measurements
		• pH of blood – acidosis

Actual diagnosis:
Acute haemorrhagic pancreatitis

Treatment and outcome

The patient was treated in intensive care with buprenorphine to control pain, blood transfusion, oxygen and insulin for the disturbed glucose metabolism.

Other measures sometimes tried but unproven in efficacy, include pancreatic inhibitors such as glucagon, calcitonin and somatostatin, antacids, anticholinergics and H_2-receptor blockers, and the antiprotease, Trasylol.

The patient recovered slowly in the next 6 weeks but was left with permanent diabetes.

7 Chronic Abdominal Pain

Introduction

Common diagnostic and management problem across the clinical board.

Frequently encountered by

> general practitioners
>
> physicians
>
> surgeons
>
> gynaecologists
>
> psychiatrists
>
> paediatricians
>
> geriatricians

In many cases no definite organic cause is found, but this should not mean that the pain is 'imaginary', 'functional' or whatever other euphemistic term is used.

The diagnostic approach must be to determine a specific cause but continuing and repeated investigative searching exercises should not go on indefinitely.

Causes of chronic abdominal pain

Abdominal

inflammatory	• chronic cholecystitis
	• chronic pancreatitis
	• chronic appendicitis
	• Crohn's disease
'chemical'	• peptic ulcer
	• oesophagitis (hiatus hernia)
mechanical	• intestinal obstruction
	• biliary obstruction

- ureteric obstruction
- liver congestion e.g. heart failure, tumours

neoplastic
- carcinoma stomach
- carcinoma colon
- carcinoma pancreas
- hepatic metastases

vascular
- chronic mesenteric ischaemia
- abdominal aortic aneurysm

disturbed mobility
- irritable bowel syndrome
- functional dyspepsia
- diverticulosis

Gynaecological

(lower abdominal pain)
- 'mittelschmerz'
- chronic salpingitis
- cervical erosion
- uterine fibroids
- ovarian tumours

Extra-abdominal
- metabolic
    exogenous – lead poisoning
    endogenous
        uraemia
        diabetic coma
        porphyria
        Addison's disease
- neurogenic
    tabes dorsalis
    arthritis/radiculitis
- psychogenic
    anxiety
    depression

Grades of severity (and causes)

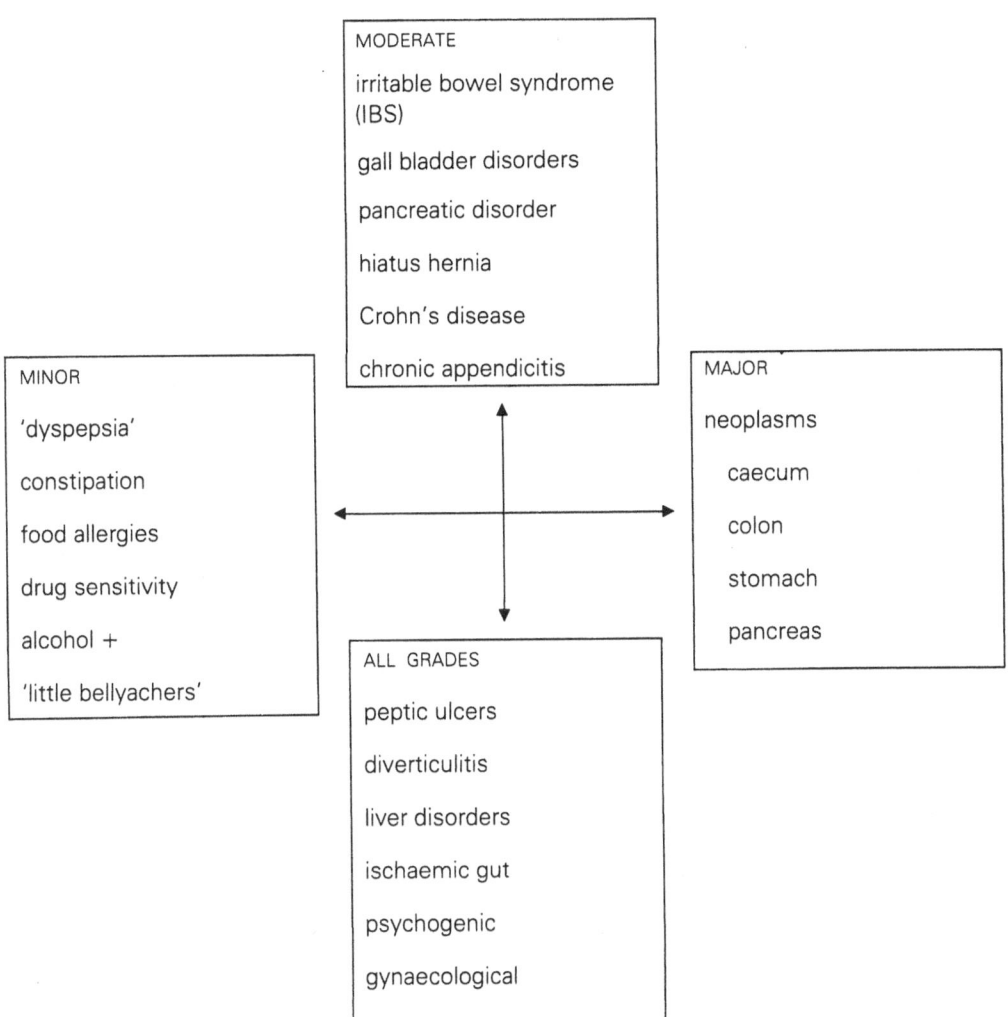

MODERATE

irritable bowel syndrome (IBS)

gall bladder disorders

pancreatic disorder

hiatus hernia

Crohn's disease

chronic appendicitis

MINOR

'dyspepsia'

constipation

food allergies

drug sensitivity

alcohol +

'little bellyachers'

MAJOR

neoplasms

  caecum

  colon

  stomach

  pancreas

ALL GRADES

peptic ulcers

diverticulitis

liver disorders

ischaemic gut

psychogenic

gynaecological

Frequency

Annual prevalence of 'chronic abdominal pain' in a general practice population of 2500	
no discoverable cause	60
minor causes	20
IBS	15
gynaecological	10
peptic ulcers	5
hiatus hernia	5
diverticulitis	3
cancers	2
gall bladder disease	2
Less than 1 per year	
Crohn's disease	
pancreatic disease	
liver disease	
ischaemic gut	

Age incidence

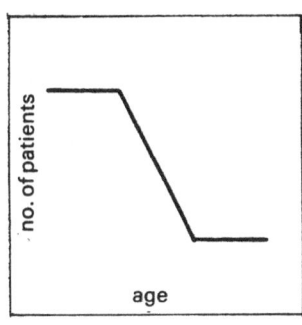

- 'little bellyachers'
- Crohn's disease
- gynaecological causes
- 'chronic appendicitis'

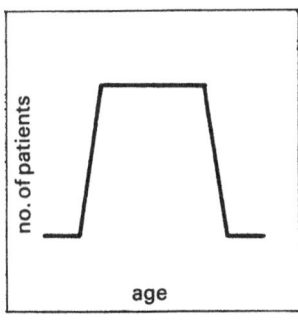

- peptic ulcers
- hiatus hernia
- IBS
- psychogenic
- gall bladder disease

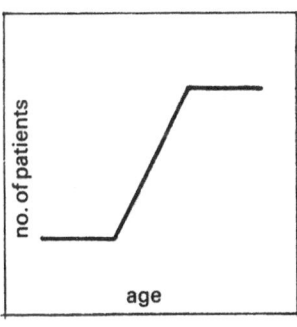

- cancers
- diverticulitis
- ischaemic gut

Diagnostic approach

History

A detailed history is of importance in deciding the cause of the chronic abdominal pain and should be the part of the diagnostic process on which the doctor should spend most time.

Abdominal pain – diagnosis depends on

- site
- character
- radiation
- aggravating factors
- relieving factors

Site – the value of the site of the pain on deciding its origin is shown in Fig. 7.1

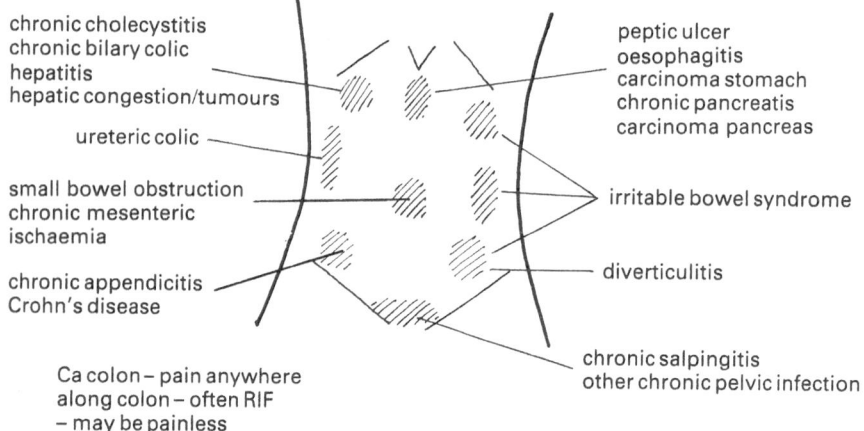

chronic cholecystitis
chronic bilary colic
hepatitis
hepatic congestion/tumours

peptic ulcer
oesophagitis
carcinoma stomach
chronic pancreatis
carcinoma pancreas

ureteric colic

small bowel obstruction
chronic mesenteric
ischaemia

irritable bowel syndrome

chronic appendicitis
Crohn's disease

diverticulitis

Ca colon – pain anywhere
along colon – often RIF
– may be painless

chronic salpingitis
other chronic pelvic infection

Fig. 7.1   *Value of site of chronic abdominal pain in deciding its cause*

Character

deep-seated gnawing
pain   →   • peptic ulcer

retrosternal burning →   • oesophagitis

colicky pain   →   • intestinal obstruction

- intestinal ischaemia
- ureteric colic
- lead poisoning

burning pain →	• causalgia due to nerve root irritation (referred pain)
momentary stabbing pain →	• functional
'grumbling' pain →	• irritable bowel syndrome

Radiation

epigastrium → back	• duodenal ulcer
	• chronic pancreatitis
	• carcinoma pancreas

epigastrium → R. hypochondrium
       interscapular area } → gall bladder disease
       tip of R. shoulder

epigastrium → retrosternal/ left arm	• oesophagitis
loin → groin	• renal colic
lower abdomen → low back	• chronic salpingitis
differing abdominal sites	• irritable bowel syndrome

Aggravating factors

eating →	• gastric ulcer
not eating →	• duodenal ulcer
night-time →	• duodenal ulcer
lying flat →	• oesophagitis, chronic pancreatitis
bending/stooping →	• oesophagitis
movement →	• root pain (arthritis)
anxiety/stress →	• irritable bowel syndrome

Relieving factors

eating →	• duodenal ulcer
alkalis →	• gastric ulcer
	• duodenal ulcer
	• oesophagitis
sitting up →	• chronic pancreatitis
standing →	• oesophagitis

passing flatus →   ● colonic disease

bowel evacuating →   ● colonic disease

Associated symptoms

rumbling, flatulence →   ● irritable bowel

anorexia →   ● carcinoma stomach

weight loss →   ● carcinoma stomach

    ● carcinoma pancreas

    ● carcinoma colon

    ● chronic pancreatitis

symptom of anaemia →   ● carcinoma stomach

    ● carcinoma colon

    ● lead poisoning

'heartburn' →   ● oesophagitis

waterbrash →   ● duodenal ulcer

dysphagia →   ● oesophagitis with stricture

itching →   ● gall bladder disease

painful eyes
athralgia   } →   ● Crohn's disease
back pain

thirst →   ● diabetes

    ● uraemia

'lightning pains' in the
limbs →   ● tabes dorsalis

Other relevant associations

bowels

increasing
constipation →   ● carcinoma colon

diarrhoea →   ● carcinoma colon

    ● Crohn's disease

diarrhoea 30 min after
eating →   ● mesenteric ischaemia

constipation/diarrhoea → ● irritable bowel syndrome

stools

blood	occult →	• peptic ulcer
		• carcinoma stomach
		• carcinoma colon
	frank →	• carcinoma colon
		• Crohn's disease
pus/mucus →		• Crohn's disease
		• diverticulitis

bulky, offensive, floating →	• chronic pancreatitis
pale →	• gall bladder disease
ribbon-like, pellets →	• irritable bowel syndrome

micturition

dysuria →		• urinary tract infection
polyuria →		• uraemia
		• diabetes
dark urine →		• gall bladder disease
urine	dark→	• gall bladder disease
	protein →	• uraemia
	pus →	• ureteric colic, pyelitis
	sugar →	• diabetes
	'port-wine' →	• porphyria

menstruation

pelvic pain worse with period →	• chronic salpingitis
pelvic pain between periods →	• 'mittelschmerz' (due to painful ovulation)

Family history

The relevant associations which may be of diagnostic help include:

peptic ulcer

Crohn's disease – family history of

• bowel disease

• rheumatoid arthritis

- Hashimoto's thyroiditis
- pernicious anaemia
- diabetes

bilirubin gallstones

- congenital spherocytosis
- thalassaemia
- sickle cell anaemia

carcinoma stomach

- pernicious anaemia

Diet

Diet is of no significance in the development of peptic ulcer

Inadequate roughage predisposes to irritable bowel syndrome

Inadequate fluid intake may encourage the formation of renal stones

Alcohol

Alcohol is relevant in

- chronic pancreatitis
- probably duodenal ulcer

Smoking

This may be relevant in

- gastric ulcer
- mesenteric ischaemia due to atherosclerosis

Psychological state

The irritable bowel syndrome is more likely to occur with an anxiety state

Clinical examination

The signs which may be helpful in determining the cause of chronic abdominal pain are shown in Fig. 7.2

In the large majority of cases of chronic abdominal pain no abnormal signs are found in the abdomen and no cause can be discovered.

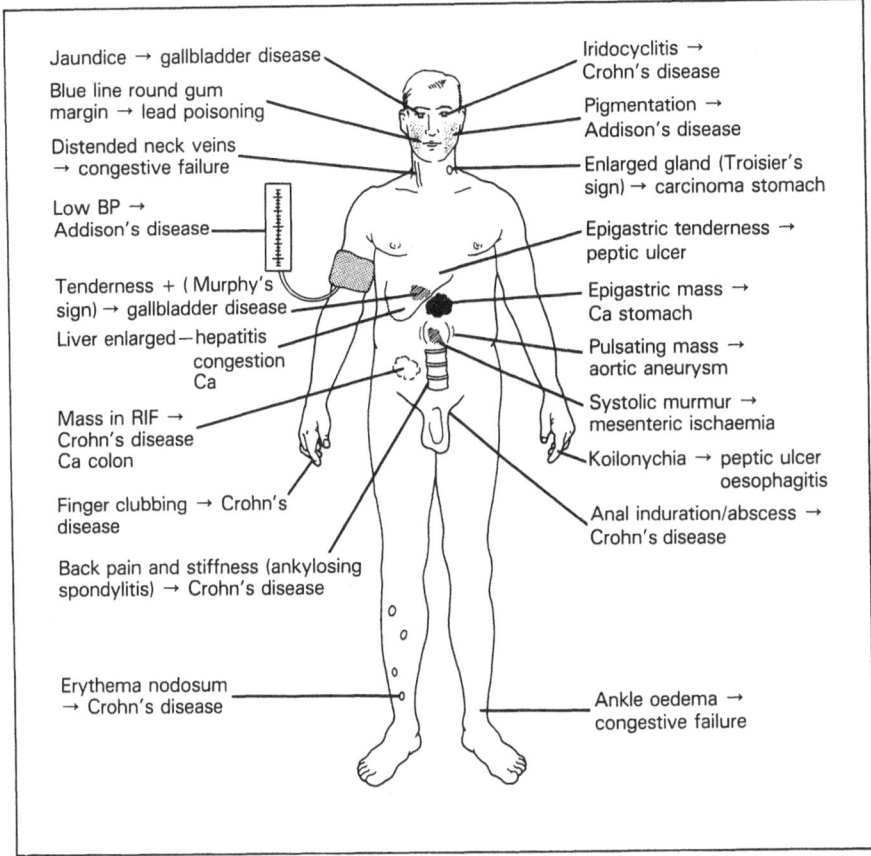

Jaundice → gallbladder disease

Blue line round gum margin → lead poisoning

Distended neck veins → congestive failure

Low BP → Addison's disease

Tenderness + (Murphy's sign) → gallbladder disease

Liver enlarged — hepatitis
congestion
Ca

Mass in RIF → Crohn's disease
Ca colon

Finger clubbing → Crohn's disease

Back pain and stiffness (ankylosing spondylitis) → Crohn's disease

Erythema nodosum → Crohn's disease

Iridocyclitis → Crohn's disease

Pigmentation → Addison's disease

Enlarged gland (Troisier's sign) → carcinoma stomach

Epigastric tenderness → peptic ulcer

Epigastric mass → Ca stomach

Pulsating mass → aortic aneurysm

Systolic murmur → mesenteric ischaemia

Koilonychia → peptic ulcer
oesophagitis

Anal induration/abscess → Crohn's disease

Ankle oedema → congestive failure

Fig. 7.2   *Helpful signs in chronic abdominal pain*

Investigations

Before embarking on investigation of chronic abdominal pain consider:

over-investigation can do irreparable psychological harm in reinforcing the patient's fear that he has serious physical disease.

on the other hand some patients need the reassurance of thorough investigation to allay their anxieties – the GP will have to decide.

it is desirable therefore to have at least one full and adequate investigation, and if negative, it should not be repeated at other times and in other places.

children – only 10% will have evience of organic disease underlying their recurrent abdominal pain.

elderly – diagnosis of organic disease becomes more difficult:

    they will complain less

    symptoms may be non-specific

    inflammatory pyrexia may be absent

    more than one disease is often present

perspicacious investigation is therefore more necessary.

watch out for *stomach cancer* in

- pernicious anaemia
- first symptoms > 50 years old
- after gastrectomy
- Peutz–Jegher's syndrome –
  brown-black spots on lips, hands, mouth
  abdominal pain
  GI bleeding due to polyposis

if symptoms are *severe* and especially if *persistent* always investigate.

Investigations of value in diagnosing abdominal pain

Radiology

plain X-ray

gall bladder disease	• stones (10–30%)
	• limey bile
	• 'porcelain' gall bladder
Crohn's disease	• mass in RIF
renal stones (70% radio-opaque)	
intestinal obstruction	• gas distension
	• fluid levels
mesenteric ischaemia	• 'thumbprinting'

barium studies

barium meal	• oesophagitis
	• peptic ulcer
	• carcinoma stomach
	• carcinoma pancreas
small bowel enema	• Crohn's disease

large bowel enema	• carcinoma colon
	• diverticulosis
	• Crohn's disease
cholecystogram	• gall bladder disease
intravenous cholangiogram	• gall bladder disease
endoscopic retrograde cholangio-pancreatography	• gall bladder disease
intravenous pyelogram	• renal stones
computerized tomography	• tumours
	• gall bladder disease
	• hepatic metastases

Blood tests

Hb – anaemia	• peptic ulcer
	• oesophagitis
	• carcinomata stomach/colon
abnormal red cells	• thalassaemia
	• sickle cell disease

$$\left.\begin{array}{c}\text{thalassaemia}\\\text{sickle cell disease}\end{array}\right\} \rightarrow \begin{array}{l}\text{gallstones}\\\text{(bilirubin)}\end{array}$$

raised ESR	• carcinoma
	• Crohn's disease
liver function abnormal	• gall bladder disease
blood sugar ↑	• diabetes
blood urea ↑	• uraemia

Urine tests

bile pigments	• gall bladder disease
sugar	• diabetes
protein	• uraemia
porphobilinogen	• porphyria

Ultrasound

	• abdominal tumours
	• gall bladder disease
	• chronic pancreatitis
	• hepatic metastases

Re-investigation

If the initial investigation is thorough and negative it is better *not* to re-investigate chronic abdominal pain because of the risk of reinforcing the patient's anxieties about serious underlying disease.

Re-investigation *should* be considered however if:

- the symptoms remain severe
- the symptoms remain persistent
- a trial of simple symptomatic treatment is unsuccessful
- the character of the pain changes
- a new development occurs
- the patient progressively loses weight

Specific conditions

'Little bellyachers'

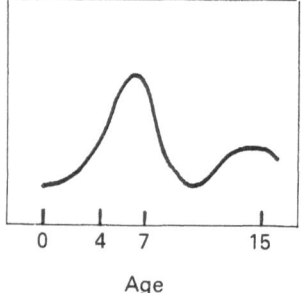

Age

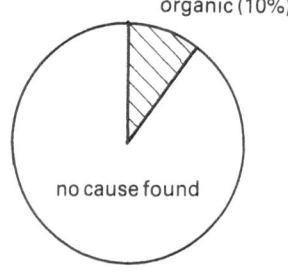

- age 4–7 boys and girls

    12–15 in girls

- recurring bouts of central abdominal pain of variable intensity last minutes or hours, child may become pale.
- may be accompanied by pains in legs, vomiting or headache.
- no abnormalities found on examination
- often positive family history of abdominal disorders or migraine.
- 90% – no organic cause found
- 10% – 'mesenteric adenitis'

    renal disease

- most disappear after 8 years
- girls 12–15 recurring RIF pains (possibly related to menses)

Chronic abdominal pain

Non-ulcer dyspepsia

- typical ulcer pain
    related to food
    relieved by antacids
- no evidence of peptic ulcer
    barium meal
    endoscopy
- 'cause unknown' – possibilities
    pre-ulcer phase
    variant of irritable bowel syndrome
    pylorospasm
    psychogenic
- treat symptomatically with antacids
- response to H_2-receptor blockers is poor

Chronic pancreatitis

- most cases in developed countries due to alcoholism
- M > F
- 35–45 years old
- recurrent epigastric pain lasting days or weeks radiating through to the back
- worse on lying, better on sitting/standing
- bout of pain may follow bout of drinking
- diarrhoea ($\frac{1}{3}$) – stools large, bulky, offensive, difficult to flush away
- features of malabsorption
    weight loss
    anaemia from deficiency of:
        iron
        vitamin B12
        folate
    tetany (hypocalcaemia)
    bleeding (vitamin K)

vitamin deficiency

> sore tongue
>
> stomatitis
>
> cracked skin
>
> oedema (hypoalbuminaemia)

- tests

> X-ray abdomen – calcification in pancreas (rare)
>
> ultrasound – abnormal pancreas
>
> barium meal – deformed duodenum
>
> stool – excessive fat
>
> blood
>
> > flat glucose-tolerance test
> >
> > low calcium
>
> ERCP
>
> > stones
> >
> > dilatation of pancreatic ducts

Irritable bowel syndrome

- cardinal symptoms

> abdominal pain
>
> abnormality of bowels

- the various sites of pain:

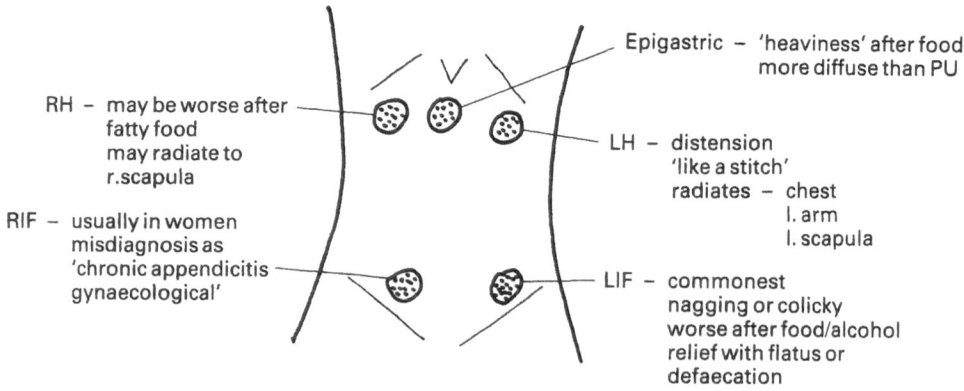

Epigastric – 'heaviness' after food more diffuse than PU

RH – may be worse after fatty food may radiate to r.scapula

LH – distension 'like a stitch' radiates – chest l. arm l. scapula

RIF – usually in women misdiagnosis as 'chronic appendicitis gynaecological'

LIF – commonest nagging or colicky worse after food/alcohol relief with flatus or defaecation

Chronic abdominal pain

- associated symptoms
    - anorexia
    - flatulence
    - post-prandial fullness
    - general
        - fatigue +
        - palpitations
        - left mammary pain
- bowels
    - constipation
    - diarrhoea
    - alternating constipation/diarrhoea
- stools
    - no blood
    - ribbon-like
    - small pellets
- tests – sigmoidoscopy and barium enema necessary *once* to
    - reassure patient } not cancer
    - reassure doctor

Carcinoma stomach

- common in UK, Japan
  uncommon in USA
- M : F = 3 : 1 peak age 50–60 years
- main sites
    - prepyloric (70%) → obstruction
    - body → few symptoms
    - fundus → oesophageal obstruction
    - diffuse infiltration → rare
- may develop as chronic gastric ulcer
- symptoms
    - anorexia – may be late
    - epigastric pain unrelated to food
    - weight loss
    - vomiting

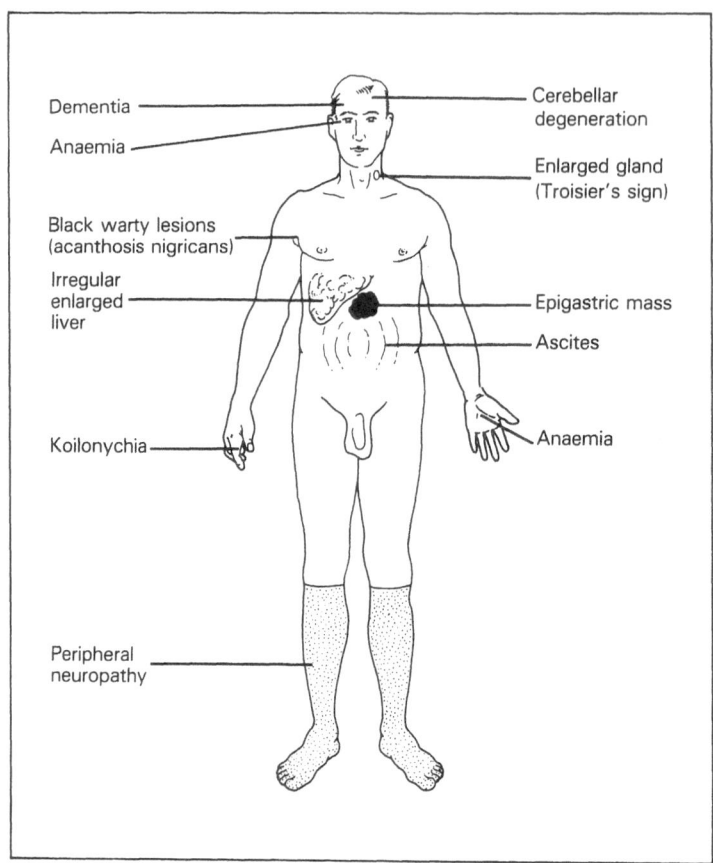

Fig. 7.3 *Possible signs in carcinoma stomach*

- signs – see Fig. 7.3
- tests

  gastroscopy and biopsy – *essential*

  barium meal

  malignant ulcer

  proliferative tumour

  diffuse infiltration – rare

  blood – iron-deficiency anaemia

  stool – occult blood

NB. Remember the possibility of gastric carcinoma in patients with pernicious anaemia (Fig. 7.4)

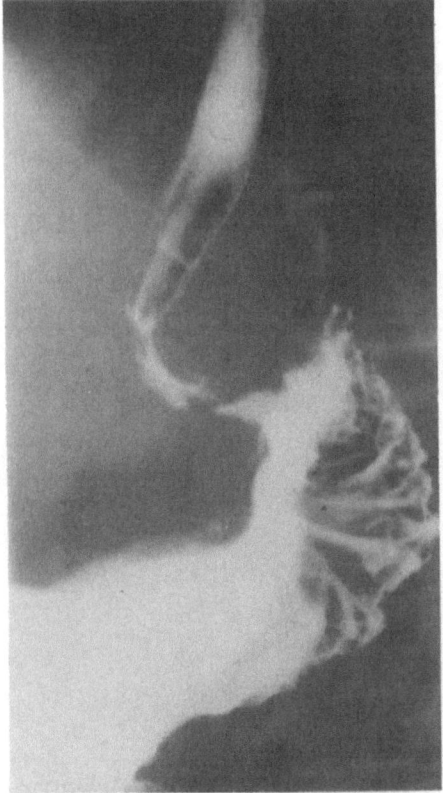

Fig. 7.4 *Barium meal showing filling defect of the stomach due to carcinoma*

Carcinoma of colon

- commonest carcinoma in alimentary tract in UK
- men > women: peak over 50 years
- affects descending colon/rectum in two thirds of patients
- types of tumour

  proliferative

  ulcerative

  constricting

- symptoms

  bowels

  increasing constipation – usually carcinoma descending colon

  diarrhoea – usually carcinoma ascending colon

195

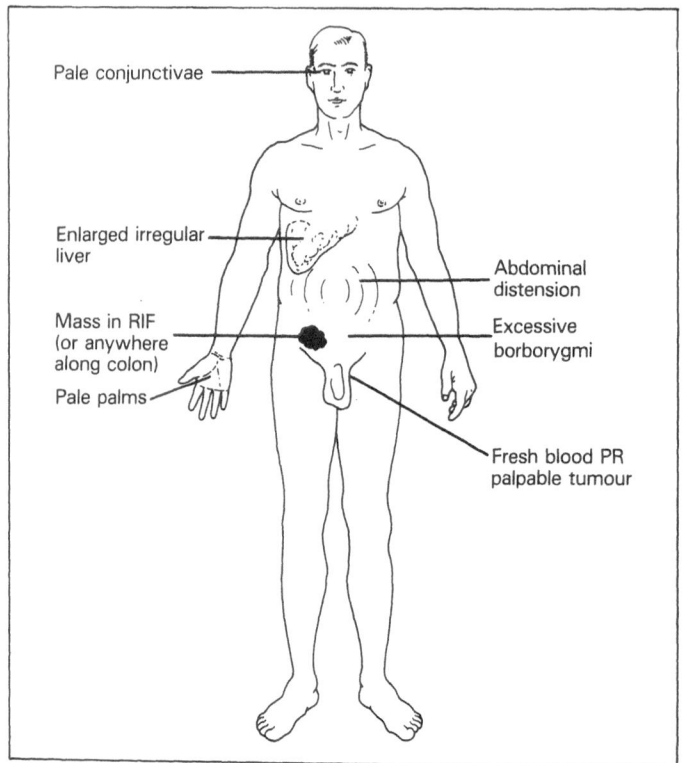

Fig. 7.5 *Possible signs in carcinoma of colon*

    colicky abdominal pain

    rectal bleeding – especially rectal carcinoma

    tenesmus – carcinoma rectum

    weight loss

    symptoms of anaemia

- signs – shown in Fig. 7.5
- tests

    sigmoidoscopy – detects 50% colonic tumours

    barium enema

    colonoscopy – useful for proximal tumours

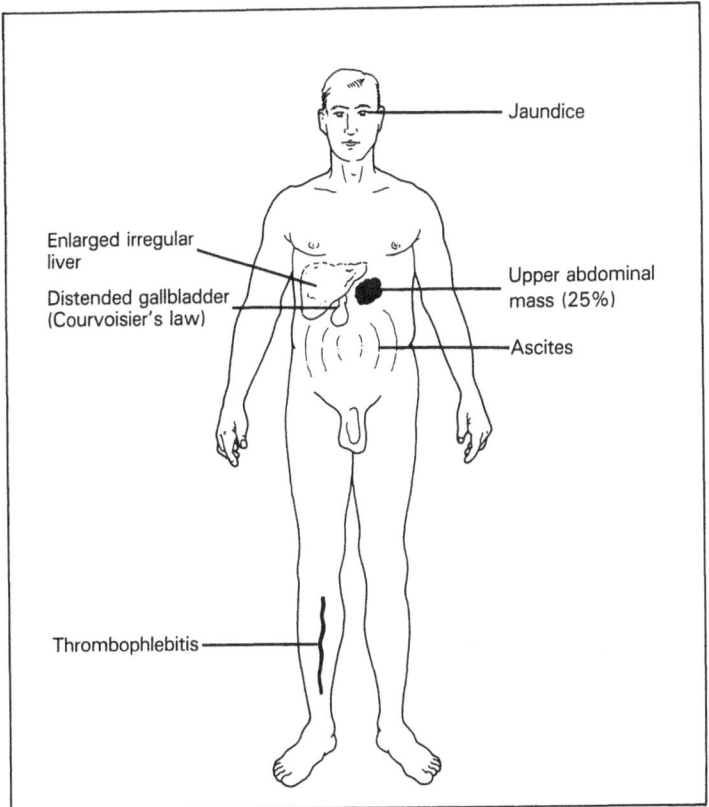

Fig. 7.6 *Possible signs in carcinoma of pancreas*

Acute intermittent porphyria
- 5–10 cases per 100 000 population
- due to a deficiency in an enzyme responsible for synthesis of haemoglobin (uroporphyrinogen synthetase)
- precipitating factors

    drugs

      barbiturates

      sulphonamides

      tranquillizers

      antidepressants

      phenytoin

      methyl dopa

      oral hypoglycaemics

Carcinoma of pancreas

- M > F: peak 55–70 years
- cigarette smoking may be aetiological factor
- usually scirrhous adenocarcinoma involving head (two thirds)
- symptoms

  may be symptomless until advanced

  vague abdominal discomfort

  more definite

  dull boring pain

  goes through to the back

  worse after food

  worse lying down

  anorexia, nausea, vomiting

  weight loss with rapid emaciation

  jaundice – painless, progressive

  diabetes – rare

  thrombophlebitis anywhere
- signs – shown in Fig. 7.6
- tests

  ultrasound

  CT scan – best test if available

  barium meal – may show distorted duodenal loop

  ERCP

  urine – may show

  sugar

  bile pigments

  blood sugar may be unstable

  liver function tests

  bilirubin ↑

  alkaline phosphatase ↑

  angiography – useful to determine operability

excessive dieting

female sex hormones

  contraceptives

  menopause

infections

- the clinical manifestations are shown in Fig. 7.7
- tests

  urine – normal on passing – port-wine colour in a few hours (increased porphobilinogen found)

  blood – profound hyponatraemia
              amylase ↑

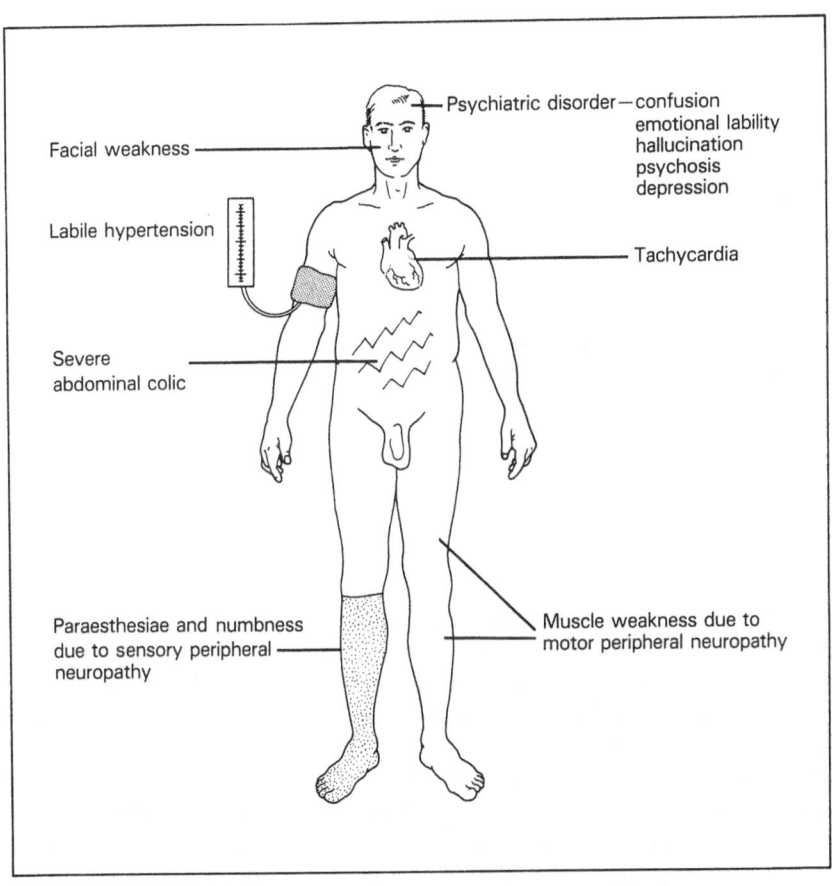

Fig. 7.7 *Acute intermittent porphyria*

Pitfalls in diagnosis

- A negative barium meal does not exclude carcinoma of stomach.
- Carcinoma of colon may be overlooked in a patient with known diverticulosis.
- Small renal stones may be easily overlooked in a straight X-ray of the abdomen.
- Forgetting carcinoma of stomach, caecum or colon as a cause of unexplained anaemia in a middle-aged or elderly patient.
- Not considering lead poisoning as a cause of chronic intestinal colic, e.g. a young child perhaps living in an old house where lead paint is still evident.
- Omitting to test the pupils in a patient with unusual abdominal pain (Argyll–Robertson pupils in tabes dorsalis).

Useful practical points

- The history is the most important part of the diagnostic process in chronic abdominal pain.
- If the possibility of gastric carcinoma is being considered then gastroscopy and biopsy are mandatory.
- If a patient with 'peptic ulcer' fails to improve with treatment always consider gastric carcinoma.
- A change in the established pattern of indigestion in gastric ulcer should also suggest carcinoma.
- 'Chronic appendicitis' is not a pathological entity – it is really recurrent attacks of acute appendicitis.
- Always consider chronic mesenteric ischaemia when abdominal pain after meals is periumbilical rather than epigastric.

Case challenge

A 63-year-old female patient presented with upper abdominal pain for the previous 3 months. The pain was a dull aching pain in the epigastrium sometimes, but not invariably, occurring about 30 min after eating; the pain was often worse at night in bed; recently it had started to go through to the back. She was losing weight but thought this was due to being afraid to eat because of the pain though she also admitted that her appetite was deteriorating. She had also started to vomit recently. There was a past history of gall bladder trouble and she had not long finished a 2 year course of chenodeoxycholic acid for gallstones. The only other problem she had was swelling of her legs over the past few weeks worse on the right side.

The examination findings are shown in Fig. 7.8.

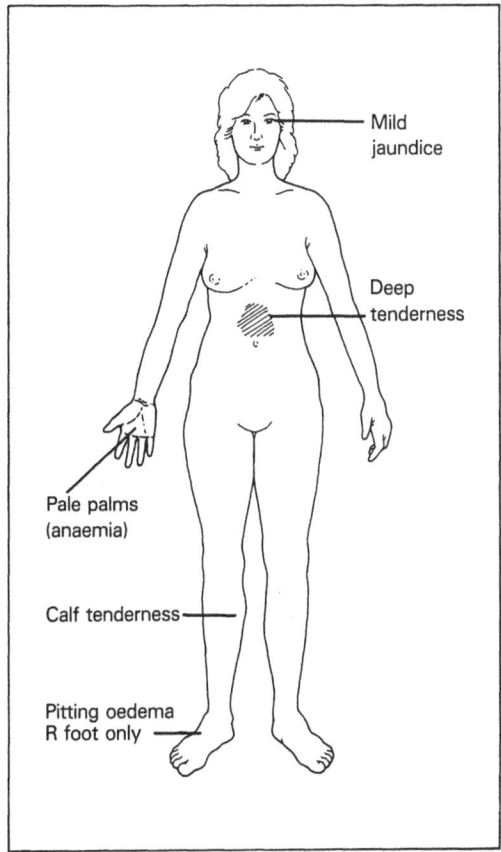

Fig. 7.8 *Examination findings in case challenge*

Questions	Give four possible diagnoses
	What tests would you do to establish the correct diagnosis?

Possible diagnoses

- peptic ulcer
- carcinoma of stomach
- chronic gall bladder disease
- carcinoma of pancreas

The clinical considerations in these diagnoses and the tests required are shown.

Peptic ulcer

For	history	• epigastric pain $\frac{1}{2}$ hour after meals, occurs at night (esp. DU)
	exam	• epigastric tenderness
Against	history	• not always related to meals
		• anorexia
		• weight loss – but could be due to fear of eating
Tests		• endoscopy
		• barium meal

Gastric carcinoma

For	history	• epigastric pain not related to food
		• anorexia
		• weight loss
	exam	• evidence of thrombophlebitis
Against	exam	• no epigastric mass
		• no hepatomegaly
		• no enlarged glands (Troisier's sign)

Gall bladder disease

For	history	• previous history
	exam	• mild jaundice
Against	history	• no biliary colic
		• anorexia
		• weight loss
	exam	• not tender in R hypochondrium
Tests		• ultrasound for biliary dilatation
		• intravenous cholangiography
		• oral cholecystogram – less reliable
		• urinary bile pigments ⎫
		serum bilirubin ⎬ may help
		liver function tests ⎭

Carcinoma pancreas

For history
- dull epigastric pain → back
- pain worse lying down
- anorexia, vomiting, loss of weight

exam
- anaemia
- jaundice
- evidence of thrombophlebitis

Against exam
- no mass (but mass only present in ¼)
- liver not enlarged (late development)

Tests
- ultrasound
- barium meal for distorted duodenal loop
- CT scan – best if available
- urine – bile pigments/sugar
- blood

  sugar ↑

  bilirubin ↑

  alkaline phosphatase ↑
- angiography

Actual diagnosis:
Carcinoma of head of pancreas

Treatment and outcome

The condition was found to be inoperable on angiography since the tumour had already invaded the portal vein.

A combination of cytotoxic drugs and/or radiotherapy has been claimed to prolong life expectancy but was not tried in this case.

She died in 4 months.

8 Constipation

Introduction

Definition – infrequent passage of excessively hard faeces.

Constipation is a universal experience, at some time.

The understanding of 'constipation' is a compromise between what the patient believes and what the doctor knows – there may be great differences.

The range of normal frequency of bowel emptying is wide – from once a week to 4–5 times daily.

As a symptom of clinical importance it is recent constipation rather than a longstanding habit that is significant.

Causes

Functional

dietary
- low food intake
    anorexia (any cause)
    slimming
- inadequate bulk/fibre
    green leafy vegetables
    fruit
    wholemeal products

bad habit – ignoring call
- hurrying from home to work
- shift work
- holidays
- overcrowded lavatories
- children – dislike lack of privacy and cleanliness in some schools
- prolonged travelling

dyschezia	• follows repeatedly ignoring calls to defaecate rectum becomes insensitive to faecal content
immobility	• post-operative
	• prolonged bed rest due to illness
	• lack of exercise

Gastrointestinal disorders

Organic

painful ano-rectal condition	• piles
	• fissure
	• abscess
intestinal obstruction	• carcinomata colon/rectum
	• diverticular disease
	• inflammatory bowel disease

Mobility disorders
- irritable bowel syndrome
- diverticulosis
- Hirschsprung's disease
- acquired megacolon
- pregnancy
- old age

Endocrine
- hypothyroidism
- diabetes
- hyperparathyroidism – high calcium

Metabolic
- dehydration
- hypokalaemia
- porphyria

Systemic
- scleroderma

Constipation

Drugs (iatrogenic)
- aluminium- or bismuth-containing antacids
- iron preparations
- analgesics containing opiate/codeine
- tricyclic antidepressants
- anticholinergics, e.g. Pro-Banthine
- ganglion-blockers for hypertension
- anticonvulsants
- lead poisoning (toxic, *not* iatrogenic)

Neurological
- paraplegia
- cauda equina tumour
- multiple sclerosis
- cerebral palsy
- autonomic/peripheral neuropathy

Psychiatric
- depression
- psychosis
- anorexia nervosa

Grades of severity

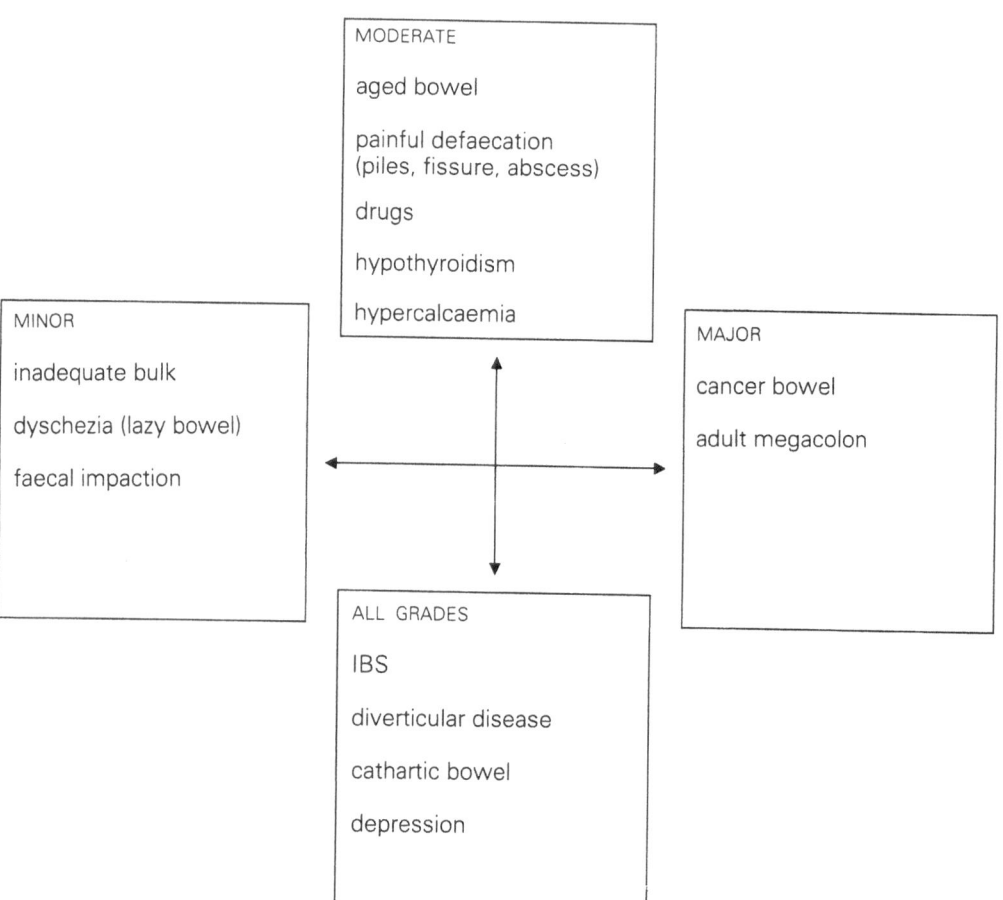

Frequency

Up to 20% of British adults take *regular laxatives*

'*Constipation*' is not a frequent direct presentation for consultation

Annual rate of consulting in general practice of 2500 persons	
consulting for constipation	20–25

Constipation is a more common incidental feature in other diagnoses

Often females in early adult life – may ease during periods or pregnancy – possible hormonal factor involved

Age incidence

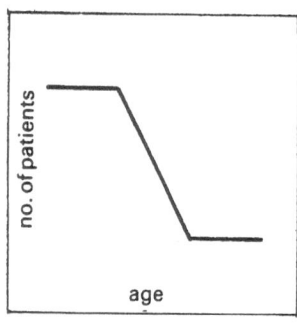

- bad habits
- painful defaecation
- imaginary (parental)

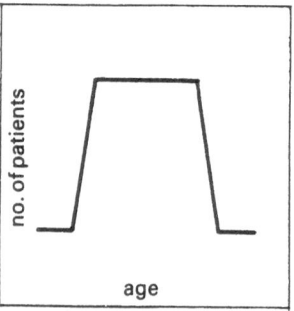

- inadequate bulk
- dyschezia (lazy bowel)
- IBS
- depression
- hypothyroidism
- piles, fissure
- cathartic bowel

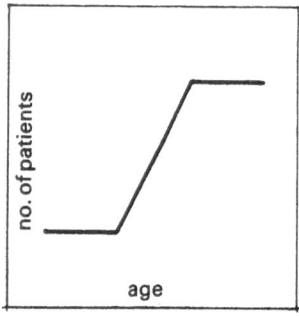

- faecal impaction
- carcinomata of large bowel
- diverticular disease

Significance

Beware of recent onset of constipation in elderly/middle aged

Beware of alternating diarrhoea/constipation

Do not let 'familiarity breed contempt':

   organic disease may develop

   non-GI causes may be responsible

Often iatrogenic

Constipation becomes significant:

   when it causes undue discomfort or alarm

   when it leads to excessive self-medication with laxatives

   when the patient feels he needs medical attention

The doctor's aims in treating constipation:

   to exclude organic disease

   to satisfy the patient about the frequency of bowel action

   to dissuade him from over-use of laxatives

Diagnostic approach

General

Obtain a clear understanding of what patient means by 'constipation'. Get on patient's 'wave-length' – he may mean

- infrequent defaecation
- daily defaecation but with difficulty
- insufficient amount of stool
- sensation of incomplete emptying – keep carcinoma of rectum in mind

Appreciate that it may be a difficult and sensitive matter to the patient so a sympathetic approach by the doctor is helpful

History

Bowel habit
- ask about circumstances in which bowel habit lapsed
- how much time is currently allowed and when
- how often bowels are open – can still be 'normal' if once a week or less

Stools
- assess size – a normal size and normal consistency even if infrequent is not constipation – should be small and hard in true constipation
- shape

  ribbon-like → irritable bowel syndrome

  small pellets → irritable bowel syndrome
- blood present →

  carcinoma rectum/sigmoid/colon

  piles

  diverticular disease

  inflammatory bowel disease (especially Crohn's)
- slime (mucus) present →

  irritable bowel syndrome

  inflammatory bowel disease – often mixed with blood

Duration
- acute onset should always suggest organic disease
- onset in middle-aged or elderly – look for carcinoma colon
- if constipation in an adult goes back to childhood

  faulty bowel habit most likely

  Hirschsprung's disease possible but less likely

Pain
- local peri-anal

  piles

  fissure

  abscess
- abdominal

  colic

    intestinal obstruction

    lead poisoning

    porphyria

  grumbling (esp. LIF)

    irritable bowel

    diverticulosis

General symptoms

there are no symptoms directly attributable to chronic constipation – headache, nausea, malaise, fatigue are likely to be psychogenic

there may be symptoms due to a general disease which is causing the constipation

weight loss must always be taken seriously, especially in the middle-aged or elderly, and should be regarded as due to carcinoma until proven otherwise

myxoedema	• mental and physical slowing
	• cold intolerance
	• increasing weight
	• hoarse voice
	• hair falling out
diabetes	• excessive thirst
	• polyuria
	• loss of weight
hyperparathyroidism	
GI tract	• anorexia
	• nausea
	• vomiting
kidney	• renal colic
	• dysuria
musculoskeletal	• weakness
	• back pain
psychiatric	• depression
	• personality change
porphyria	• recurrent abdominal colic
	• muscle weakness (polyneuropathy)
	• paraesthesiae, numbness (polyneuropathy)
	• psychiatric
	depression
	confusion
	emotional lability
scleroderma	• polyarthritis
	• dysphagia
	• Raynaud's disease

lead poisoning
- symptoms of anaemia
- weakness of wrists
- mental disturbances

neurological
- leg weakness or paralysis
- numbness, paraesthesiae legs
- urinary retention or incontinence

Drug history

the complete list of drugs likely to cause constipation is shown on page 207

the most frequent preparations in practice are:

- iron preparations
- aluminium and bismuth antacids
- codeine-containing analgesics
- tricyclic antidepressants

Mental state

children – constipation is often an expression of psychological stresses in the family

adults
- depression, don't forget this itself can be due to myxoedema
- anorexia nervosa

    anorexia

    restlessness

    amenorrhoea

    constipation
- true psychosis

Past history – relevant factors which might help in diagnosing the cause of the constipation are:

- polyarthritis ⎫
  iridocyclitis ⎪ inflammatory bowel
  erythema nodosum ⎬ → disease with
  ankylosing spondylitis ⎭ stricture →
  constipation
- mental disturbances →

    hyperparathyroidism

    porphyria
- diabetes

Constipation

- thyroid trouble

    operation for thyrotoxicosis

    radioactive iodine treatment for thyrotoxicosis → myxoedema

    goitre – may be Hashimoto's thryoiditis → myxoedema

- Raynaud's disease – scleroderma
- peptic ulcer – aluminium- and bismuth-containing antacids
- epilepsy – anticonvulsants may cause constipation
- anaemia – iron preparations

Family history

The conditions which may be associated with the occurrence of constipation in a patient include:

- auto-immune disease →

    inflammatory bowel disease

    (Crohn's, ulcerative colitis)

    rheumatoid arthritis

    Hashimoto's myxoedema

    pernicious anaemia

    collagen disease

    hypoparathyroidism

- psychiatric disease → depression in the patient
- acute porphyria (rare)

Examination

abdomen – the abdominal findings which may be relevant are shown in Fig. 8.1

ano-rectal

anal
- piles
- fissure
- abscess
- purple induration → Crohn's disease
- tight sphincter → Hirschsprung's disease

215

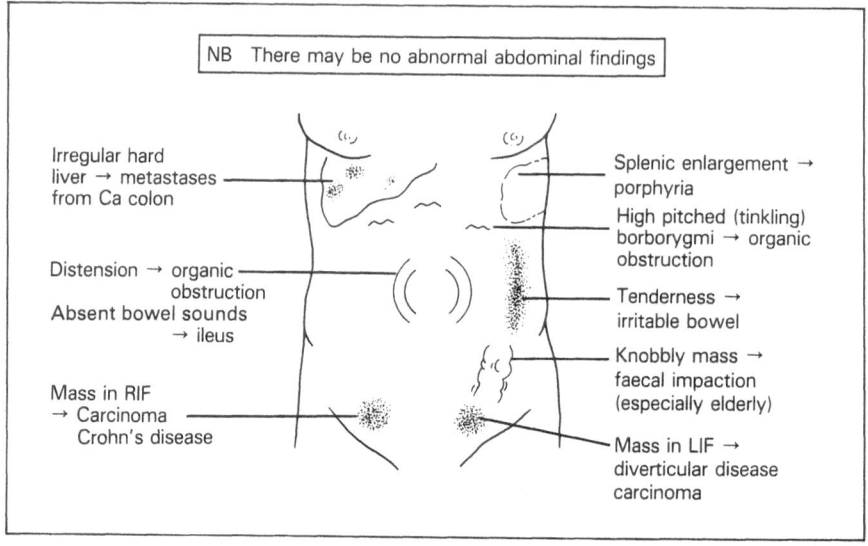

NB   There may be no abnormal abdominal findings

Irregular hard
liver → metastases
from Ca colon

Splenic enlargement →
porphyria

High pitched (tinkling)
borborygmi → organic
obstruction

Distension → organic
             obstruction
Absent bowel sounds
          → ileus

Tenderness →
irritable bowel

Knobbly mass →
faecal impaction
(especially elderly)

Mass in RIF
→ Carcinoma
   Crohn's disease

Mass in LIF →
diverticular disease
carcinoma

Fig. 8.1   *Possible abdominal signs in constipation*

rectum	• empty → intestinal obstruction Hirschsprung's disease
	• hard faeces → faecal impaction
	• tumour → carcinoma rectum
blood in stool	• carcinomata rectum/sigmoid
	• diverticular disease
	• Crohn's disease

general – the systemic signs which may be of diagnostic help are shown in Fig. 8.2

Investigations

indications

• recent onset constipation especially elderly

• blood in the stools

• weight loss

• progressive anaemia

• no response to treatment

• systemic disease suspected

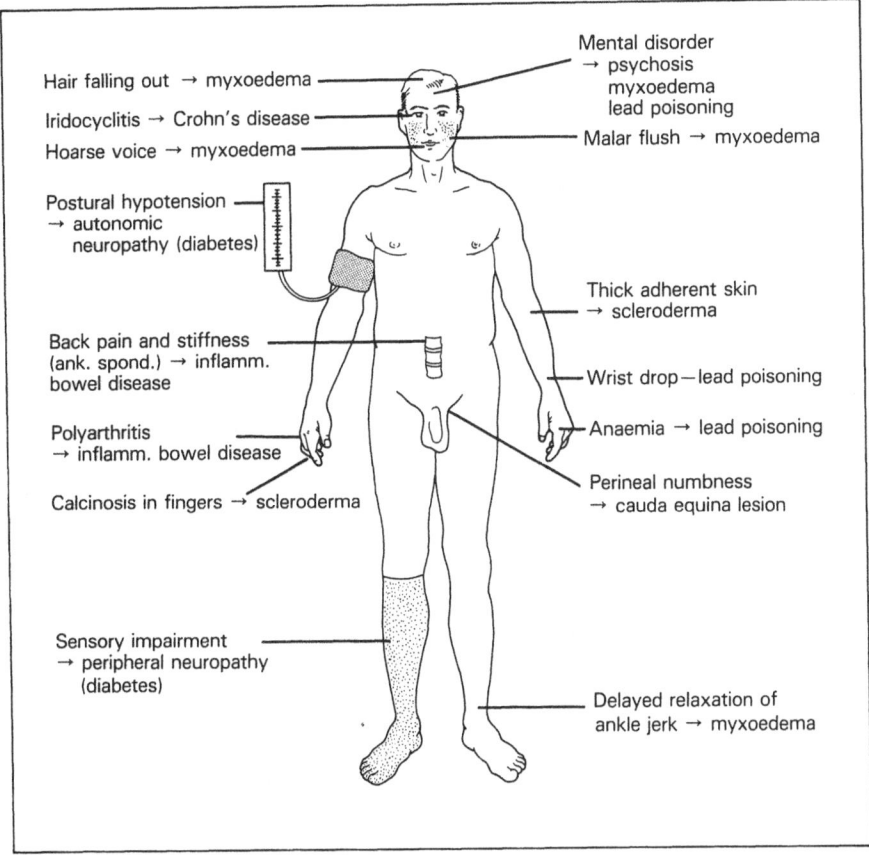

Fig. 8.2 *General signs of value in the diagnosis of constipation*

stools – for occult blood

- carcinomata rectum/colon
- piles
- diverticular disease
- Crohn's/ulcerative colitis

sigmoidoscopy

    local

- piles
- fissure
- stricture
- abscess

rectum
- tumour (carcinoma)
- faecal impaction
- narrow ampulla with dilatation above → Hirschsprung's disease
- melanosis coli – laxative abuse

radiological tests

  plain X-ray abdomen
- obstruction
    air/fluid levels
    distended bowel loops proximal to obstruction
- ileus – air in small and large bowel

  barium enema for
- obstruction
    carcinoma
    diverticular mass
    benign polyp
- stricture
    carcinoma
    Crohn's/ulcerative colitis
- Hirschsprung's disease
    narrowed distal segment
    dilated proximal segment

  small bowel enema for Crohn's disease

colonoscopy – indications
- occult blood in faeces
- sigmoidoscopy normal
- small and large bowel enemas normal

blood tests

  Hb – anaemia
- carcinoma colon
- Crohn's/ulcerative colitis
- lead poisoning

  red cells – punctate basophilia
- lead poisoning

ESR ↑	• carcinoma
	• active inflammatory bowel disease
	carcinoma
	Crohn's/ulcerative colitis
	diverticular disease
	• scleroderma
thyroid function ↓	• myxoedema
sugar ↑	• diabetes
calcium ↑	• hyperparathyroidism
urea ↑	• uraemia → ileus
potassium ↓	• hypokalaemia
lead level ↑	• lead poisoning

Urine tests

lead excretion ↑	• lead poisoning
porphobilinogen present	• porphyria
red cells/pus cells	• spread of carcinoma colon to urinary tract
	• diverticular disease

Specific conditions

Carcinoma of colon

- commonest malignancy in alimentary tract in UK
- good prognosis if diagnosed early
- usually > 50 years: M > F
- predisposing factors
    long-standing ulcerative colitis
    familial polyposis of colon
- 2/3 in descending colon and rectum
- presentation
    left side → early obstruction
    right side → anaemia from bleeding

- symptoms

    most important is *recent change* of bowel habit

    colicky abdominal pain if obstructing

    rectal bleeding

    loss of weight

    symptoms of anaemia

    tenesmus in rectal carcinoma

- examination – see Fig. 8.3

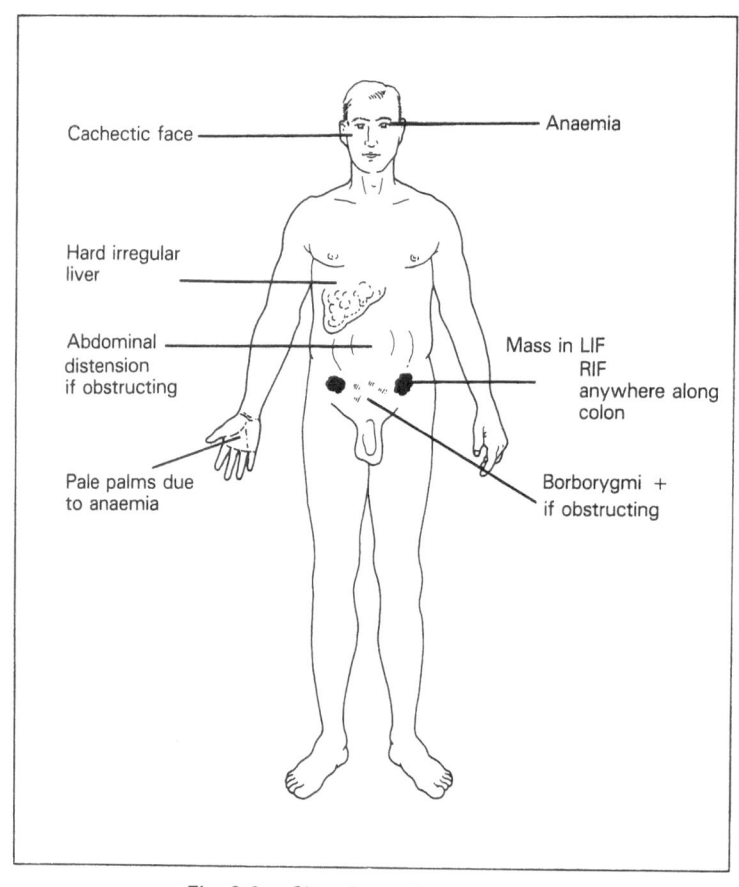

Fig. 8.3   *Signs in carcinoma of colon*

Constipation

- tests

    sigmoidoscopy is the best test for
    carcinoma rectum/sigmoid colon

    barium enema for more proximal cancer but
    may miss the tumour

    colonoscopy better than barium enema for
    proximal cancer

Megacolon

Hirschsprung's disease (aganglionosis)

- congenital
- failure of development of nerve plexus in rectum/
  pelvic colon
- boys : girls 8 : 1
- symptoms from birth

    total constipation

    abdominal distension

    vomiting

- sometimes milder forms present later in childhood
- rectal examination – empty rectum
- tests

    barium enema – narrow distal segment
                           dilated colon above
                           retained faeces +

    rectal biopsy – absence of nerve plexus

Acquired megacolon

- older children and adults
- most due to persistent failure to empty the rectum
  properly for various reasons (see page 205)
- other causes

    milder form of Hirschsprung's disease

    hypothyroidism (cretinism)

    Chagas' disease (Latin America)

    scleroderma

    laxative abuse especially anthracenes

221

- clinical

    gross abdominal distension

    rectal examination – loaded rectum
                                                lax sphincter
- barium enema
    gross dilatation of rectum extending down
    to anus

    no narrowed segment

    rectum loaded with faeces

Faecal impaction
- elderly particularly prone
- spurious diarrhoea often – fluid leaking round impacted faeces
- urinary incontinence may also occur
- abdominal mass in LIF – 'nobbly'
- rectal examination

    hard faeces

    easily indented with finger
- always exclude carcinoma rectum

    sigmoidoscopy

    barium enema

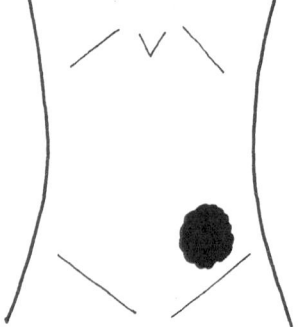

NB Faecal impaction may also occur in young children

Irritable bowel syndrome
- usually women 20 – 40 years
- cardinal symptoms

    abdominal pain

    alteration in bowel habit
- abdominal pain

    variable site   • often left side

                                      • often LIF

    colicky, constant, 'grumbling'

    may occur after eating

    relieved by   • passing flatus

                                  • defaecation

Constipation

- bowel change
  variable
  - constipation commonest
  - diarrhoea sometimes
  - may get both
- stools
  - ribbon-like
  - pellets
  - mucus sometimes
- other symptoms
  - flatulence, distension
  - stomach rumbling
  - post-prandial fullness
  - nausea, anorexia
  - headache, tiredness
- tests – necessary to
  exclude organic disease, especially carcinoma
  reassure patient
  sigmoidoscopy
  - normal mucosa
  - colonic spasm

  barium enema

Diverticular disease

- 90% in descending colon
- occurs over 40 years of age – increases with age
- may be symptomless diverticulosis; when infected
  → diverticulitis
- recurring attacks of pain
  LIF
  colicky
  settles in 1–2 days
- bowel disturbance
  constipation usual
  diarrhoea occurs with diverticulitis
- rectal bleeding may occur

- diverticulitis –   fever

          severe pain in LIF

          tender mass on LIF

          rectal tenderness

          complications

              abscess

              perforation

              peritonitis

              intestinal obstruction

              fistula – bladder

                       vagina

- tests

    WBC and ESR will distinguish painful diverticular disease from diverticulitis

    sigmoidoscopy

    barium enema

Myxoedema

- constipation is one of the cardinal symptoms
- other important symptoms

    mental slowing

    physical slowing

    increasing weight

    hoarseness of voice

    cold intolerance

    loss of hair

- examination findings are shown in Fig. 8.4

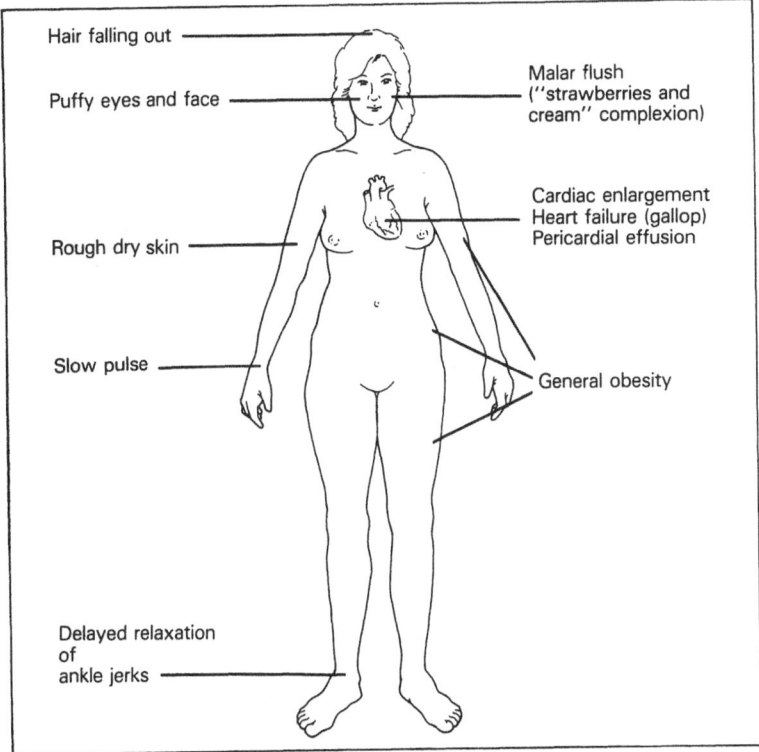

Fig. 8.4 *Signs of myxoedema*

- tests
    - thyroid function
        - serum thyroxine (T4) ↓
        - thyroid-stimulating hormone (TSH) ↑
    - serum cholesterol ↑
    - anaemia
        - normocytic normochronic
        - macrocytic
    - ECG
        - sinus bradycardia
        - generally low voltage
        - flat T waves
- thyrotropin-releasing hormone test useful in doubtful cases

225

Depression

- may be

    reactive – a result of external trauma

    endogenous – personality defect

- women more frequent than men

- predisposing factors

    women –   over 30 years:

                      puerperium

                      menopausal

                      gynaecological operations

    parental loss in childhood

    heavy domestic responsibilities

    lack of job satisfaction

    struggle with income

- constipation is a predominant symptom

- other symptoms –   insomnia

                        waking early

                        lack of concentration

                        loss of interest

                        loss of libido

                        loss of appetite

                        loss of weight

- tests

    a trial of antidepressive drugs is always worth-while

    always exclude carcinoma colon as cause of constipation before attributing it to depression

Pitfalls in diagnosis

- Spurious diarrhoea in faecal impaction in the elderly may result in a misdiagnosis of the underlying problem.
- An elderly patient not eating may think constipation is 'normal' and a diagnosis of carcinoma of colon is then missed.
- Omitting to do a rectal examination in a patient with vague abdominal pain – 'if you don't put your finger in it you will put your foot in it!'
- Lead poisoning, though rare, is often forgotten as a cause of colic and constipation – look for the blue line round the gum margin.
- Attributing rectal bleeding to piles and so missing a rectal carcinoma.
- Attributing alteration in bowel habits to 'gastro-enteritis' in the elderly patient especially if bedridden and confused – carcinoma of colon must always be considered and investigated.

Useful practical points

- Before making a diagnosis of functional bowel disturbance as a cause of constipation always arrange sigmoidoscopy and barium enema to exclude organic disease, especially carcinoma.
- If blood is present in the stool it is not enough to have a negative sigmoidoscopy and barium enema – a colonoscopy should also be done if possible.
- In an elderly patient with constipation always *look* into the drug cupboard to see if there are any constipating drugs.
- Don't forget that patients with functional bowel disturbances, e.g. irritable bowel, can also develop carcinoma so always investigate any *change* in long-standing symptoms.
- An elderly patient on diuretic treatment can soon become hypokalaemic resulting in constipation so check serum potassium level.
- Don't rely on a negative rectal examination to exclude rectal carcinoma – sigmoidoscopy is mandatory.

Case challenge

A 45-year-old painter and decorator presented with a 3-month history of increasing constipation. He also gave a long history of abdominal pain going back over several years: sometimes the pain was epigastric occurring about 1 hour after meals and sometimes in the left hypochondrium or left iliac fossa. He said his bowels had never been right since childhood when he never seemed to have any time to spare to go to the lavatory but he was able to cope until a few months ago when the bowels began to get more 'stubborn'. He had noticed occasional streaks of blood in the stools but said he had suffered with piles for a long time. He had recently been put on Aludrox for his 'indigestion' but claimed he had not had much relief. He thought his appetite was getting poor and he had lost about ½ (3 kg) stone since the bowels had been giving him trouble.

The abnormalities on examination were few and are shown in Fig. 8.5.

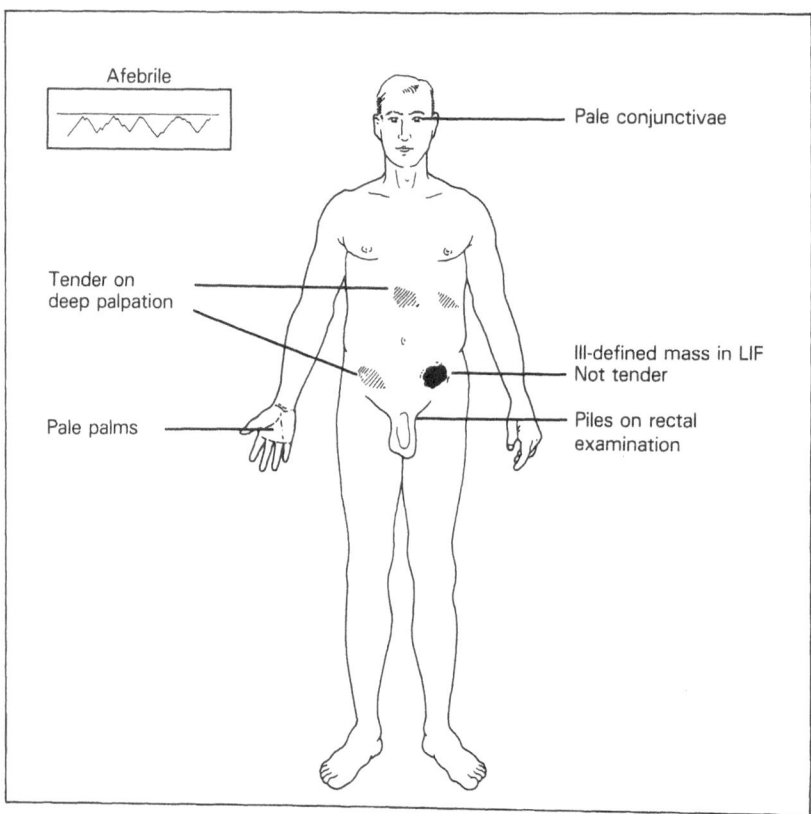

Afebrile

Pale conjunctivae

Tender on deep palpation

Ill-defined mass in LIF
Not tender

Pale palms

Piles on rectal examination

Fig. 8.5 *Signs in case challenge*

Questions	Give the differential diagnosis
	How would you decide the correct diagnosis?
Differential diagnosis	• irritable bowel syndrome
	• diverticulosis
	• dyschezia
	• carcinoma of colon
	• peptic ulcer
	• lead poisoning

Constipation

Irritable bowel syndrome

For history
- long history of abdominal pain
- long history of bowel trouble

exam
- tenderness in various abdominal sites

Against history
- blood in stools – never occurs in uncomplicated irritable bowel syndrome
- loss of weight

exam
- localized mass in LIF
- anaemia

Tests
- sigmoidoscopy
   mucus sometimes
   bowel spasm

Diverticulosis

For history
- long history of abdominal pain and constipation

exam
- mass in LIF – could be diverticulitis
- blood-streaking of stools

Against history
- loss of weight – not a feature of diverticulosis

exam
- no temperature – against diverticulitis

Tests
- sigmoidoscopy
- barium enema

Dyschezia

For history
- long history of constipation going back to childhood

Against history
- blood-streaked stools
- loss of weight and anorexia

exam
- mass in LIF
- anaemia

Tests
- rectal examination – loaded rectum
- barium enema
   dilated rectum
   loaded with faeces

229

Carcinoma of colon

For	history	• recent increasing constipation
		• loss of weight and anorexia
		• blood in stools
	exam	• mass in LIF
		• anaemia
Against	history	• long history of abdominal pain and constipation – if this is related to the current problem
		• piles could account for blood in stools
Tests		• sigmoidoscopy
		• barium enema
		• colonoscopy if these two tests are negative

Peptic ulcer

For	history	• long history of epigastric pain 1 h after meals
		• constipation caused by aluminium-containing antacid (Aludrox)
	exam	• epigastric tenderness
Against	history	• loss of weight – unless afraid to eat
		• increasing constipation – not a feature of uncomplicated peptic ulcer
	exam	• mass in LIF
Tests		• barium meal
		• gastroscopy – better – allows biopsy of any suspicious lesion

Lead poisoning

For	history	• works as a painter – might contact lead-paints especially stripping woodwork in old houses
		• constipation
	exam	• anaemia – feature of lead poisoning

Constipation

Against	exam	• no mental changes or peripheral neuropathy (wrist-drop) – two important manifestations of lead poisoning
		• mass in LIF
		• no blue line along gum margins
Tests		• punctate basophilia in red cells
		• increased blood lead level
		• increased urinary excretion of lead

Actual diagnosis:
Ulcerating carcinoma of sigmoid colon causing obstruction

Treatment and outcome

After pre-operative bowel lavage and antibiotic combination a one-stage sigmoid colectomy was carried out.

There were no postoperative complications and his subsequent progress was satisfactory with no recurrence.

The 5 year survival is 30–50%.

9 Cough

Introduction

Cough is the most frequent of symptoms – everyone coughs sometimes.

Since we breathe continuously, it should not be surprising that inhaled irritants and infections produce reflex coughs in attempts to remove them.

As well as reacting to external irritants, cough may result from intrinsic disorders of the respiratory tract.

The range of causes is wide; although the great majority are minor and self-limiting, more serious possibilities have to be kept in mind.

Causes of cough

Respiratory

infections	acute	• laryngitis
		• tracheitis
		• bronchitis
		• pneumonia
		• lung abscess
		• whooping cough
	chronic	• chronic bronchitis
		• bronchiectasis
		• tuberculosis
bronchospasm		• bronchial asthma
neoplastic		• bronchial carcinoma
		• alveolar cell carcinoma
hereditary		• fibrocystic disease

233

mechanical
- inhaled foreign body
- pneumoconiosis

idiopathic
- fibrosing alveolitis

Cardiovascular

pulmonary oedema
- left ventricular failure
- mitral stenosis

pulmonary embolism

Grades of severity

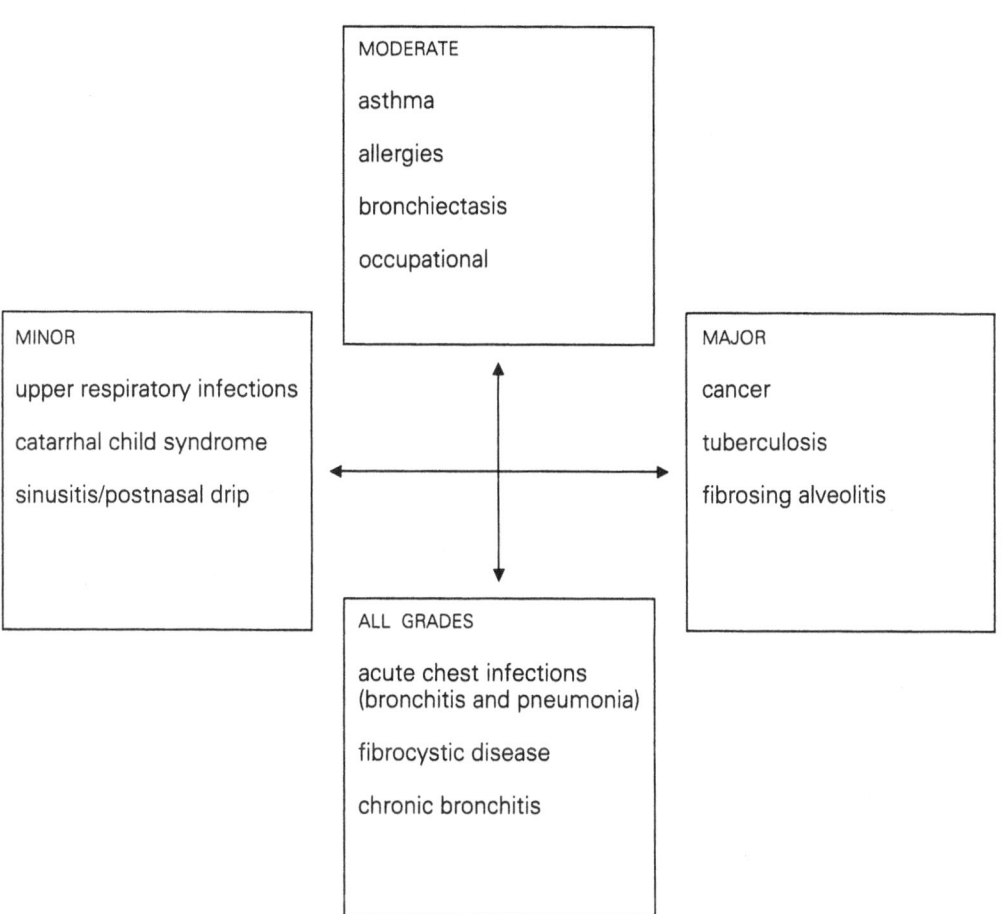

MODERATE

asthma

allergies

bronchiectasis

occupational

MINOR

upper respiratory infections

catarrhal child syndrome

sinusitis/postnasal drip

MAJOR

cancer

tuberculosis

fibrosing alveolitis

ALL GRADES

acute chest infections
(bronchitis and pneumonia)

fibrocystic disease

chronic bronchitis

Frequency

Annual prevalence of 'cough' in a general practice population of 2500	
upper respiratory infections	350
(catarrhal children 100)	
acute chest infections	155
(acute bronchitis 145)	
(pneumonia 10)	
chronic bronchitis	33
asthma	25
nasal (sinusitis, etc.)	42
'influenza'	
(interepidemic years)	12
cancer of lung	3
fibrocystic disease	1
bronchiectasis	1
tuberculosis	1 every 5–10 years

Age incidence

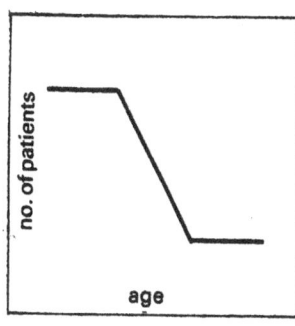

- catarrhal children
- upper respiratory infections
- measles/whooping cough
- fibrocystic disease
- acute chest infections (some)

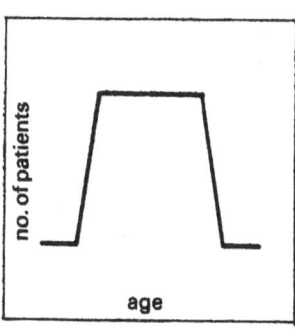

- asthma
- sinusitis
- acute chest infections (some)

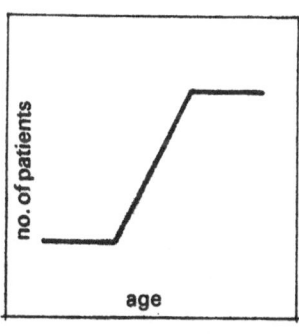

- carcinoma lung
- chronic bronchitis
- acute chest infections (some)

Diagnostic approach

History

Relevant factors
- acute or chronic cough
- character of cough
- productive (loose) unproductive (dry)
- timing of the cough
- character of sputum
- associated symptoms

Acute cough

viral infection
- common cold
- laryngitis
- tracheobronchitis
- pneumonitis

bacterial infection
- laryngitis
- tracheobronchitis
- bronchopneumonia
- pneumonia

inhalation
- foreign body
- irritant substance

Chronic cough
- chronic bronchitis
- tuberculosis
- bronchiectasis
- carcinoma lung
- lung abscess
- bronchial asthma

Character

brassy →
- involvement trachea/major bronchi

barking →
- laryngeal disease

bovine (no power) →
- vocal cord paralysis (recurrent laryngeal nerve)

paroxysmal with
whoops between →
- whooping cough

croupy (with stridor) →
- laryngeal disease

Cough

painful front of chest →   • tracheitis

Dry cough→   • viral infections

     • pleurisy

     • inhaled foreign body

     • inhaled irritants

     • left ventricular failure

     • tuberculosis

     • interstitial fibrosis

        fibrosing alveolitis

        pneumoconiosis

Loose cough →   • chronic bronchitis

     • bronchopneumonia

     • pneumonia

     • tuberculosis (when cavitating)

     • bronchiectasis

     • carcinoma lung

     • bronchial asthma (sputum with difficulty)

Timing of cough

   on waking →   • bronchiectasis

     • chronic bronchitis

   changing posture →   • bronchiectasis

     • lung abscess

   meal time →   • hiatus hernia (irritating lung)

     • oesophageal diverticulum

     • tracheo-oesophageal fistula (carcinoma)

Character of sputum

   clear white or grey →   • uninfected bronchitis

   green or yellow →   • bacterial infection

   'rusty' sputum →   • pneumococcal pneumonia

   thick and sticky →   • bronchial asthma

   profuse, watery →   • alveolar cell carcinoma

   thin, clear mucoid →   • viral infection

   'redcurrant jelly' →   • bronchial carcinoma

profuse, purulent,
offensive →
- bronchiectasis
- lung abscess

pink and frothy –
pulmonary oedema →
- LV failure
- mitral stenosis

frank blood →
- pulmonary embolism

Associated symptoms

wheezing →
- bronchospasm (asthma)

breathlessness →
- asthma
- LVF
- chronic obstructive airways disease

stridor (especially in
bed) →
- obstruction of – larynx
                       trachea

night sweats →
- tuberculosis

fever, rigors →
- acute infection

weight loss →
- carcinoma
- tuberculosis

recurrent severe lung
infections →
- carcinoma
- bronchiectasis
- inhaled foreign body

hoarseness →
- laryngeal involvement

vomiting after coughing →
- whooping cough

epileptic fit after coughing
(cough epilepsy) →
- chronic obstructive lung disease

diarrhoea →
- secondary amyloidosis in bronchiectasis

Other relevant factors in history

smoking habits →
- carcinoma of bronchus
- chronic bronchitis

occupation

    miner →   ● pneumoconiosis

    aircraft making →   ● berylliosis

    insulation (building) → ● asbestosis

    farmer →   ● 'farmer's lung (allergic pneumonitis from mouldy hay)

hobby

    pigeons
    budgerigar } →   ● 'bird-fancier's lung' (allergic alveolitis)

    contacts →   ● tuberculosis

past history

    recurrent lung infections
    since childhood →   ● bronchiectasis

                              ● fibrocystic disease

    hay fever, eczema →   ● asthma

    family history →   ● asthma

                              ● fibrocystic disease

                              ● emphysema – α_1-antitrypsin deficiency

                              ● tuberculosis

Examination

General – the general findings which may be helpful in the diagnosis of the cause of a cough are shown in Fig. 9.1

Lungs – many conditions can be diagnosed by carefully examining the chest following the age-old precepts

                    ● inspection

                    ● palpation (don't forget lymph glands)

                    ● percussion

                    ● auscultation

the abnormal chest signs in various conditions causing cough are shown in Fig. 9.2.

Cardiovascular system – pulmonary oedema is an important cause of nocturnal cough; the signs are shown in Fig. 9.3.

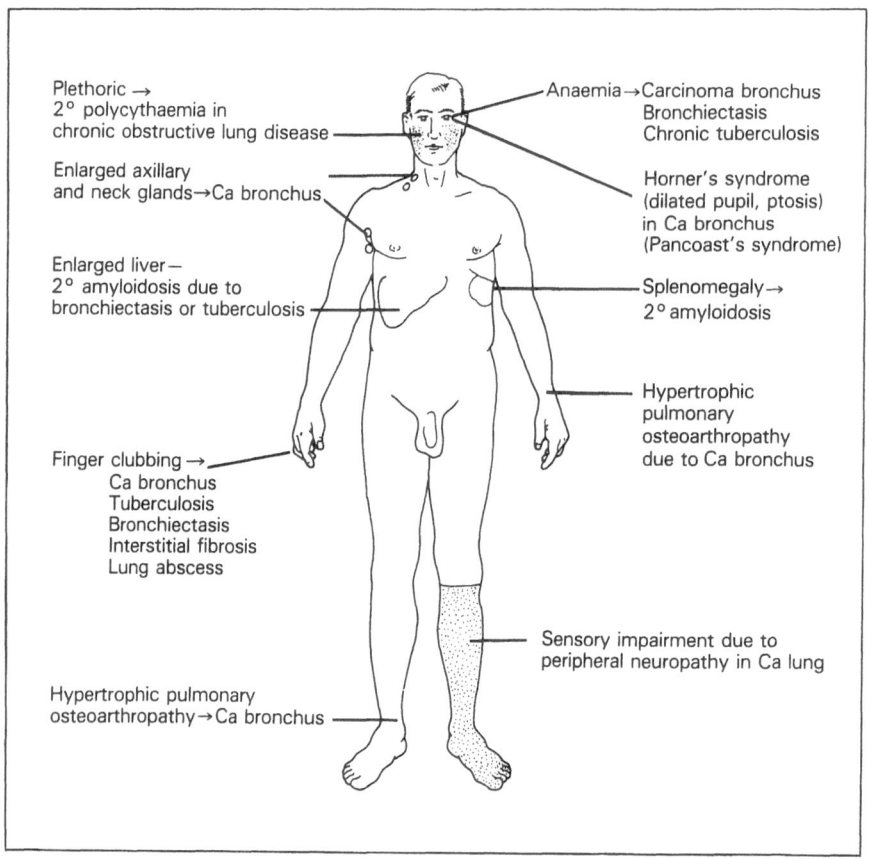

Plethoric →
2° polycythaemia in
chronic obstructive lung disease

Enlarged axillary
and neck glands→Ca bronchus

Enlarged liver—
2° amyloidosis due to
bronchiectasis or tuberculosis

Finger clubbing →
Ca bronchus
Tuberculosis
Bronchiectasis
Interstitial fibrosis
Lung abscess

Hypertrophic pulmonary
osteoarthropathy→Ca bronchus

Anaemia→Carcinoma bronchus
Bronchiectasis
Chronic tuberculosis

Horner's syndrome
(dilated pupil, ptosis)
in Ca bronchus
(Pancoast's syndrome)

Splenomegaly→
2° amyloidosis

Hypertrophic
pulmonary
osteoarthropathy
due to Ca bronchus

Sensory impairment due to
peripheral neuropathy in Ca lung

Fig. 9.1   *General findings in respiratory diseases causing cough*

CHRONIC BRONCHITIS
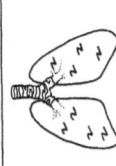
Movement—symmetrically reduced
percussion—normal in absence of emphysema
prolonged expiration
rhonchi (varying pitch) in inspiration and expiration

BRONCHOPNEUMONIA
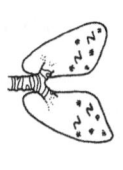
Movement—symmetrically reduced
percussion—patchy dullness
harsh vesicular breathing
rhonchi and coarse crepitations
—lung bases often
may be generalised

LOBAR PNEUMONIA
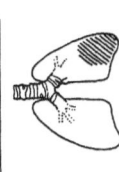
Reduced movement on affected side
vocal fremitus increased
percussion dull
high pitched bronchial breathing
fine crepitations
whispering pectoriloquy

BRONCHIAL ASTHMA
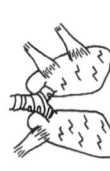
Accessory muscles used
—sterno-mastoids pectorals
movement symmetrically reduced
hyper-resonant percussion
prolonged expiration
many high-pitched rhonchi (musical chest)

INHALED FOREIGN BODY
Ca BRONCHUS (no collapse)
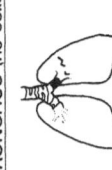
Persistent localised wheeze

TUBERCULOSIS
with CAVITATION
(also LUNG ABSCESS)
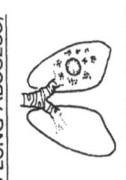
Reduced movement on affected side
dull percussion over lesion
amphoric breathing if cavity is linked with bronchus
coarse crepitations surrounding
NB. Early non-cavitating Tb either no signs or fine crepitations usually at apex—often only after coughing (post-tussive)

CARCINOMA of BRONCHUS with COLLAPSE
Trachea deviated to affected side
reduced movement affected side
vocal fremitus reduced
percussion dull
breath sounds reduced or absent
no added sounds

BRONCHIECTASIS
Trachea deviated to affected side if associated fibrosis
movement reduced on affected side
dull percussion over lesion
usually at base of lung
breath sounds reduced
coarse crepitations

INTERSTITIAL FIBROSIS
Movement symmetrically reduced
percussion normal
harsh vesicular breath sounds
diffuse coarse crepitations

Fig. 9.2 *Abnormal chest signs in cough*

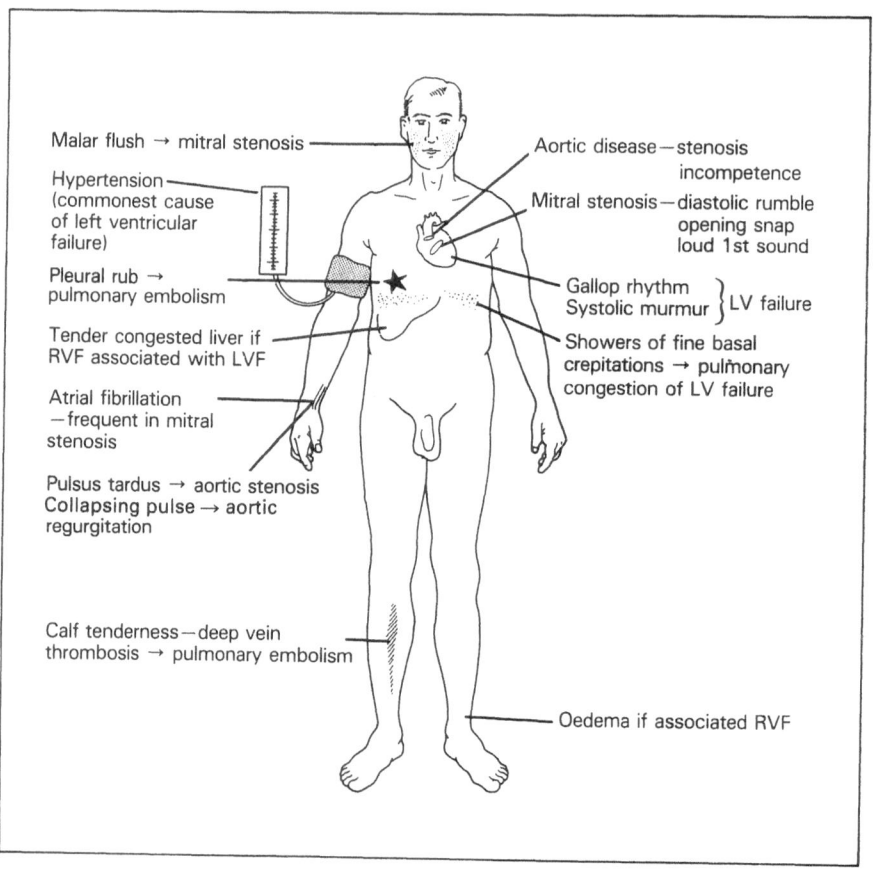

Malar flush → mitral stenosis

Hypertension
(commonest cause
of left ventricular
failure)

Pleural rub →
pulmonary embolism

Tender congested liver if
RVF associated with LVF

Atrial fibrillation
—frequent in mitral
stenosis

Pulsus tardus → aortic stenosis
Collapsing pulse → aortic
regurgitation

Calf tenderness—deep vein
thrombosis → pulmonary embolism

Aortic disease—stenosis
                incompetence

Mitral stenosis—diastolic rumble
                 opening snap
                 loud 1st sound

Gallop rhythm
Systolic murmur } LV failure

Showers of fine basal
crepitations → pulmonary
congestion of LV failure

Oedema if associated RVF

Fig. 9.3   *Possible findings in pulmonary oedema causing cough*

Investigations

Radiology

  chest X-ray

    this is the most helpful test and is mandatory in all patients with cough
    the conditions which may be seen are:

- carcinoma of bronchus (Fig. 9.4a)
- bronchopneumonia
- lobar pneumonia (Fig. 9.4b)
- bronchiectasis (Fig. 9.4c)
- tuberculosis (Fig. 9.4d)
- interstitial fibrosis
- lung abscess (Fig. 9.4e)

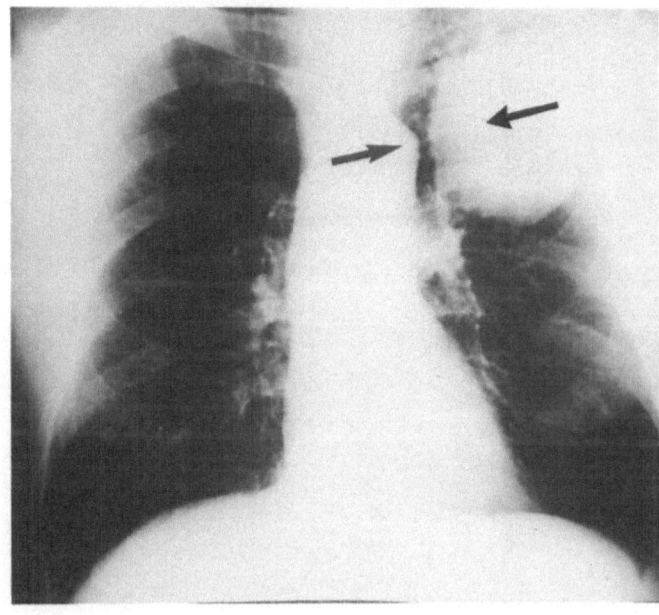

Fig. 9.4a *Chest X-ray showing bronchial carcinoma in the left upper lobe*

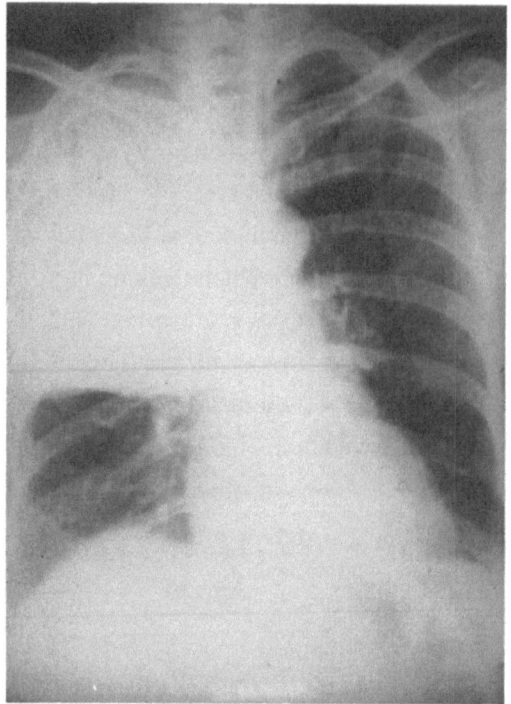

Fig. 9.4b *Chest X-ray showing right upper lobe pneumonia*

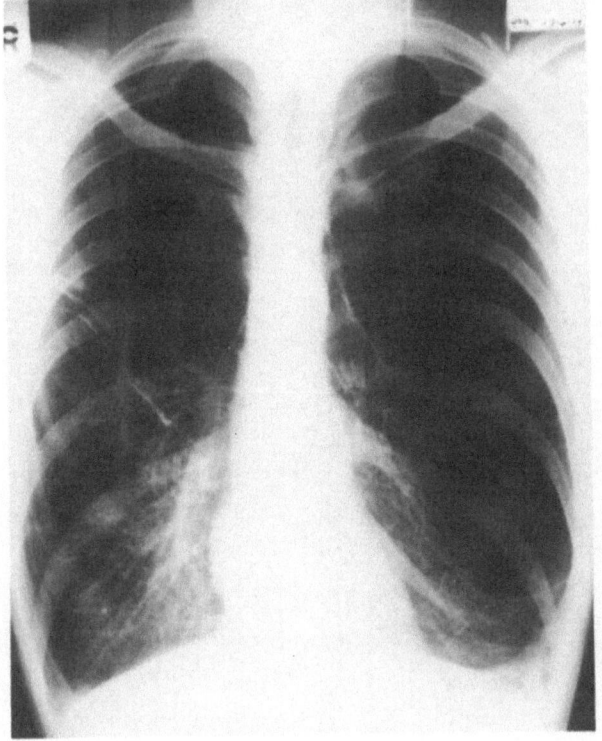

Fig. 9.4c *Chest X-ray showing bilateral basal bronchiectasis, more on the right*

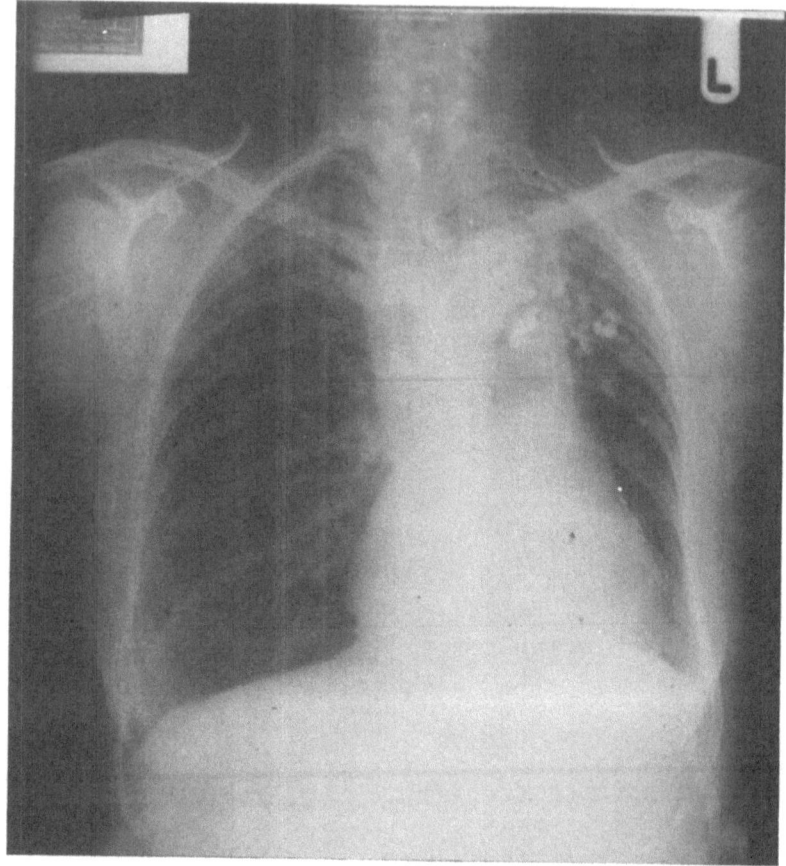

Fig. **9.4d** *Chest X-ray showing pulmonary tuberculosis with calcification at the left apex*

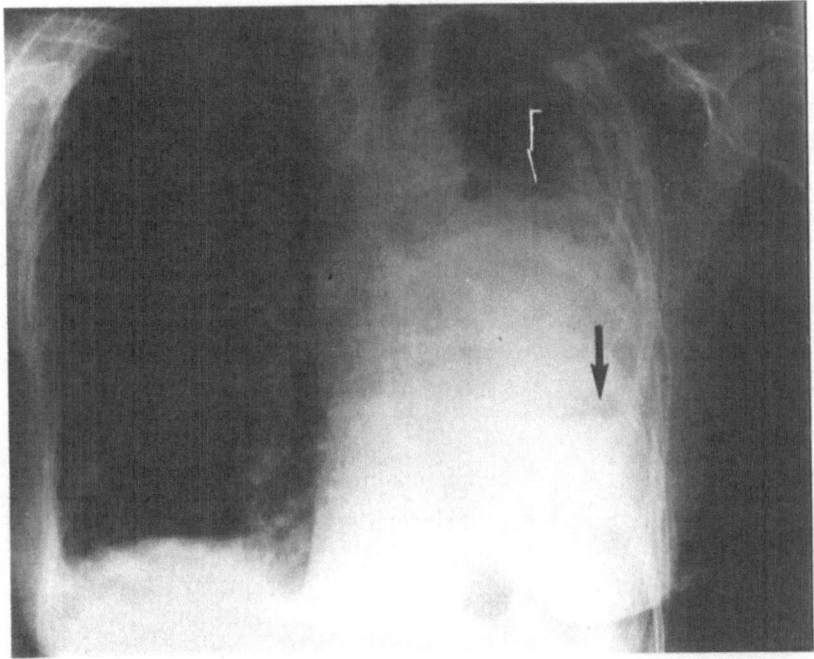

Fig. 9.4e *Chest X-ray showing fluid levels (arrowed) in two lung abscesses in the left lung*

tomography

helps more precise localization of a pulmonary lesion

may show unsuspected cavitation

may show bronchial obstruction from carcinoma

bronchography – shows bronchiectasis but it is an unpleasant examination and should only be used if surgery is being considered for localized disease.

CT scanning

more sensitive than chest X-ray

can diagnose intrapulmonary lesions in presence of pleural effusion

can detect calcification in a lesion better than with chest X-ray

sputum examination

for blood
- carcinoma bronchus
- bronchiectasis
- tuberculosis
- pneumonia
- lung abscess
- pulmonary infarction

for malignant cells
- cancer bronchus

for eosinophils
- asthma

Blood tests

anaemia
- carcinoma bronchus
- bronchiectasis
- chronic tuberculosis

polycythaemia
- chronic obstructive lung disease

eosinophilia
- asthma

ESR ↑
- any acute bacterial infection
- carcinoma bronchus
- bronchiectasis
- tuberculosis
- lung abscess

Respiratory function tests

the simplest test for chronic small airway obstruction in chronic bronchitis or asthma is the *mini-peak flow meter* which can be easily used in general practice

Vitalograph – this is a more useful but more expensive test and gives more information about the type of ventilatory defect

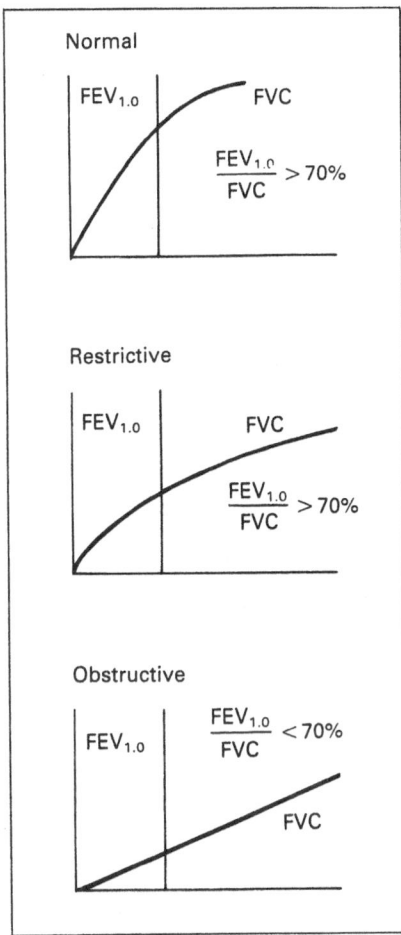

restrictive defect – generalized parenchymatosis, lung disease, ankylosing spondylitis

- fibrosis
- collapse
- congestion
- effusion
- weak respiratory muscles, e.g. myopathy

obstructive defect

- chronic bronchitis
- asthma

More complex respiratory function tests are available in respiratory units

static lung volumes

transfer factor for demonstrating interstitial lung disease

lung plethysmography for more accurate determination of small airway obstruction

In the figure:

Normal: $FEV_{1.0}$, FVC, $\frac{FEV_{1.0}}{FVC} > 70\%$

Restrictive: $FEV_{1.0}$, FVC, $\frac{FEV_{1.0}}{FVC} > 70\%$

Obstructive: $FEV_{1.0}$, $\frac{FEV_{1.0}}{FVC} < 70\%$, FVC

Ventilation/perfusion isotope scan – this is a very helpful test in diagnosis of a pulmonary infarction, when perfusion is reduced but ventilation maintained in the area of lung affected

Other tests

allergy testing – this is of very little diagnostic or therapeutic value in asthma and is rarely necessary

sweat test – finding an excess of sodium (> 70mEq/litre) indicates fibrocystic disease of the lungs (mucoviscoidosis)

lung biopsy may be useful on the diagnosis of:

- fibrosing alveolitis
- malignant lesions
- fungal infection, e.g. aspergillosis
- granulomatus disease
    - tuberculosis
    - sarcoidosis
    - Wegener's

Specific conditions

Catarrhal child syndrome

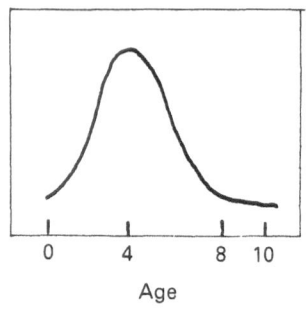

Age

- almost universal in children
- M = F
- peak 4–8 years
- probably mixture of
    - infections – mostly viral
    - individual immunological responses
    - hypersensitivities
- clinical features
    - cough
    - colds (nasal)
    - catarrh (stuffy nose)
    - wheezy chests (in 20%)
    - sore throats
    - earaches/deafness
    - cervical glands/tonsils +
- natural remission after age of 8

'Croup' (acute laryngitis)

- characteristic cough
  - barking
  - some breathing difficulty
- children 9 months–3 years
- usually 11 p.m.–2 a.m.
- recurring attacks – cease after age of 3
- occur in small local epidemics
- caused by R.S. or parainfluenza viruses
- *beware : acute epiglottitis* – may present similarly but child more ill, cannot swallow, drooling saliva, increasing difficulty in breathing

Acute chest infections

- 'acute bronchitis' and 'pneumonia' are the pathological labels but clinical presentation is different.
- main clinical types

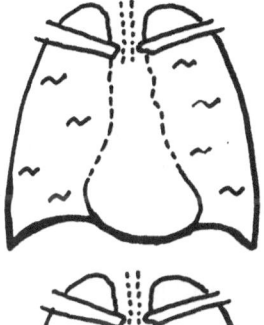

  acute wheezy chests (bronchitis)
  - diffuse and bilateral wheezes
  - common +
  - continual cough and breathlessness

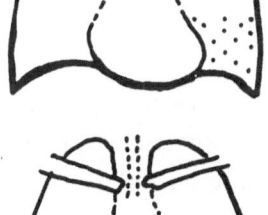

  local crackles
  - usually at one base or both bases
  - common +
  - productive – irritating cough

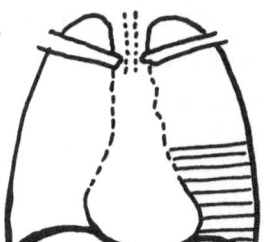

  consolidation/effusion
  - rare
  - productive cough, distressing +

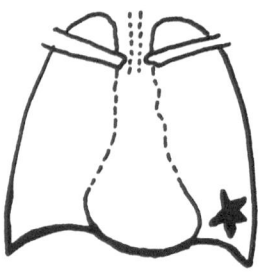

pleurisy

rare

painful dry cough

Tuberculosis

- may be symptomless – picked up on mass X-ray
- may be recent TB contact
- often insidious onset with
  anorexia
  loss of weight
  excessive fatigue
  fever
  night sweats
- respiratory symptoms
  cough
  sputum –   initially mucoid
                  later purulent
  haemoptysis
  breathlessness – late if due to TB
                  early if spontaneous pneu-
                  mothorax or pleural effusion
  pleuritic pain
- signs in lungs (see Fig. 9.2)
  may be none
  medium/coarse crepitations usually over apex –
  may be only after coughing (post-tussive)
  later – dull percussion (fibrosis)
  amphoric breathing (cavitation)
- finger clubbing

- *tests*

  chest X-ray most important

  - ill-defined apical opacities

  - pneumonic consolidation

  - cavitation

  - fibrosis

  other findings

  - pleural effusion

  - pneumothorax

  search for tubercle bacilli

  - sputum

  - gastric juice

  - laryngeal swab

- blood tests

  normocytic normochromic anaemia – not very helpful

  raised ESR

  - non-specific

  - not an index of disease activity

- *tuberculin tests*

  Mantoux test most sensitive

  Heaf test more widely used for epidemiological study

  induration at least 10mm diameter 48–72 h is positive

  may be false-negative in active TB (5–10%)

  previous BCG vaccination → misleading positive

tuberculin response suppressed in

sarcoidosis

Hodgkin's disease

advanced carcinoma or lymphoma

after measles and glandular fever – temporary

elderly patients

immunosuppressive drug treatment

- *complications of TB*

pleurisy – dry

with effusion

with empyema

pneumothorax – uncomplicated

pyopneumothorax

tuberculous laryngitis

ischiorectal abscess/fistula

mycetoma (*Aspergillus*) in lung

miliary spread → tuberculous meningitis

Bronchiectasis

- causes

obstructed bronchus

severe bacterial infection

after measles, whooping cough

tuberculosis

bronchial carcinoma

inhaled foreign body

cystic fibrosis

congenital ciliary dysfunction – Kartagener's syndrome

bronchiectasis

sinusitis

transposition viscera

pulmonary eosinophilia

- presentation

  chronic cough – worse on waking

  profuse purulent offensive sputum – related to posture

  haemoptysis

  general – lassitude, malaise, fever, rigors, sweating, weight loss

- examination – the signs are shown in Fig. 9.5.

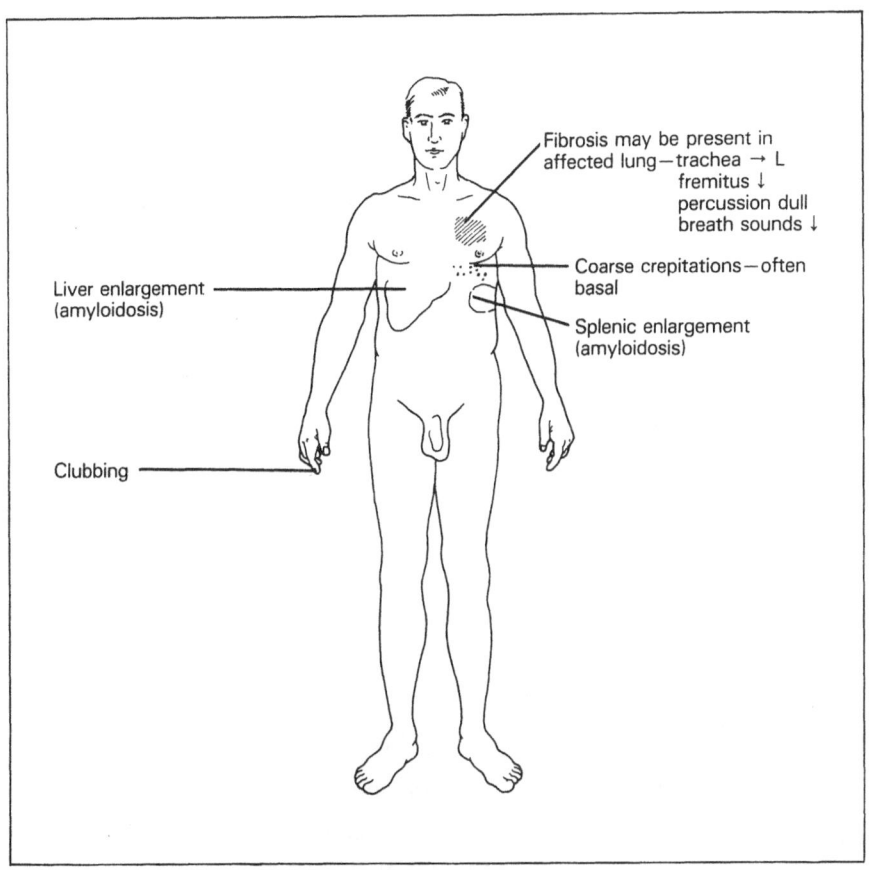

Fig. 9.5 *Signs of bronchiectasis*

- tests

    chest X-ray – dilated bronchi

                  associated fibrosis

                  active infection

                  pulmonary collapse

    bronchography –   unpleasant test

                    only if

                      unilateral disease

                      surgery contemplated

    sputum examination –   to exclude TB

                      for resistant patho-gens

    rectal biopsy –   if amyloid suspected

Bronchial carcinoma

- 50% of all male deaths from malignancy
- M : F = 4 : 1
- cigarette smoking main cause in most cases: incidence – heavy smoker: non-smoker 40 : 1
- asbestosis is another topical risk factor
- presentation

    lung symptoms

    symptoms from metastases, Fig. 9.6

      thoracic

      extra-thoracic

    non-metastatic symptoms

    local (Fig. 9.7)

- cough

    haemoptysis

    dyspnoea

    deep-seated poorly localized pain on side of lesion

    wheezing – may be localized

    a small number are picked up on routine screening

    general – see Fig. 9.8

Cough 80%
Haemoptysis 70%
Breathless 60%
Pain 40%
Wheezing 15%
Routine X-ray 5%

258

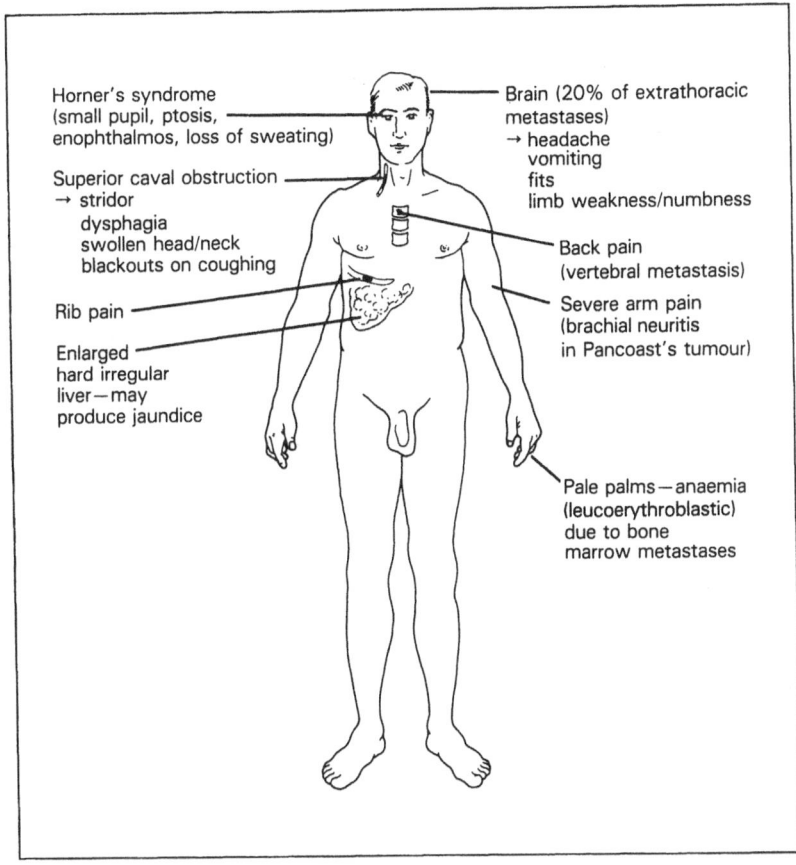

Horner's syndrome
(small pupil, ptosis,
enophthalmos, loss of sweating)

Superior caval obstruction
→ stridor
   dysphagia
   swollen head/neck
   blackouts on coughing

Rib pain

Enlarged
hard irregular
liver—may
produce jaundice

Brain (20% of extrathoracic
metastases)
→ headache
   vomiting
   fits
   limb weakness/numbness

Back pain
(vertebral metastasis)

Severe arm pain
(brachial neuritis
in Pancoast's tumour)

Pale palms—anaemia
(leucoerythroblastic)
due to bone
marrow metastases

Fig. 9.6 *Symptoms/signs from metastases in bronchial carcinoma*

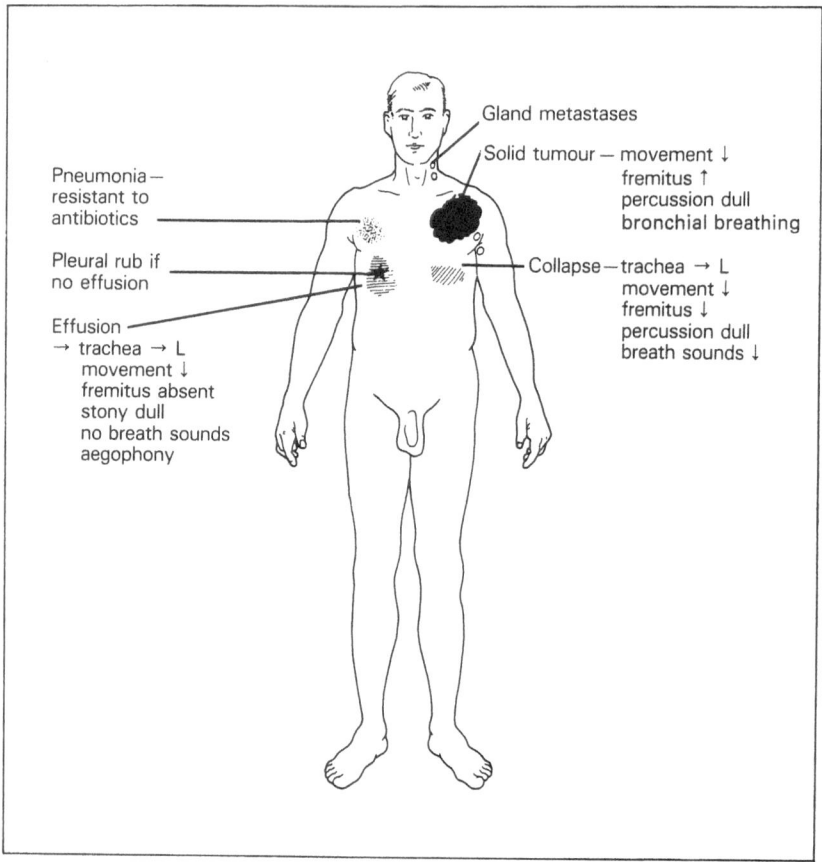

Fig. 9.7   *Local signs of bronchial carcinoma*

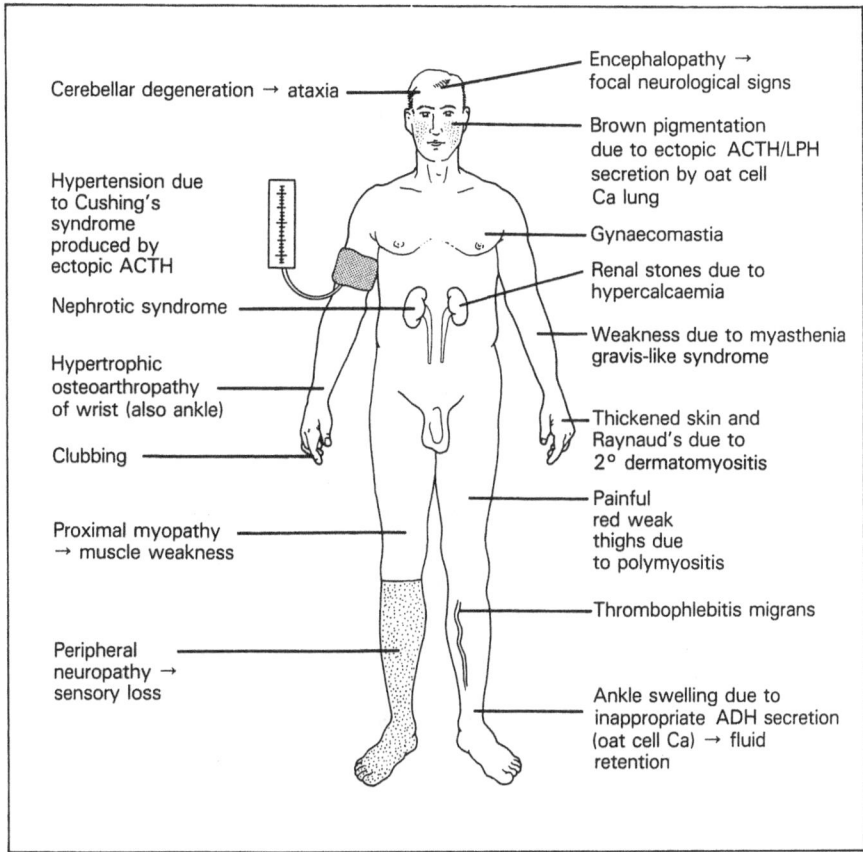

Fig. 9.8 *Non-metastatic extrapulmonary manifestations of bronchial carcinoma*

- tests

  chest X-ray – peripheral carcinoma

  hilar gland enlargement

  hilar carcinomatous mass

  collapse/consolidation

  pleural effusion

  diaphragmatic paralysis (phrenic nerve involvement)

  lung abscess

> bronchoscopy – best test
>
>> positive 60–70% of all cases
>
> biopsy of suspicious lesions essential
>
> sputum cytology less sensitive – positive 40% of confirmed cases of lung cancer

Fibrosing alveolitis

- may be

  primary ? cause

  secondary to collagen disease – rheumatoid

  SLE

  scleroderma

  secondary to drugs

  cytotoxic agents – cyclophosphamide

  methotrexate

  busulphan

  bleomycin

  others – carbamazepine

  gold

  nitrofurantoin

  methysergide

  penicillamine

  amiodarone

- symptoms – dry cough

  progressive dyspnoea on exertion

- signs – gross clubbing

  general reduction of chest expansion

  widespread crackling crepitations

- tests

  X-ray – diffuse opacities in lungs

  high diaphragm

  respiratory function

  restrictive defect FEV $\downarrow$

  vital capacity $\downarrow$

  carbon monoxide transfer factor low

Cough

> lung biopsy
> blood tests
> > antinuclear factor may be present
> > rheumatoid factor may be present

- prognosis – few months to 5 years
  > > steroids may help

Pitfalls in diagnosis

- Tuberculosis is often overlooked in the elderly by ascribing minor symptoms to old age or 'bronchitis'.
- It is easy to accept a vague, ill-defined, ill-localized, deep-seated unilateral chest pain as 'functional' – always remember bronchial carcinoma as a possible cause.
- Attributing a cough due to bronchial carcinoma to smoking, i.e. a 'smoker's cough'.
- Forgetting the possibility of bronchial carcinoma developing in a patient with known tuberculosis or chronic bronchitis.
- Not considering amyloidosis in a bronchiectatic patient who develops oedema (nephrotic syndrome) or diarrhoea (intestinal involvement).
- Overlooking serious underlying lung disease by not having a chest X-ray in a patient with pleurisy.

Useful practical points

- Anorexia, nausea and vomiting may be early symptoms in tuberculosis due to swallowing infected sputum.
- Always consider bronchial carcinoma in any unexplained cough in the middle-aged or elderly especially if they are or have been smokers.
- Never accept 'bronchitis' – acute or chronic – as an adequate explanation for haemoptysis until you are sure, on the basis of full investigation including bronchoscopy, that bronchial carcinoma has been excluded.
- A chest X-ray is not an adequate test to exclude bronchial carcinoma – bronchoscopy is mandatory.
- Always follow up – clinically and radiologically – any middle-aged or elderly patient who develops a severe lung infection 'out of the blue'.
- A single episode of haemoptysis in a smoker may mean carcinoma of the lung.
- Simple pneumoconiosis does not cause any significant deterioration in lung function tests.
- Always have an expert laryngeal examination in any patient with persistent hoarseness of the voice to pick up a recurrent laryngeal palsy due to bronchial carcinoma.

Case challenge

A 48-year-old Irish dockworker presented with a history of long-standing chronic cough and recent haemoptysis. He had been 'chesty' for at least 10 years and subject to frequent attacks of winter bronchitis: he had a chronic cough productive of white or grey sputum for most of the year and he attributed this to smoking 40 cigarettes daily for as many years. He was also fond of drinking, about 8–10 pints of beer for 4–5 nights/week. Recently his cough had got worse, he was feeling ill and sweaty, and had coughed up some bright red blood mixed with green phlegm on two occasions. On direct enquiry he admitted to loss of weight and loss of appetite.

The findings on examination are shown in Fig. 9.9.

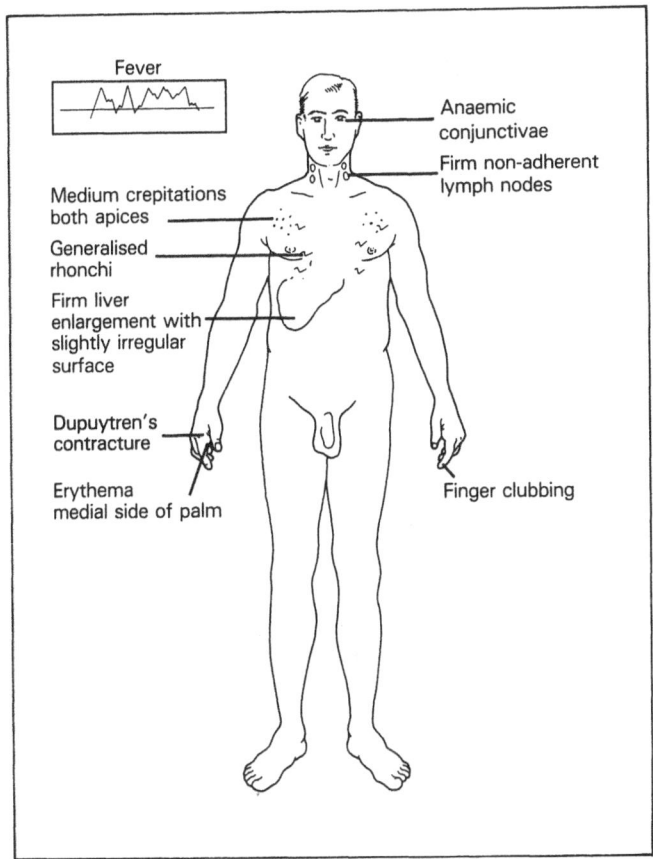

Fig. 9.9 *Examination findings in case challenge*

Questions		Give three likely diagnoses for the lung problem.
		What tests would you do to distinguish?
		What treatment would you advise?
		Is there any other diagnosis?
		How would you confirm this?
		What treatment would you suggest?

Possible diagnoses

- chronic bronchitis
- carcinoma of bronchus
- tuberculosis

Chronic bronchitis

For	history	• long history of productive cough
		• heavy smoker
	exam	• generalized rhonchi
Against	history	• recent haemoptysis
		• loss of weight
	exam	• apical crepitations – not a feature of chronic bronchitis
		• finger clubbing
Tests		• chest X-ray
		• respiratory function – obstructive defect

Carcinoma bronchus

For	history	• haemoptysis
		• anorexia and loss of weight
	exam	• neck glands – though rarely generalized as in this case
		• finger clubbing
		• anaemia
Against	exam	• *bilateral* apical crepitation
		• nil else otherwise
Tests		• chest X-ray
		• bronchoscopy – mandatory

Tuberculosis

For	history	• Irishman – reduced resistance to TB
		• alcoholism – increases susceptibility to TB
		• haemoptysis
		• sweats – very suggestive
		• anorexia and loss of weight
	exam	• apical crepitations – often post-tussive
		• neck glands – could be extension TB
		• finger clubbing
Against		• nil
Tests		• chest X-ray
		• sputum for TB – several specimens
		• tuberculin test – limited value
		• blood count and ESR – of no diagnostic value – too non-specific

---

Actual diagnosis:
Tuberculosis
X-ray showed ill-defined apical opacities with early cavitation
sputum – many tubercle bacilli

Treatment

Rifampicin   600mg daily ⎫
Isoniazid   300mg daily   ⎬   for two months
Ethambutol   25mg/kg body weight ⎭

then Rifampicin ⎫
      Isoniazid   ⎬ for a further 7 months

This 9 month course of treatment is usually 100% effective

10 Acute Sore Throat

Introduction

The syndrome of pain and soreness on swallowing accompanied by fever, malaise and tender neck glands is common in the community.

It is common but confusing, since symptoms and appearances are no guides to causation and since treatment should be based on knowledge of cause this also is confused.

However, sound 'guesses' can be made with attention to clinical presentation and a knowledge of the natural history of the condition.

Grades of significance

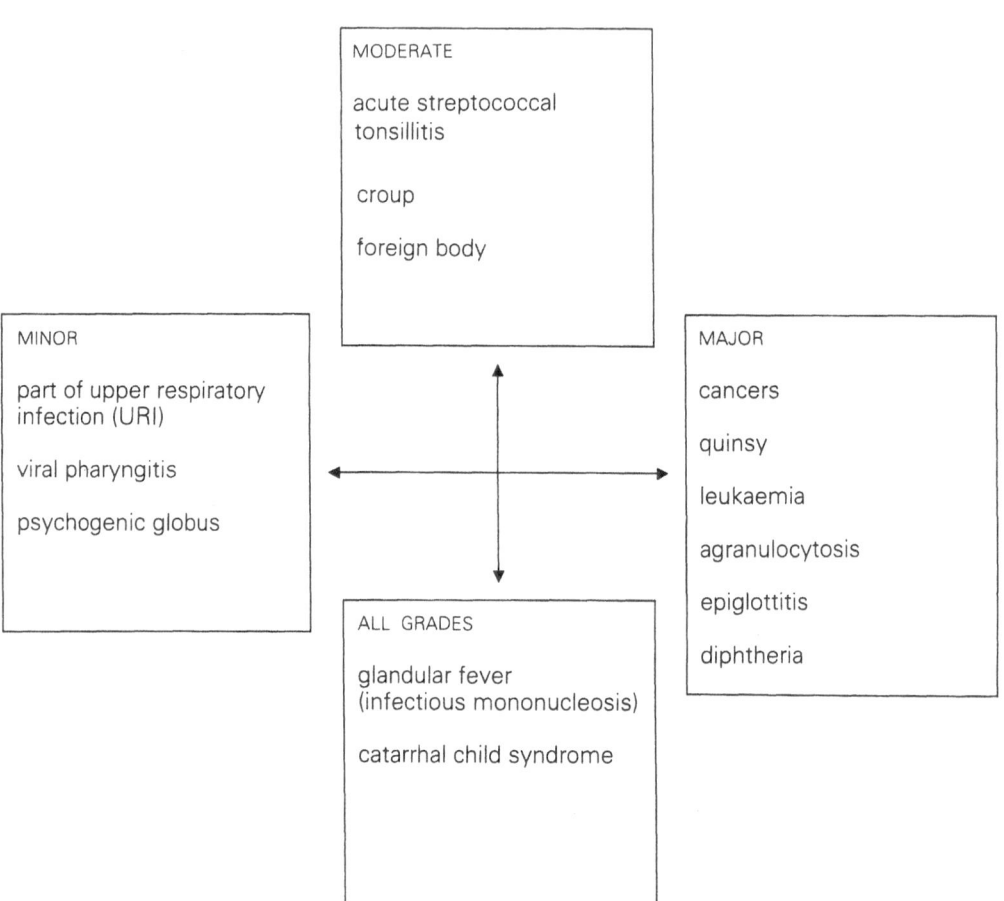

Frequency

Acute sore throat is a disease of primary care, seen only coincidentally in hospital practice

Annual prevalence of acute sore throat
in a general practice of 2500 persons

Common U R I	100+
Acute streptococcal tonsillitis	30
Acute 'viral' tonsillitis	50
Glandular fever	3
Croup	5
others	less than 1 per year
Total	188

Age incidence

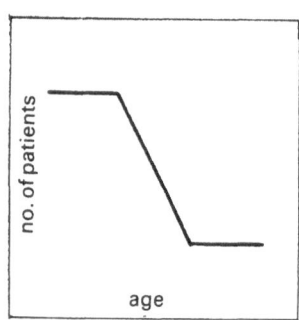

- catarrhal child syndrome
- croup
- epiglottitis

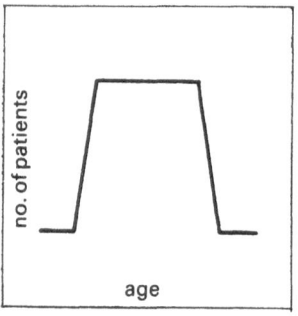

- streptococcal tonsillitis
- glandular fever
- quinsy
- leukaemia

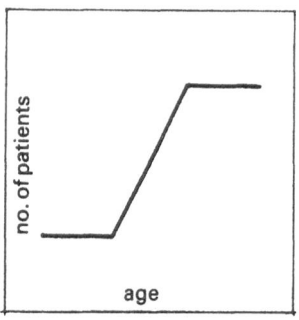

(rare)
- carcinoma of pharynx and larynx
- foreign bodies (in edentulous)

Significance

Painful condition lasting up to one week (average 4–5 days)

In itself benign but very rarely streptococcal infections may lead to

- acute nephritis (possibly 1 in 1000 attacks)
- rheumatic fever (about 1 in 2500 attacks)

May present as feature of underlying serious disease

(rare)

- leukaemia
- agranulocytosis (from drug reactions)
- carcinoma

Diagnostic approach

History

Onset
- sudden within an hour or so with much pain in streptococcal tonsillitis
- slower, over a day or two, in viral throats
- slow and prolonged in glandular fever
- persistent – chronic laryngitis, cancers and globus hystericus

General systemic upset
- individual variability
- more severe illness usually in streptococcal infections
- adults tend to be more ill than children

Associated
- earache, usually referred pain with normal eardrums, but there may be accompanying otitis media
- abdominal pain and fever may be presenting features in young children
- hoarseness in laryngitis and cancers

Examination
- *fever* + in streptococcal throat.
- *tongue* more furred in streptococcal throat – may be a 'strawberry' tongue white with red papillae.
- *smell of breath* – unpleasant + in streptococcal and Vincent's infections.

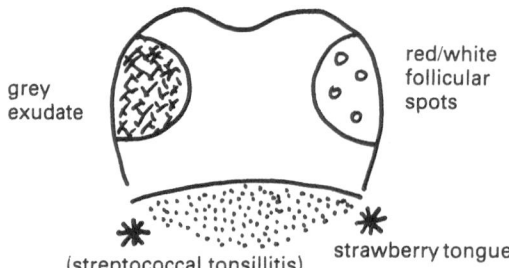

grey exudate

red/white follicular spots

(streptococcal tonsillitis)   strawberry tongue

- *fauces*

    streptococcal

    tonsils +

        red white follicular spots

        greyish exudate

    '*viral*'

    tonsils +

        red

        greyish exudate may be present

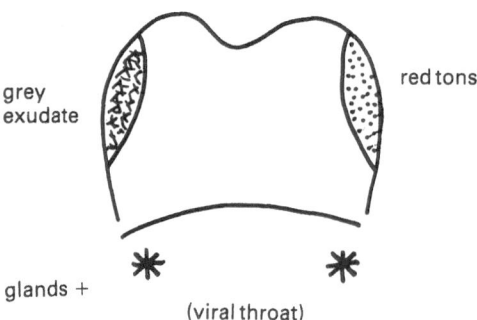

grey exudate

red tonsil

glands +

(viral throat)

Acute sore throat

- '*quinsy*' (peritonsillitis)

  unilateral

  redness and swelling + of peritonsillar tissues extending into soft palate

  trismus +

  cervical glands +

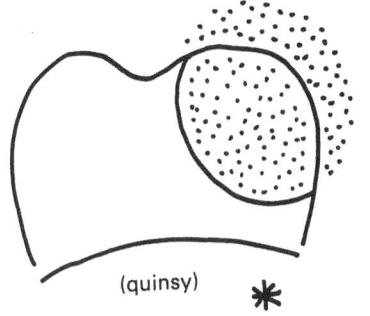

swollen red tonsils and peritonsillar area

(quinsy) ✳

- *diphtheria*

  white tough exudate over tonsils and palate adherent to tissues

  glands enlarged + giving bull-neck appearance

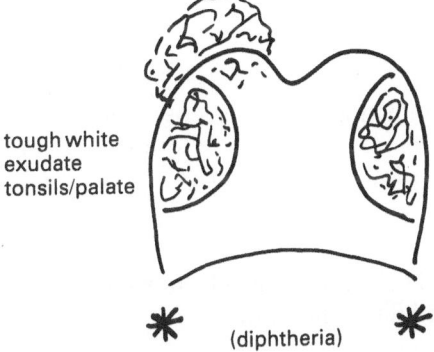

tough white exudate tonsils/palate

✳ (diphtheria) ✳

- *gums*

  may be ulcerated + in Vincent's angina and in leukaemia

275

- *cervical glands*

    note cervical glands are palpable in normal child from 3–10 years

    may be tender only

    may be tender and swollen

    may be extremely swollen with surrounding cellulitis of neck tissues

- *skin*

    erythematous rashes may accompany streptococcal or viral infections or may be due to drug sensitivities such as to ampicillin in glandular fever

Investigations

'Routine' tests are not necessary; only use investigations for a good reason

Throat swab for bacteriology: these have limitations –

    there is at least a 24 hour delay in reporting

    in majority 'no pathogenic organisms' are detected

    usually an immediate decision on treatment has to be taken, i.e. to use antibiotics or not and it may be impractical to wait for result of swab

    throat swabs are of value in epidemics of throat infections in closed communities; in unusual appearances of throat to exclude diphtheria, gonococcal infection, *Candida*, or other organisms

    are of value in early years in practice to test one's ability to spot the 'specific' case

Blood tests

    not required routinely.

    main value in diagnosis of glandular fever (infectious mononucleosis), but usually this diagnosis is not considered until condition has been present for longer than a week: positive findings are presence of atypical mononuclear cells and positive specific immunological tests.

Urine

    acute nephritis is a very rare consequence of a streptococcal infection and a check for albuminuria is indicated when any possibility is present.

Specific conditions

Streptococcal tonsillitis

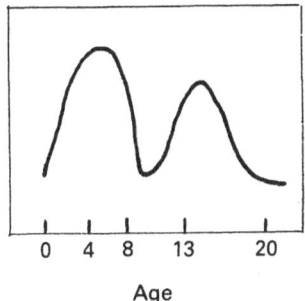

Age

- biphasic peak incidence at 4–8 years and in teens
- sudden onset
- quite ill – high fever
  headache (adults)

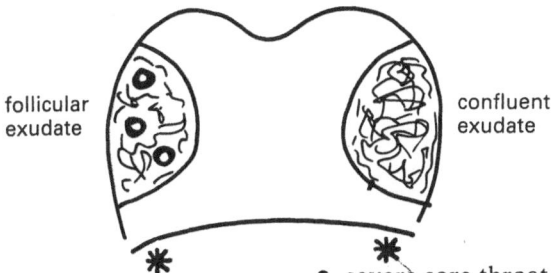

follicular exudate

confluent exudate

- severe sore throat
- tonsils + red
- follicular or confluent exudate
- cervical glands + and tender
- coated tongue and offensive smell
- may be erythematous rash
- abdominal pain and vomiting (in children)
- settles in under one week; resolution speeded with antibiotics by 1 or 2 days.
- note that in only ⅓ of acute follicullar tonsillitis is *Streptococcus pyogenes* isolated

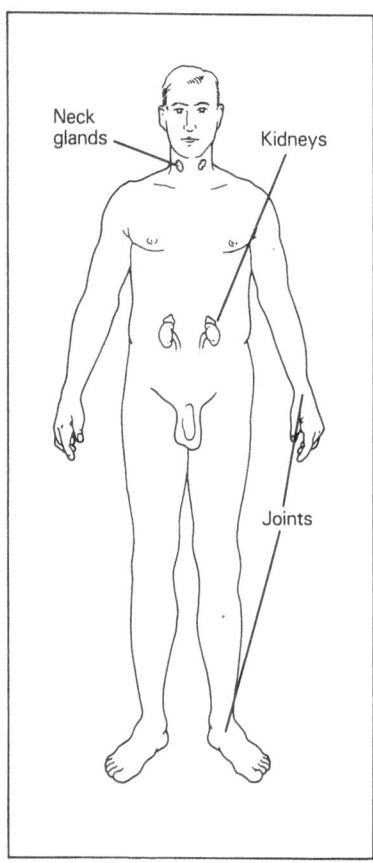

Neck glands

Kidneys

Joints

- *complications*

    rare — cervical adenitis

    otitis media

    very rare — acute nephritis

    rheumatic fever

    erythema nodosum

- *investigations*

    throat swab if unusual presentation, i.e. possible diphtheria

    blood tests if unusual course – possible glandular fever or blood disorders

Quinsy (peritonsillitis)

- usually streptococcal
- adults (very rare in children)
- sudden onset of sore throat

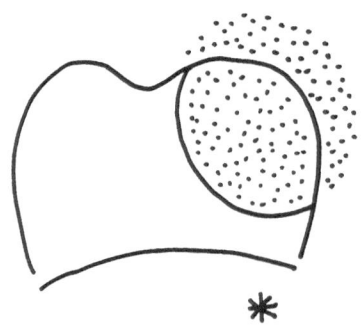

swollen red tonsils and peritonsillar area

Acute sore throat

- prolonged course – does not improve after 4–5 days
- unilateral
- swelling + of peritonsillar region extending to soft palate, often difficult to differentiate the tonsil
- increasing general illness with fever and dehydration
- difficulty in swallowing ++
- trismus
- cervical glands ++
- investigations not helpful

Glandular fever (infectious mononucleosis)

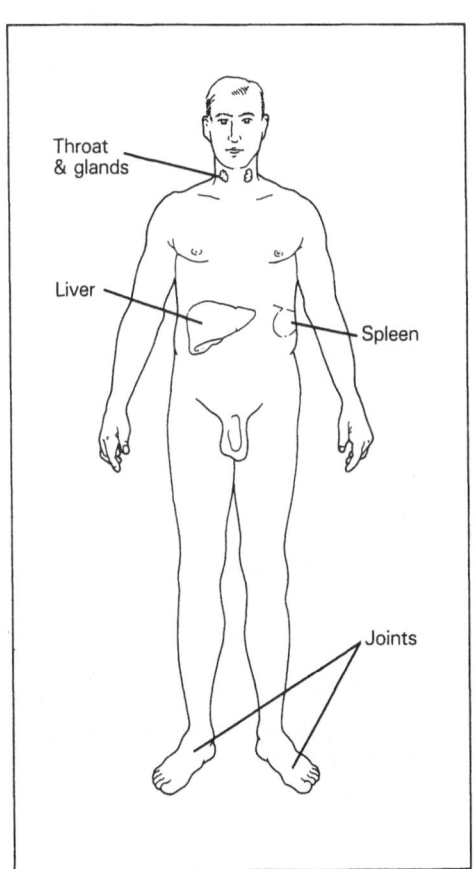

- teenagers or young adults
- sporadic and endemic
- epidemics and case-to-case contacts unusual, except in closed communities
- sore throat persisting for a week or longer
- swollen red tonsils with white follicular or grey exudates; petechiae may be noted on hard palate
- lymph glands : enlarged and tender

    anterior and posterior cervical

    inguinal and axillary (sometimes)
- spleen enlarged (rarely felt +)
- variable degrees of illness – from minor subclinical condition to severe illness and very rarely death
- erythematous rash – more often following ampicillin
- *rarely*

    jaundice

    joint pains and swellings

    heart failure due to myocarditis, may cause sudden death

    second attacks rare but can occur.
- *diagnosis*

    blood

    atypical GF mononucleated cells

    positive Paul – Bunnell or Monospot tests
- *family history*

    siblings may suffer from glandular fever when they reach vulnerable age period

Acute epiglottitis

- rare
- dangerous + + + possible death from suffocation
- acute infection of throat – epiglottitis and adjacent structures causing much swelling
- caused by *Haemophilus influenzae*
- infants 6–24 months

Acute sore throat

- sudden onset
- croupy cough
- difficulty in breathing with stridor
- fever
- child still, not crying, distressed +
- afraid to swallow because of pain and drooling of saliva from mouth
- cherry red epiglottis – *but do not try and examine throat with spatula at home* because of risk of increasing respiratory obstruction
- investigations – nil
- *get to a unit with facilities for intubation as soon as possible*

Pitfalls in diagnosis

- Young children do not complain of a 'sore throat' but present with fever and tummy ache.
- High fever, headache and pain in neck may also occur in meningitis.
- Appearance of fauces is no help in making a specific pathogenic diagnosis.
- 'Scarlet fever' may be an antibiotic rash.
- Glandular fever may be a multi-system disease and sore throat may not be prominent.
- Gonococcal throat infections not unknown in male homosexuals.
- Diphtheria still occurs in some countries and in returning travellers.

Useful practical points

- Most acute throat infections are *not* caused by streptococci or other specific pathogens.
- A clinical diagnosis has to be made as to how ill is the patient, what is likely course and does he/she need antibiotics or can it be left to resolve naturally?
- The commonest causes of trismus are quinsy and infection around unerupted lower molars and not tetanus.
- Consider glandular fever (infectious mononucleosis) in a sore throat in a teenager *but* most acute sore throats in teenagers are not glandular fever but viral or streptococcal.
- Following an attack of glandular fever some teenagers suffer recurring bouts of non-specific acute tonsillitis that require tonsillectomy.
- Think of acute epiglottitis in a sick infant with croup.

Case challenge

G. J., 29-year-old college lecturer consults for a sore throat and cough for 5 days. Neck glands are swollen. Feels unwell. Tired + because of heavy work load. Wife is 4 months pregnant with her first child. He states that he had 'glandular fever' when he was an undergraduate.

Examination

On examination his tonsils are swollen and red

Tongue is black and teeth are stained yellow

He does not appear very ill but is agitated and anxious

No enlargement of neck glands

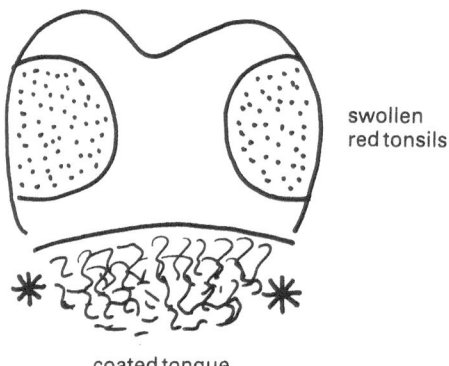

swollen
red tonsils

coated tongue

Acute sore throat

Questions

What further questions would you ask?

What is likely diagnosis?

What investigations may be helpful?

How would you manage the case?

Further questions

- smoking habits?
- was past diagnosis of 'glandular fever' confirmed by blood test?
- any possible contact cases of infections among his students?
- is he concerned over possibility of his wife becoming infected and the effects on the unborn baby?
- enquire on work and other personal problems?

Possible diagnoses

- non-specific pharyngitis in a heavy smoker with an anxious personality
- glandular fever
- streptococcal tonsillitis

Consideration of pros/cons in diagnosis

Non-specific pharyngitis in worried man?

- anxious personality
- pregnant wife, for first time
- insignificant symptoms
- few signs
- heavy smoker – black tongue and yellow teeth (probably pipe smoker)

Glandular fever?

- has contacts with young students who are the at-risk group
- has a previous history of 'glandular fever' – may not have been confirmed and therefore not a true infection
- second attacks rare but do occur
- symptoms have been present for 5 days and his neck glands are painful and swollen

283

Streptococcal tonsillitis

- not very ill
- no exudate on tonsils
- accompanying cough suggests a more general upper respiratory infection

Management

Tests

- arrange for blood test to exclude glandular fever
- take throat swab as he is so worried over his infectivity for his pregnant wife

Results

- blood test – no evidence of glandular fever
- throat swab – no pathogenic organisms

Actual diagnosis:
Viral pharyngitis

Treatment

Strong reassurance on his own health and that there are no risks for his wife

Strong advice to stop smoking

No specific medication

Resolved within a week

11   Earache

Introduction

Earache is a symptom of all ages but most prevalent in children.

Earache may be caused by disorders of the ear or from other structures.

Precise diagnosis of earache may be difficult.

Common, may be difficult but usually benign and self-limiting.

Grades/causes of significance

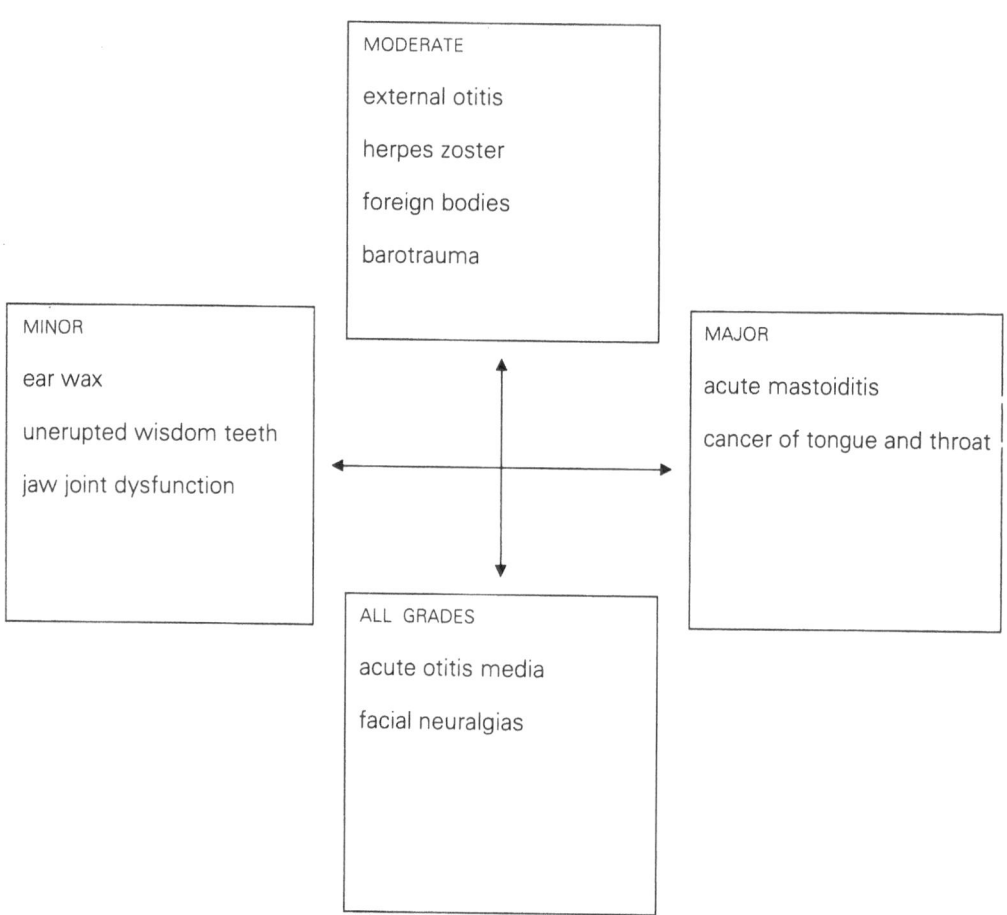

MODERATE

external otitis

herpes zoster

foreign bodies

barotrauma

MINOR

ear wax

unerupted wisdom teeth

jaw joint dysfunction

MAJOR

acute mastoiditis

cancer of tongue and throat

ALL GRADES

acute otitis media

facial neuralgias

Frequency

Earache is largely a condition of primary care

*Annual prevalence of earache in a general
practice of 2500 persons*

	Patients consulting
Common	
Acute otitis media	75
Wax	30
External otitis	20
Dental causes	5
Facial neuralgias	2
Barotrauma	2
Rare	
Herpes zoster	1 in 5 years
Acute mastoiditis	1 in 25 years
Cancer of throat/mouth	1 in 30 years

Age incidence

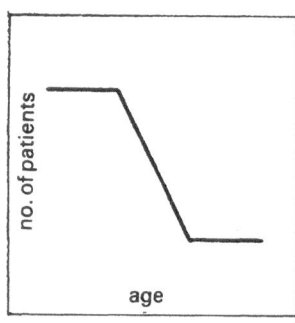

- acute otitis media
- foreign body in external meatus

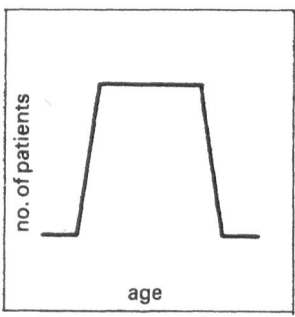

- external otitis
- dry wax
- dental causes (wisdom teeth etc.)
- barotrauma
- facial neuralgias

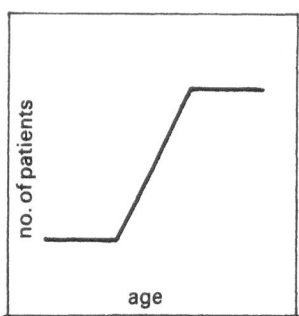

- herpes zoster
- cancers
- foreign bodies in throat

Significance

Most cases are otitis media or external otitis

Acute otitis media – severe earache

    now a relatively benign but recurring disorder of children

    complications – persistent deafness with social consequences, especially learning problems

Note earache from outside the ear by referred pain

Note barotrauma from air travel or diving

Diagnostic approach

History

Age	• acute otitis media in children
	• external otitis in young adults
	• wax at all ages
	• dental causes in young and middle age
Onset	
hours	• sudden, often overnight in acute otitis media
days	• progressive over 2–3 days in external otitis
weeks	• neuralgias, referred pains and cancers – over a few weeks
General systemic upset	• may be severe in acute otitis media
	• external otitis may be severe locally but little general upset unless appreciable secondary infection
Preceding	• upper respiratory infections in acute otitis media
	• swimming/hair washing in wax and external otitis
Previous history	• recurrences in acute otitis media and external otitis
Pain character	• dull, aching, throbbing in acute otitis media
	• sore, tender in external otitis
Associated features	• pain on eating and swallowing with dental and throat causes
Deafness	• in acute otitis media, external otitis and wax

Examination

General
- appearance and composure
- fever, often higher in otitis media in young children

External ear

pinna
- swelling → otitis externa
- vesicular rash → herpes
- redness → cellulitis spread from external otitis

meatus
- swelling
- redness
- scaling $\Bigg\} →$ otitis externa – various degrees
- wax/debris
- weeping/discharge

Middle ear

drum
- colour – dull/pink/red/calcareous
- thickening/bulging
- perforation $\Bigg\} →$ otitis media
- discharge
- mobility impaired

Mouth and throat
- tongue – ulcers
- teeth – caries, unerupted wisdom
- gums – gingivitis, ulceration, dental abscess
- pharynx – ulcers, redness, exudate
- tonsils – swelling, ulceration, exudate

Neck/head
- mastoid – tender/swelling
- face and neck – rash/palsy
- eyes – pupils/lids
- scalp – rash
- cervical glands – swelling/tender

Investigations

Few investigations necessary in most cases

Hearing tests	• essential as test of function
	• crude – speech or tuning fork
	• sophisticated – audiometers
	• checks of recovery

Swabs from meatus if discharge for bacteriology

Radiology	• of mastoid/middle ear for expert assessment
Computerized tomography	• very special indications

Specific conditions

Acute otitis media
- condition of childhood with maximal prevalence at 4–8 years
- part of 'the catarrhal child syndrome'
- *causes* may be:

  most cases no specific cause found

  bacterial

  pneumococci

  H. influenzae

  streptococci

  staphylococci

  viral

  non-infective – immunological responses
- sudden onset
- considerable systemic upset
- may be preceded by cough/cold/catarrh
- *symptoms*

  earache only 75%

  discharge 20%

  deafness only 5%

- *signs*

  external meatus usually normal but may be secondarily infected if ear discharge

  drum may be dull-opalescent, pink, red.

  drum may be perforated with or without discharge

  'safe' perforation where some drum tissue between it and bony walls

  'unsafe' perforated where bone is part of its wall.

- *course*

  drum may take 2 weeks to 2 months to return to normal

  deafness may persist for weeks (**note**: glue ear)

  persisting discharge (chronic otitis media) is rare

  complications are very rare

    mastoiditis

    chronic otitis media

    intracranial sepsis

- *management*

  antibiotics *not* required in most attacks, decisions have to be made on clinical grounds

External otitis

- a disease of skin and not of middle ear
- may be *acute dermatitis* caused by irritants or sensitizers
- may be part of a *general eczematous diathesis*
- may be *local skin infection* (boils etc)
- may be secondary to self-inflicted *trauma* – cleansing, scratching

Earache

- *symptoms*

  itching

  soreness – pain

  discharge – usually thin/non-purulent

  deafness – due to swelling of external
  meatal walls and not to damage to drum

- *signs*

  swelling of meatal walls and drum often
  not visible

  meatal skin red, sealing, crusted

- *treatment*

  local cleansing

  local steroid/antibiotics

  systemic antibiotics/steroids

Pitfalls in diagnosis

- Difficulties in differentiating between external otitis and otitis media
- Difficulties in examination
- 'Non-ear' earache from referred causes

Practical points

- Try and see the drums, but may be impossible.
- Examine possible referral sites, e.g. mouth, throat, teeth, particularly in adults

Case challenge

Debra C. aged 11, earache for 2 days (both ears). Previous attacks since age of 3

On examination

Marked swelling of both external meati with discharge

Pain on moving pinnae

Drums seen with difficulty look red

Hearing loss

Questions	What further questions would you ask?
	What is likely diagnosis?
	What investigations may be helpful?
	How would you manage the case?

Further questions

- details of previous attacks
- what hobbies and leisure pursuits?

    she is a swimmer of championship standards and swims daily for over 1 hour

- what toilet habits?

    does she clean ears, how, and with what?

- toothache, sore throat?
- recent cough/cold?
- recent air travel?

Possible diagnoses

- external otitis
- acute otitis media

Diagnostic pros/cons

External otitis

For

- previous attacks
- swimmer +

    irritation from water/chlorine

- local trauma from excessive cleansing or use of ear plugs
- bilateral
- soreness
- swelling of external meati
- red drum may be part of external otitis

Acute otitis media

For

- previous attacks
- red drum

Test

- swab for causal pathogenic organisms?

> ## Actual diagnosis:
> Acute otitis externa

Treatment

Gentle toilet of external ears by nurse or doctor

Systemic antibiotics

Local steroid ear drops

Advice on future care of ears, especially for swimmers

Settled slowly but recurred

12 Headache

Introduction

Occasional headache is almost universal and acceptable as 'normal'.

Problematical headaches are those that are severe, constant or recurring at frequent intervals.

Causes of 'headache' range far beyond the head.

The individual with headaches is worried over possibilities of 'blood pressure', 'stroke' and 'brain tumour'.

Pain-sensitive structures causing headaches

- basal intracranial arteries
- intracranial venous sinuses
- meningeal arteries
- basal dura mater
- scalp muscles

Causes of headache

Vascular
- migraine
- hypertension
- systemic infection, e.g. flu
- drugs
    - nitrates and nifedipine for angina
    - hydrallazine for hypertension
    - alcohol

Inflammatory
- meningeal irritation
    - meningitis
    - subarachnoid haemorrhage

297

- any systemic infection (including flu)
- cranial (temporal) arteritis

Raised intracranial pressure
- space-occupying lesion
    - abscess
    - haematoma
    - tumour
- benign intracranial hypertension
- infections, e.g. encephalitis
- bleeding – stroke

Trauma
- immediate post-traumatic
- chronic subdural haematoma
- anxiety ('compensationitis')
- dysautonomic cephalgia

Local disease
- eyes
    - refractive
    - retrobulbar neuritis
    - glaucoma
- sinuses – sinusitis
- teeth
    - impaction
    - infection
    - malocclusion
- neck – spondylosis
- skull
    - Paget's disease
    - myelomatosis
    - carcinomatosis

Psychogenic
- anxiety (tension headache)
- depression

Miscellaneous	• anaemia ($< 10\,g\%$)
	• chronic lung disease – hypercapnia
	• after coughing or sneezing
	• after sexual intercourse
	• endocrine disease
	myxoedema
	Addison's disease
	Conn's syndrome

Grades of severity of underlying disorder

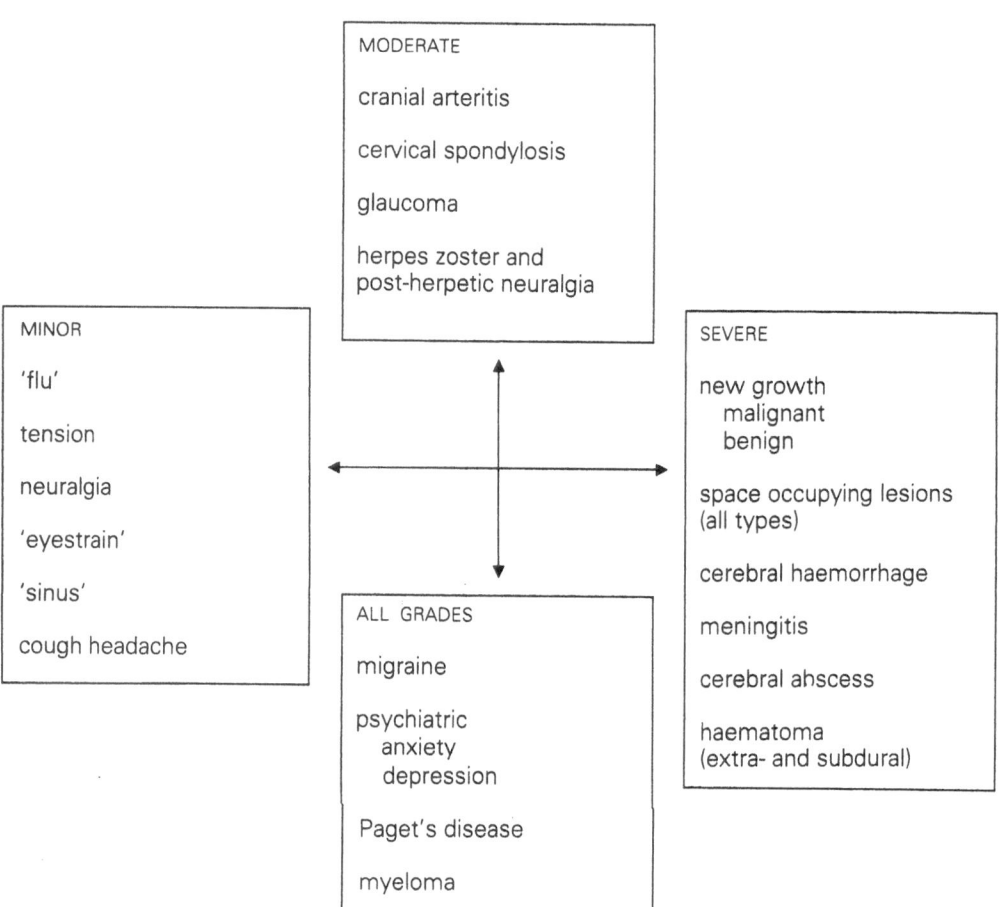

MODERATE

cranial arteritis

cervical spondylosis

glaucoma

herpes zoster and
post-herpetic neuralgia

MINOR

'flu'

tension

neuralgia

'eyestrain'

'sinus'

cough headache

SEVERE

new growth
  malignant
  benign

space occupying lesions
(all types)

cerebral haemorrhage

meningitis

cerebral ahscess

haematoma
(extra- and subdural)

ALL GRADES

migraine

psychiatric
  anxiety
  depression

Paget's disease

myeloma

high BP

Frequency

*Annual prevalence of headaches
in a population of 2500*

general infections (flu etc.)	
– headache as major feature	100
migraine	25
psychogenic	25
cervical spondylosis	10
(facial) neuralgia	5
high blood pressure (headache +)	5
less than 1 per year	
stroke (subarachnoid haemorrhage)	1 in 2y
secondary brain tumour	1 in 5y
cranial arteritis	1 in 7y
primary brain tumour	1 in 10y
subdural/extradural haematoma	1 in 15y

Age prevalence

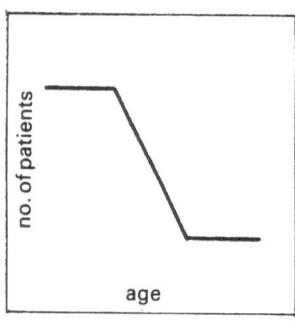

- migraine
- meningitis
- hydrocephalus

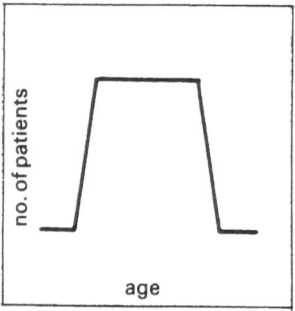

- migraine
- subarachnoid haemorrhage
- psychogenic

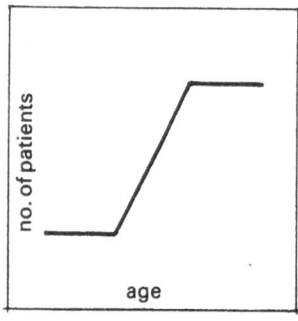

- neoplasms
- cranial arteritis
- cervical spondylosis
- high blood pressure
- neuralgia

Diagnostic approach

History

Onset

abrupt →
- subarachnoid haemorrhage
- intracerebral haemorrhage
- cluster headache
- infection
    meningitis
    encephalitis
    systemic, e.g. flu

over a few days →
- glaucoma
- purulent sinusitis
- brain abscess
- retrobulbar neuritis
- ophthalmic herpes
- malignant hypertension

over a few weeks →
- brain tumour
- subdural haematoma
- temporal arteritis
- skull deposits
    myeloma
    carcinoma

chronic/recurrent
(episodic) →
- migraine
- tension headache
- cervical spondylosis
- depression
- refractive eye problems ('eye strain')

Character

throbbing →
- migraine
- severe hypertension
- raised intracranial pressure
- chronic bronchitis (hypercapnia)

intense unilateral boring	
pain →	• cluster headache (migrainous neuralgia)
burning →	• temporal arteritis
'worse headache ever' →	• subarachnoid haemorrhage
	• acute anxiety
bizarre	• pressure
	• weight on head
	• band round head
	• continuous for days, weeks or months

Brace grouping (pressure / weight on head / band round head / continuous for days, weeks or months) → anxiety ('tension head-ache')

Site

hemicranial
- sides vary → • migraine
- same side always → • brain tumour
  - • angioma/arteriovenous malformation

frontal →
- • supratentorial brain tumours
- • local disease
  - eyes
  - sinuses
  - dental disease
- • ophthalmic herpes zoster

orbital-frontal → • cluster headache

retro-orbital → • retrobulbar neuritis

temporal →
- • giant cell arteritis
- • arthritis temporo-mandibular joint

fronto-temporal → • migraine

occipital →
- • infratentorial brain tumours
- • hypertension
- • cervical spondylosis

vertex → • anxiety/depression

Timing

night →
- • cluster headache (repetitive nightly)
- • brain tumour
- • severe hypertension

on waking →
- brain tumour
- severe hypertension
- frontal sinusitis

early afternoon →
- maxillary sinusitis

Aggravating factors

coughing/straining/
sexual intercourse →
- brain tumour especially posterior fossa
- other conditions with raised intracranial pressure
- hypertensive headache
- migraine
- meningitis
- cough headache

change of position →
- obstructive hydrocephalus, e.g. tumour
- vascular headache
- post-concussional headache

bright light →
- meningitis/encephalitis
- migraine
- subarachnoid haemorrhage

neck flexion →
- meningitis
- subarachnoid haemorrhage

other neck movements →
- cervical spondylosis

emotional stress →
- migraine
- tension headache

having a period →
- migraine

eating cheese, chocolate,
drinking wines, beer →
- migraine

Relieving factors

rest →
- vascular headache

darkness →
- migraine
- meningitis
- subarachnoid haemorrhage

sitting/standing →
- brain tumour

pregnancy →
- migraine

vomiting →
- migraine

Associated symptoms

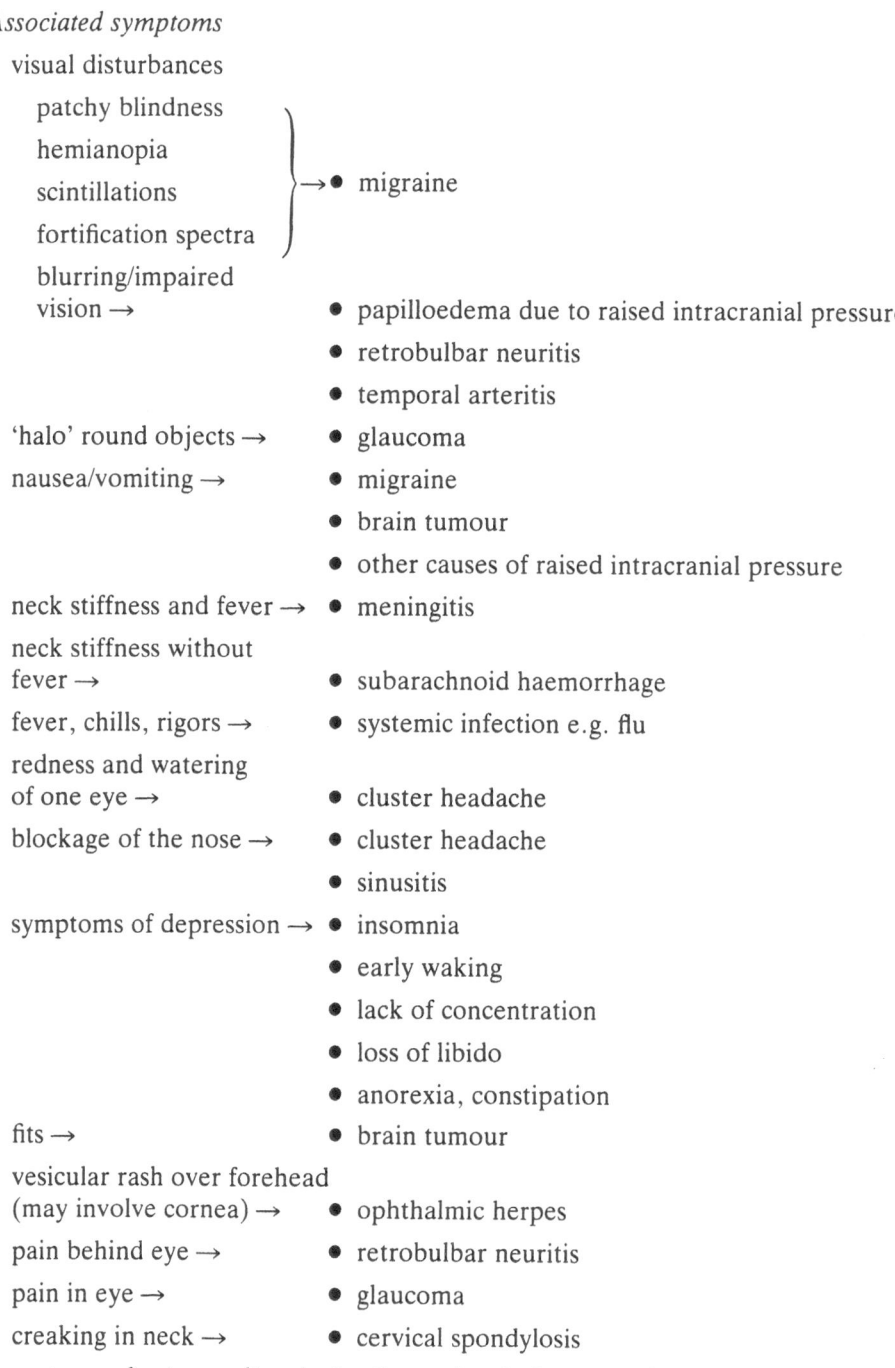

visual disturbances
  patchy blindness
  hemianopia
  scintillations   → ● migraine
  fortification spectra
  blurring/impaired
  vision →   ● papilloedema due to raised intracranial pressure
                      ● retrobulbar neuritis
                      ● temporal arteritis

'halo' round objects →   ● glaucoma

nausea/vomiting →   ● migraine
                      ● brain tumour
                      ● other causes of raised intracranial pressure

neck stiffness and fever → ● meningitis

neck stiffness without
fever →   ● subarachnoid haemorrhage

fever, chills, rigors →   ● systemic infection e.g. flu

redness and watering
of one eye →   ● cluster headache

blockage of the nose →   ● cluster headache
                      ● sinusitis

symptoms of depression → ● insomnia
                      ● early waking
                      ● lack of concentration
                      ● loss of libido
                      ● anorexia, constipation

fits →   ● brain tumour

vesicular rash over forehead
(may involve cornea) →   ● ophthalmic herpes

pain behind eye →   ● retrobulbar neuritis

pain in eye →   ● glaucoma

creaking in neck →   ● cervical spondylosis

Symptoms of *primary disorder* leading to headache – see Fig. 12.1

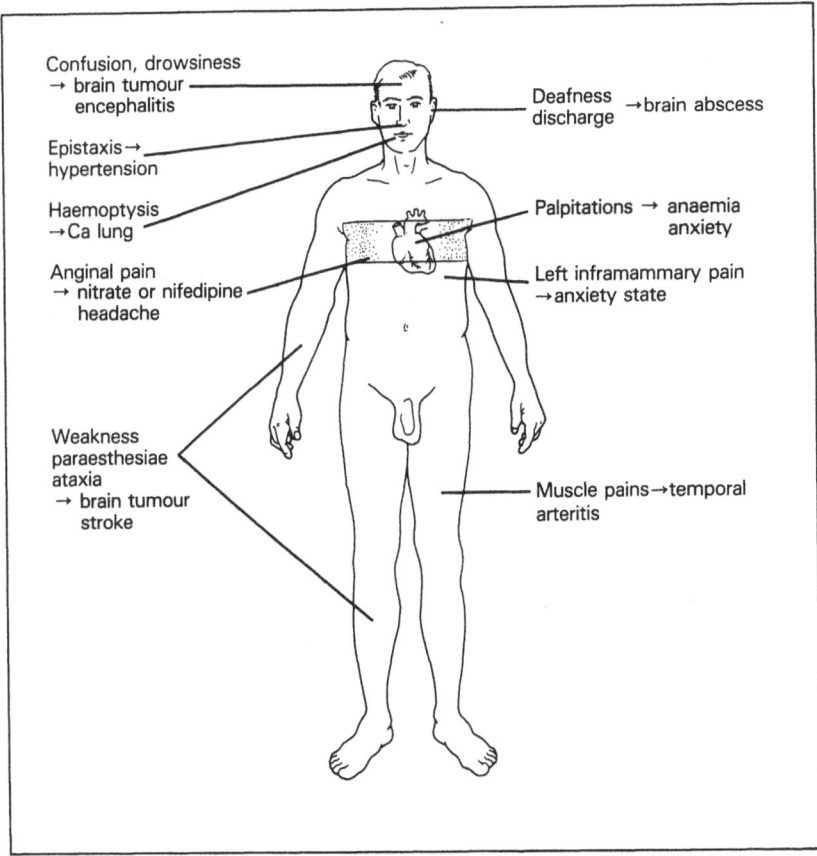

Fig. 12.1   *Symptoms of primary disorders which may lead to headache*

Past history of *head injury* – may cause various headaches

- immediate post-traumatic – due to bruising of the brain – lasts several days
- chronic subdural haematoma

    deep-seated

    unilateral or generalized

    drowsy, confused

    hemiparesis often

- 'nervous instability'
    constant headache

    giddiness

    excessive fatigue

    can't concentrate

    often linked with compensation
- dysautonomic cephalgia

    injury to sympathetic nerves in carotid sheath in neck

    episodic, throbbing

    unilateral

    small pupil

    excessive sweating

family history
- migraine – often hereditary
- hypertension
- some brain tumours

    certain gliomas

    neurofibroma

    haemangioblastoma
- anxiety

Examination

A meticulous examination of the nervous system is mandatory – this should include

mental state – mood, anxiety- tension, mental changes (dementia)

cranial nerves	I	• smell not usually tested unless olfactory groove tumour suspected
	II	• visual acuity
		• visual fields
		• fundi
III, IV and VI		• external occular movements
		• nystagmus

V	• motor – jaw clenching
	• sensation (including conjunctiva)
VII	• facial movements
	• taste – anterior 2/3 of tongue
VIII	• hearing
IX	• gag reflex
	• taste – posterior 1/3 of tongue
X	• palatal/pharyngeal movements
XI	• sterno-mastoid, trapezius
XII	• tongue movements

motor system
- muscle tone
- muscle power
- abdominal reflexes
- deep reflexes
- plantar responses

sensory system
- touch, pain, temperature
- vibration
- joint position (and Romberg's sign)

cerebellar system
- finger–nose test
- heel–knee test
- standing for truncal ataxia
- walking for veering to one side

a general examination of other systems is also essential

the possible findings on examination in patient with headache are shown in Fig. 12.2

Investigations

Blood count

leucocytosis
- bacterial meningitis
- brain abscess
- sinusitis
- systemic infections

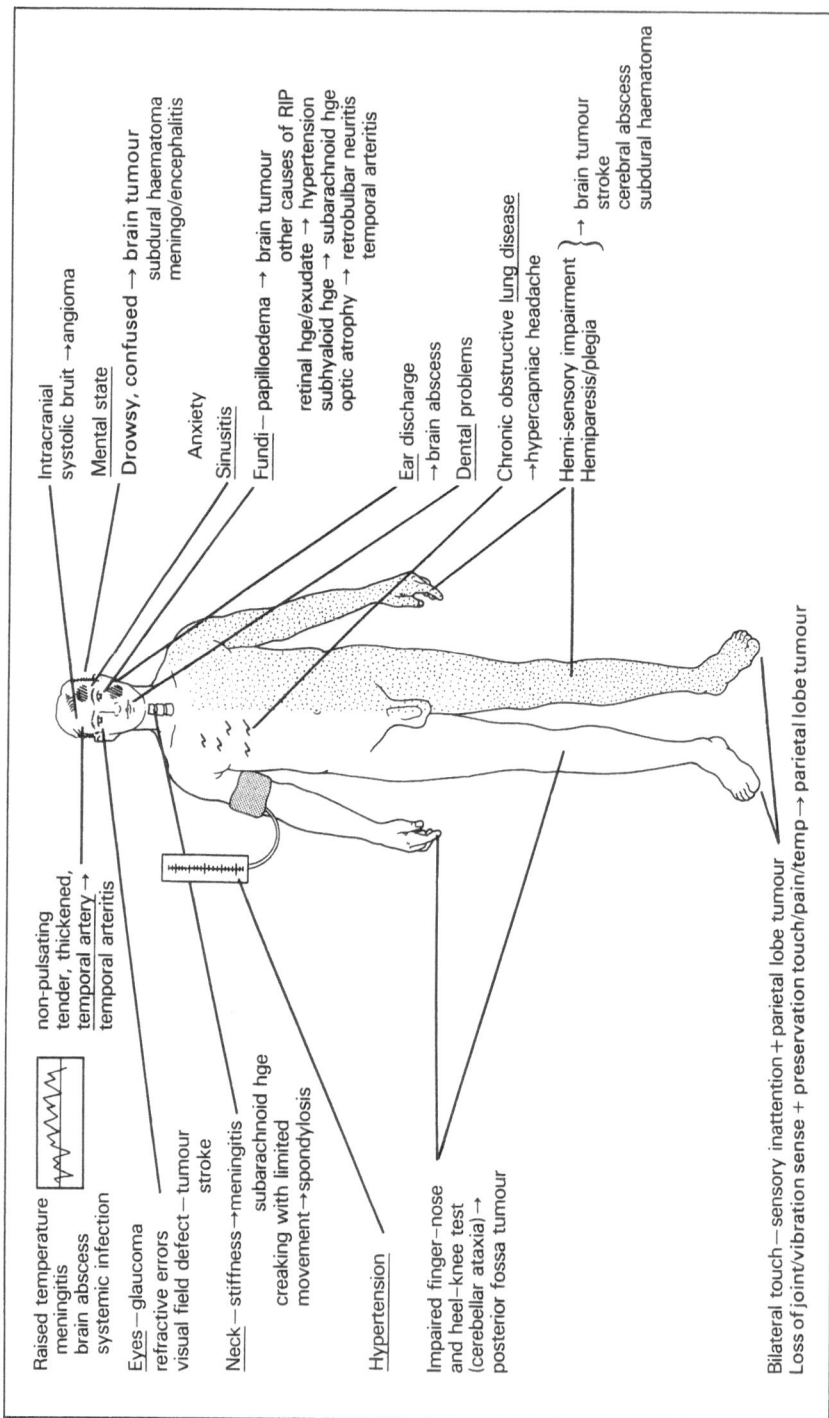

Fig. 12.2 *Possible examination findings in headache*

Intracranial
systolic bruit →angioma

Mental state

Drowsy, confused → brain tumour
                    subdural haematoma
                    meningo/encephalitis

Anxiety

Sinusitis

Fundi— papilloedema → brain tumour
       other causes of RIP
       retinal hge/exudate → hypertension
       subhyaloid hge → subarachnoid hge
       optic atrophy → retrobulbar neuritis
                       temporal arteritis

Ear discharge
→brain abscess

Dental problems

Chronic obstructive lung disease
→hypercapniac headache

Hemi-sensory impairment ⎫→ brain tumour
Hemiparesis/plegia   ⎭ stroke
                           cerebral abscess
                           subdural haematoma

Raised temperature   non-pulsating
meningitis   tender, thickened,
brain abscess   temporal artery →
systemic infection   temporal arteritis

Eyes — glaucoma
refractive errors
visual field defect — tumour
                      stroke

Neck — stiffness →meningitis
                  subarachnoid hge
       creaking with limited
       movement →spondylosis

Hypertension

Impaired finger–nose
and heel–knee test
(cerebellar ataxia) →
posterior fossa tumour

Bilateral touch — sensory inattention + parietal lobe tumour
Loss of joint/vibration sense + preservation touch/pain/temp → parietal lobe tumour

anaemia < 10 g%
- can cause headache

polycythaemia
- chronic obstructive lung disease
- cerebellar haemangioblastoma (rare)

Raised ESR
- temporal arteritis

Chest X-ray
- should be done in all cases of suspected brain tumour
- may show bronchial carcinoma – the commonest cause of brain tumour

Skull X-ray

may be helpful in
- brain tumours
- sinusitis
- malignant deposits in skull
- dental problems
- Paget's disease

possible findings in brain tumour

calcification →
- displacement of calcified pineal
- meningioma
- craniopharyngioma
- oligodendroglioma
- astrocytoma

enlarged vascular channels →
- meningioma
- angioma

increased bone density →
- meningioma

eroded sella turcica →
- pituitary tumour

eroded petrous temporal →
- acoustic neuroma

Lumbar puncture
- meningitis/encephalitis
- subarachnoid haemorrhage
- dangerous if raised intracranial pressure

Radioisotope scan (technetium-99) – can help in localization and vascularity of some tumours

vascular tumours	• meningioma
	• angioma
	• glioma
cerebral metastases	• multiple avascular defects

Electroencephalogram – very limited value in headache

Air encephalogram/ventriculogram

    painful and unpleasant test

    not for routine use in suspected brain tumour

    only of value if suspected sellar, parasellar or third ventricle tumours difficult to pick up on CT scan

CT scan

    most effective test to pick up brain tumour

    also valuable in detecting cerebrovascular episodes

indications	• recent headache in middle aged/elderly
	• progressive headache
	• nocturnal headache
	• consistently localized headache
	• associated fits
	• associated focal neurological defects
	• any suspicion of papilloedema

Specific conditions

Migraine	• F > M (for all types)
	• peaks 20–50 years
	• types
	classic migraine (neurological migraine)
	common migraine
	vertebro-basilar migraine
	hemiplegic migraine
	ophthalmoplegic migraine
	migrainous neuralgia (cluster headache)

Headache

- *classic migraine*

  3 components – neurological prodromata

  headache

  vomiting

  prodromata

    visual – scintillation

  fortification

  scotoma

  hemianopia

    sensory – paraesthesiae (unilateral)

  headache

    unilateral – varying side

    fronto-temporal or hemicranial

    severe throbbing

    1 h–several days

  vomiting $\rightarrow$ relief of headache
  trigger factors – see Fig. 12.3

- *common migraine*

  generalized throbbing headache

  no aura

  often at week-ends

  often pre-menstrual

- *vertebro-basilar migraine*

  prodromata from brain stem

    vertigo

    diplopia

    dysarthria

    ataxia

    bilateral paraesthesiae

    transient loss of consciousness

  headache often occipital

  frequent in adolescent girls

  family history common

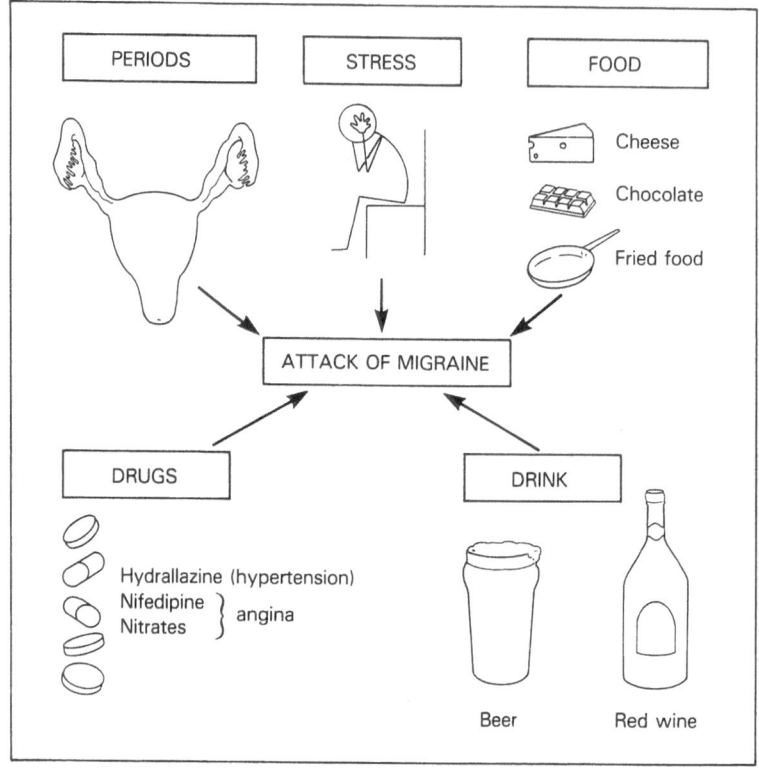

Fig. 12.3   *Trigger factors in migraine*

- *hemiplegic migraine*

    occurs in infants, children, adults

    attack of hemiplegia at onset of or during the headache

    may last several days

    frequently familial

    may account for inexplicable stroke in young adult

- *ophthalmoplegic migraine*

    children > adults

    headache periorbital

    weakness of eye movements

    consider possibility of aneurysm of posterior communicating artery

- *migrainous neuralgia (cluster headache)*

    boring, piercing pain

    in eye

    frontal area

    temple

    15 minutes–2 hours

    occurs nightly for 3–6 weeks (clusters)

    usually same time each night – 2–3 hours after falling asleep

    other features shown in Fig. 12.4

    occasional Horner's syndrome

    small pupil

    ptosis

    exophthalmos

    lack of sweating one side of face

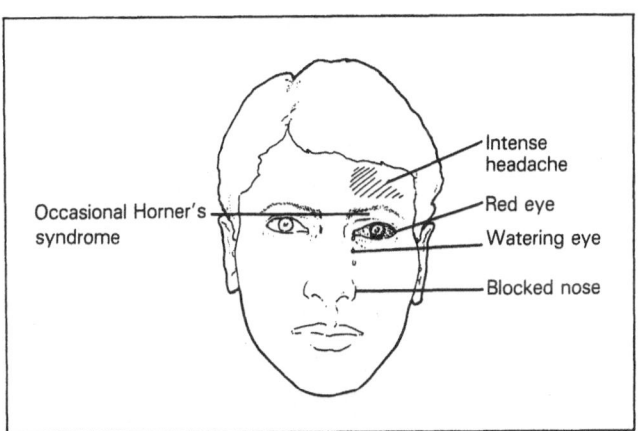

Fig. 12.4 *Migrainous neuralgia*

- investigation of migraine
    there is no need for tests in classical migraine
    indications for tests
    - always on *same* side
    - hemiplegic or ophthalmoplegic migraine
    - systolic murmur – orbital

                                                        temple

                                                        mastoid area
    tests
        arteriography best for
            angioma
            malformation arteriovenous
        isotope scan may show vascular tumour
        CT scan

Brain tumours

- incidence 5–10 per 100 000 population
- 2 peaks of incidence: children < 10 years
                                                40–60 years
- main types
    children
        medulloblastoma (posterior fossa)
        ependymoma (posterior fossa)
        cerebellar astrocytoma
        glioma of brain stem
    adults
        cerebral glioma
        cerebral metastases
        meningioma
        pituitary adenoma
- typical triad of symptoms
    headache
    vomiting
    fits

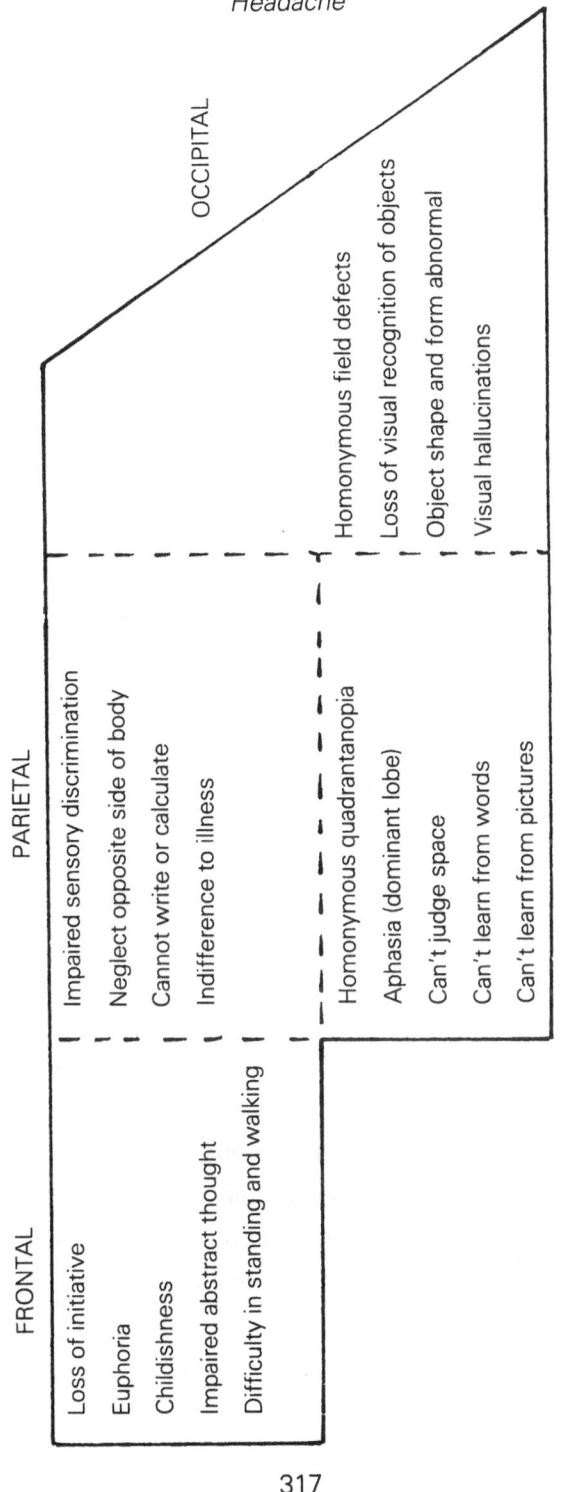

Figure 12.5 *Localization of brain tumours*

317

- localizing features – see Fig. 12.5
- examination

    papilloedema

    localizing features as in Fig. 12.5

- tests – see pages 309–12

    CT scan now supersedes all other tests in diagnostic value

    nuclear magnetic reasonance (NMR) in future may be better than CT scanning in diagnosing tumours

NB other causes of raised intracranial pressure:

- space occupying lesions

    abscess

    haematoma

- benign intracranial hypertension
- infections

    meningitis

    encephalitis

- subarachnoid haemorrhage

Temporal arteritis

- > 50 years – mean age 70 years
- more frequent in males
- the clinical features are shown in Fig. 12.6
- closely related to polymyalgia rheumatica – occurs in 50% of patients with temporal arteritis
- large arteries may be involved in 10–15% of cases
- tests

    ESR high > 50 mm/h

    temporal artery biopsy

        loss of internal elastic lamina

        giant cell infiltration

        chronic inflammatory cells

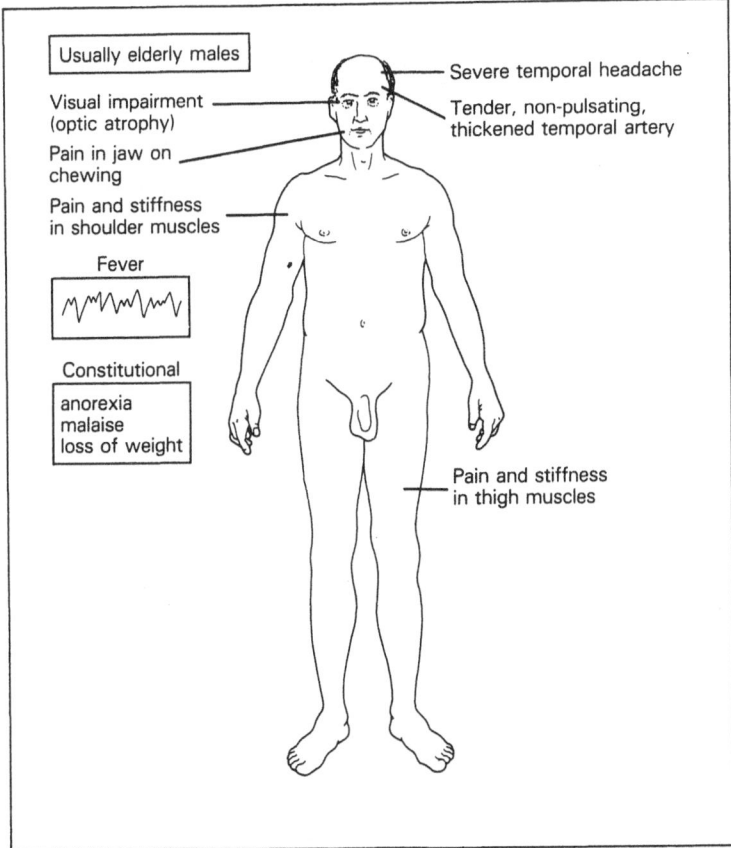

Fig. 12.6 *Features of temporal arteritis*

Tension headache	• commonest cause of headache
	• usually < 40 years old
	• bilateral – often at vertex
	may be frontal, temporal, occipital
	may be 'all over'
	• character – pressure
	weight
	tight band
	constant ache
	sharp stabbing pain
	other bizarre descriptions

319

- lasts for hours, days, weeks, months – continuous
- often related to emotional stress
- may be associated with fear of brain tumour
- associated features – anxiety

  depression

  giddiness

  insomnia
- may co-exist with migraine since emotional stress is a trigger factor for migraine also – main differentiation:

  rarely throbbing

  no prodromata

  no vomiting
- tests

  not necessary for diagnostic purposes

  skull X-ray may reassure the patient

Pitfalls in diagnosis

- It is easy to attribute a headache, wrongly, to tension or migraine when it is really the first symptom of a brain tumour.
- Headache in a hypertensive patient is often attributed to the raised blood pressure when it is really due to anxiety induced in the patient by being told he has high blood pressure
- Giving early antibiotics in a patient with fever and headache may mask an unsuspected meningitis and prevent its diagnosis.
- Subjecting a patient with headache and suspected brain tumour to a battery of expensive tests and ignoring a simple chest X-ray which might well give the diagnosis of bronchial carcinoma (with cerebral metastases).
- Paying too little attention to a relative's complaint of a personality change when assessing a patient with headache – it may well be the clue to a brain tumour.

Useful practical points

- Always suspect temporal arteritis in an elderly patient presenting with new headache – an ESR is a very useful diagnostic help.
- Migraine starting >40 years of age is unusual – it may well be symptomatic of underlying organic disease.
- If migraine always occurs on the same side of the head, consider an underlying angioma.
- Supraorbital headache with a red, watery eye, and possibly a blocked nose, indicates migrainous neuralgia (cluster headache).
- All new headache in middle age onwards should be regarded as due to a brain tumour until proved otherwise.
- If temporal arteritis is diagnosed it is essential to start steroid treatment immediately to prevent permanent loss of vision.
- The most valuable test in the diagnosis of a brain tumour is a CT scan – it supersedes all other tests.

Case challenge

A 27-year-old woman with a history of migraine since childhood presented with progressive headache over a period of 6 weeks. Her previous attacks of migraine were always heralded by fortification spectra followed by unilateral throbbing fronto-temporal headache (either side) and ending with vomiting. Her present exacerbation however was a generalized throbbing headache, which tended to wake her in the morning; she was still getting visual disturbances, transient blurring rather than fortifications; also, whereas vomiting previously relieved the pain, she found now that vomiting was not so effective and the headache persisted. Other neurological symptoms included recent giddiness, occasional double vision and transient numbness on one side of her face.

She had been taking an oestrogen pill for some years because of long-standing irregularity of her periods.

The examination findings are shown on Fig. 12.7.

Questions	Name four possible diagnoses.
	How would you distinguish between them?
Possible diagnoses	• migraine
	• brain tumour
	• hypertension
	• benign intracranial hypertension

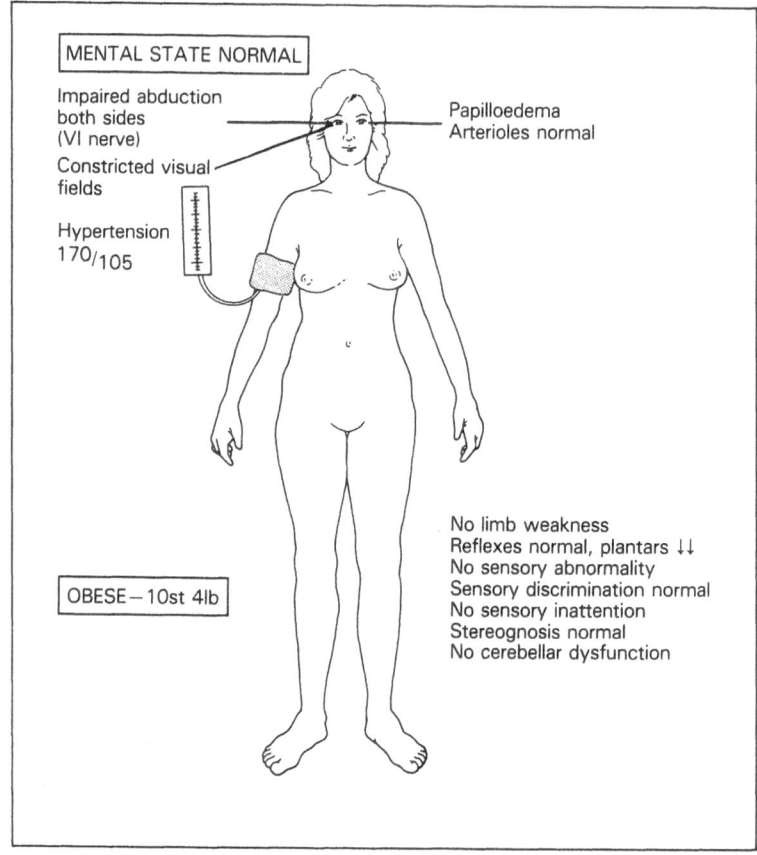

Fig. 12.7 *Examination findings in case challenge*

Migraine

For	history	• long history of migraine
		• throbbing headache
		• vomiting with headache
Against	history	• generalized, not unilateral, headache
		• transient blurring unusual in migraine
		• vomiting doesn't relieve headache
	exam	• papilloedema
		• bilateral weakness of abducens (VI) nerve
		• nystagmus

Headache

Tests		• no specific tests for migraine unless angioma or a-v malformation suspected

Brain tumour

For	history	• generalized throbbing headache
		• headache worse on waking
		• associated vomiting
		• transient blurring – suggests raised intracranial pressure
	exam	• papilloedema
		• peripheral field constriction results from papilloedema
Against	history	• no fits
		• otherwise no points against
	exam	• no focal neurological signs
		• bilateral abducens (VI) weakness is a non-specific manifestation of raised intracranial pressure
Tests		• CT scan best – supersedes all other tests
		• radio-isotope test may help if a CT scan is not possible

Hypertension

For	history	• throbbing headache
		• worse on waking
		• oestrogens can induce or aggravate hypertension (increased renin output)
	exam	• hypertension found
Against	history	• nil
	exam	• blood pressure not high enough to induce hypertensive headache
		• no arteriolar changes in fundus
Tests		• the only value of tests in this case is to show whether the hypertension has previously been severe enough to induce hypertensive headache
		• chest X-ray for cardiac enlargement
		• ECG for left ventricular strain pattern

Benign intracranial hypertension

For	history	• nature of the headache suggests raised intracranial pressure
		• the condition usually occurs in young females
		• contraceptive pill may predispose to the condition
		• menstrual irregularities are frequent in the condition
		• giddiness and diplopia may occur
	exam	• papilloedema confirms raised intracranial pressure
		• bilateral abducens (VI) nerve weakness also indicative of raised intracranial pressure
		• obesity is a feature of the condition
Against	history	• nil
	exam	• nil
Tests		• CT scan

the main value is in excluding other causes of raised intracranial pressure such as tumour

it may show: normal ventricle

small ventricle

• lumbar puncture is contraindicated because of the risk of coning

---

Actual diagnosis:

CT scan was quite normal; benign intracranial hypertension diagnosed as a diagnosis of exclusion

---

Treatment and outcome

She was treated with a thiazide diuretic and supplementary potassium and she improved within 4 weeks with almost complete disappearance of the headache. Other methods which may be tried include:

prednisolone 40–60 mg/day: dexamethasone 2–4 mg/day

oral glycerol 15–60 mg 4–6 times daily

acetazolamide 250 mg tds

theco-peritoneal shunt

13 Palpitations

Introduction

Frequent symptoms indicative of cardiac arrhythmia.

May signify little more than anxiety or may signify imminent death.

May have non-cardiac cause.

Wide range of causes and presentations with differing pathophysiological changes.

Basic causes lie in defects of the pacemaking mechanisms within the heart.

Satisfactory management requires exact diagnosis which in its turn requires confirmation by ECG or other investigations.

Types of arrhythmia causing palpitations

Sinus tachycardia

Atrial
- ectopic beats
- atrial tachycardia (also Wolff–Parkinson–White syndrome)
- atrial flutter
- atrial fibrillation

Ventricular
- ectopic beats
- ventricular tachycardia

Atrioventricular block (heart block)

Grades of severity

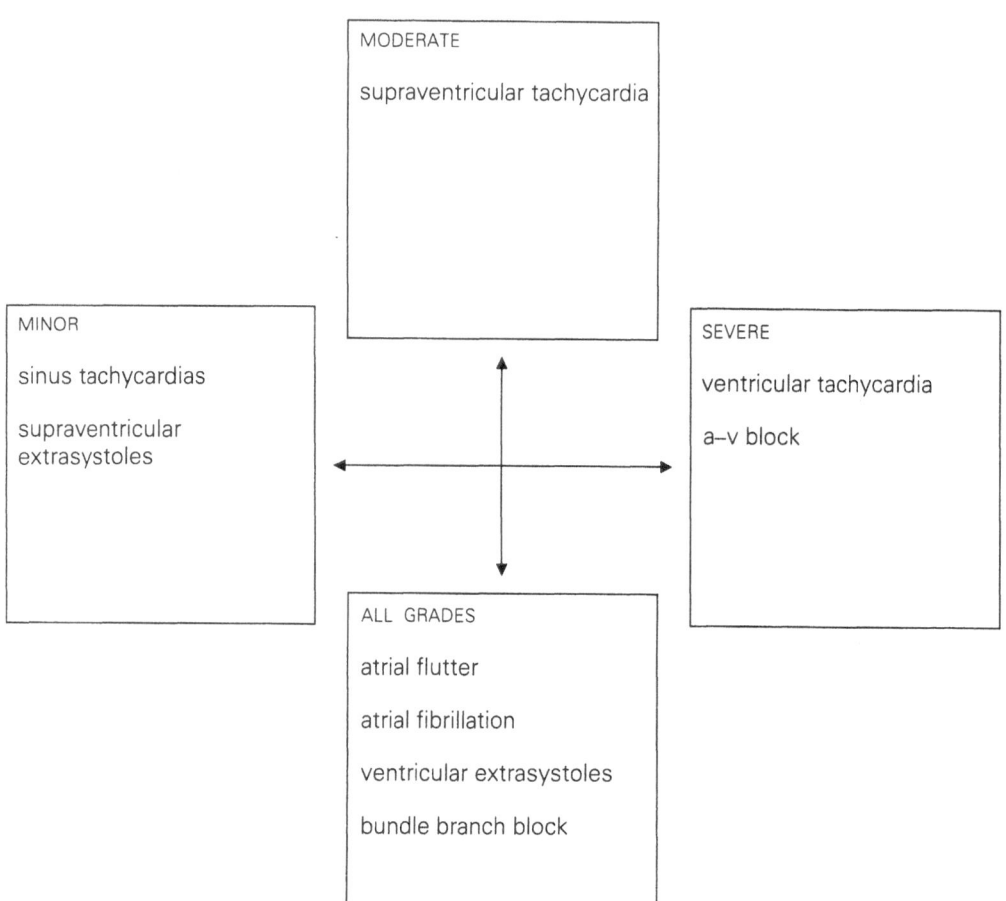

MODERATE

supraventricular tachycardia

MINOR

sinus tachycardias

supraventricular
extrasystoles

SEVERE

ventricular tachycardia

a–v block

ALL GRADES

atrial flutter

atrial fibrillation

ventricular extrasystoles

bundle branch block

Frequency

---

*Annual prevalence of cardiac arrhythmics
in a population of 2500*

Sinus tachycardia	20
Supraventricular extrasystoles	15
Supraventricular tachycardia	5
Atrial fibrillation	10
Atrial flutter	<1
Ventricular extrasystoles	10
Ventricular tachycardia	?
Sinus bradycardia	7
Heart block (AV and BBB)	5

Age incidence

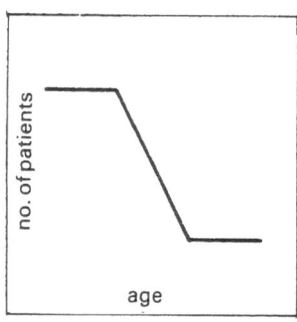

- sinus tachycardia (physiological)
- sinus bradycardia (physiological)
- Wolff–Parkinson–White syndrome

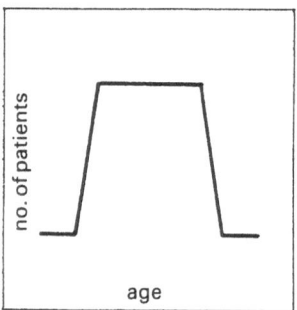

- thyroid disease
- alcoholism
- mitral stenosis
- IHD

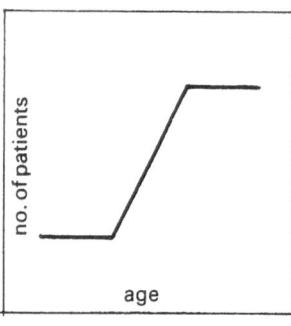

- high blood pressure
- myocardial infarction
- IHD
- iatrogenic (drug effects)
- heart block

Diagnostic approach

History

The diagnosis of the cause of the palpitations may often be made on the history of the attacks

First of all, it is important to decide whether the complaint of palpitations means

- rapid and/or irregular heartbeat
- normal rate but beats 'hard'
- slow, forceful

Relevant factors are
- rate
- rhythm
- onset of the attack
- duration of the attack
- precipitating factors
- relieving factors
- associated symptoms

Description of the attack

Rate – it is often helpful to ask the patient to tap out the palpitations either on their own chest or on the desk

$< 60 \rightarrow$
- sinus bradycardia
- complete heart block

60–90 forceful beat →
- anxiety
- anaemia
- thyrotoxicosis (usually faster)
- aortic regurgitation

90–140 →
- sinus tachycardia

150 →
- atrial flutter

$> 160 \rightarrow$
- supraventricular (atrial) tachycardia most likely
- atrial flutter/fibrillation
- ventricular tachycardia

Rhythm

    regular →
- sinus tachycardia
- atrial tachycardia
- atrial flutter
- ventricular tachycardia

    irregular → ectopic beats
- sudden thud
- missed beat
- skipped beat
- 'heart stopping'
- fleeting and repetitive

    chaotic 'all over the place' →
- atrial fibrillation

Onset

    sudden →
- paroxysmal atrial tachycardia – may end suddenly or gradually
- atrial flutter
- ventricular tachycardia

    gradual →
- atrial fibrillation

Duration

    few seconds only →
- ectopic beats

    minutes or hours →
- usually atrial tachycardia
- ventricular tachycardia – less common

    indefinite →
- atrial fibrillation

Precipitation

    emotion/stress →
- sinus tachycardia

    exercise →
- sinus tachycardia
- may be organic
  heart failure
  anaemia
  thyrotoxicosis

    smoking →
- ectopic beats
- atrial tachycardia

Relief

   exercise →   • ectopic beats

   vagal stimulation

      breathholding

      straining

      self-induced vomiting   } • paroxysmal atrial tachycardia

      eyeball pressure

      neck pressure

Associated symptoms

   dizziness →   • cerebrovascular disease

   syncope →   • severe brady/tachy-arrhythmia

                    • Stokes–Adams attack

                    • associated cerebrovascular disease

                    • associated aortic stenosis

   angina →   • ischaemic heart disease

                    • aortic stenosis

   left mammary pain →   • anxiety

                    • mitral valve prolapse

   breathlessness →   • anxiety state (hyperventilation)

                    • mitral stenosis

                    • heart failure

   lump in throat

   tingling in the fingers } → • anxiety

Other relevant symptoms   • angina

                    • thyrotoxicosis

                        weight loss

                        heat intolerance

                        excessive sweating

                        nervousness, tremors

                        neck swelling

                    • throbbing occipital headache worse on waking in the morning → hypertension

- myocarditis

    fever

    malaise

    breathlessness

    pericarditic pain

       anterior chest

       worse on inspiration

       better on sitting up

    may get preceding upper respiratory infection

Drugs
- digitalis
- diuretics → hypokalaemia
                 hypomagnesaemia
- caffeine – coffee, tea
- alcohol → cardiomyopathy
- sympathomimetic – beta-agonists (asthma)
- thyroxine (myxoedema)
- psychiatric

    trycyclic antidepressants

    mono-amine oxidase inhibitors

Past history
- rheumatic fever → rheumatic heart disease
- alcoholism → cardiomyopathy
- diphtheria (rare now) → myocarditis
- severe virus infection → myocarditis
- murmur since childhood → atrial septal defect

Family history
- hypertension
- coronary artery disease

Examination

The possible findings are shown in Fig. 13.1

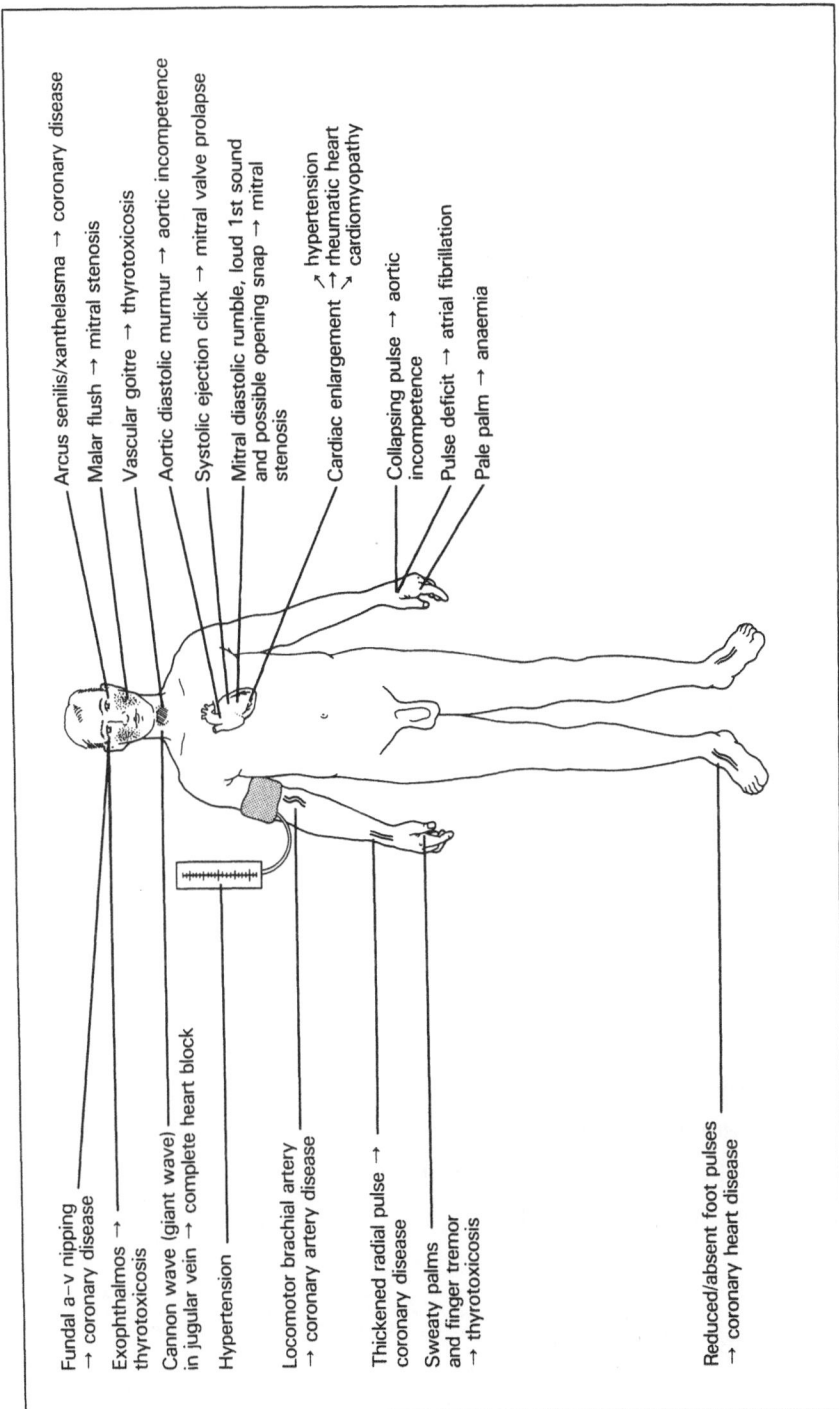

Arcus senilis/xanthelasma → coronary disease

Malar flush → mitral stenosis

Vascular goitre → thyrotoxicosis

Aortic diastolic murmur → aortic incompetence

Systolic ejection click → mitral valve prolapse

Mitral diastolic rumble, loud 1st sound and possible opening snap → mitral stenosis

Cardiac enlargement ↗ hypertension
→ rheumatic heart
↘ cardiomyopathy

Collapsing pulse → aortic incompetence

Pulse deficit → atrial fibrillation

Pale palm → anaemia

Fundal a–v nipping → coronary disease

Exophthalmos → thyrotoxicosis

Cannon wave (giant wave) in jugular vein → complete heart block

Hypertension

Locomotor brachial artery → coronary artery disease

Thickened radial pulse → coronary disease

Sweaty palms and finger tremor → thyrotoxicosis

Reduced/absent foot pulses → coronary heart disease

Fig. 13.1 *Possible signs in a patient with palpitations*

Carotid sinus massage

- produces vagal stimulation
- may help differentiation
- may stop an attack of paroxysmal atrial tachycardia
- no effect in ventricular tachycardia
- may help diagnosis of atrial flutter by temporarily increasing a-v block so that heart rate slows and the fast flutter P waves (300/min) are clearly seen

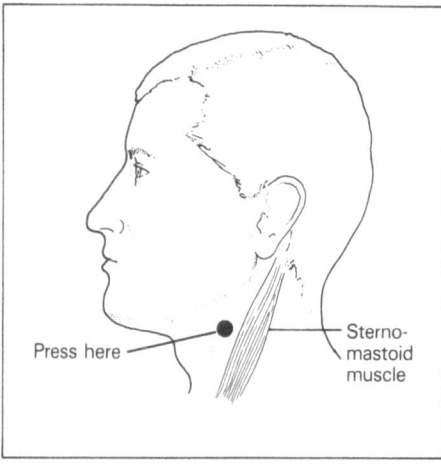

Press here — Sterno-mastoid muscle

Exercise can help

- irregularity disappears → ectopic beats
- irregularity worse → atrial fibrillation
- no increase in heart rate → heart block

Investigation

Electrocardiogram

   this is the most important test

   it is most helpful if recorded during an attack

   it may be normal between attacks

sinus tachycardia (Fig. 13.2a)	• heart rate 90–140/min • rhythm regular • normal P waves • normal QRST

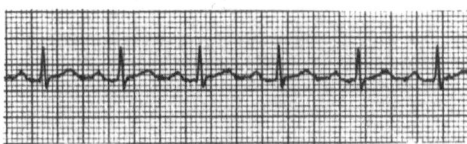

Fig. 13.2a *ECG showing sinus tachycardia with heart rate of 100/min*

atrial ectopic beats (Fig. 13.2b)	• premature beat • rhythm regular otherwise • P wave normal or abnormal depending on origin in atrium or a-v node • QRST normal

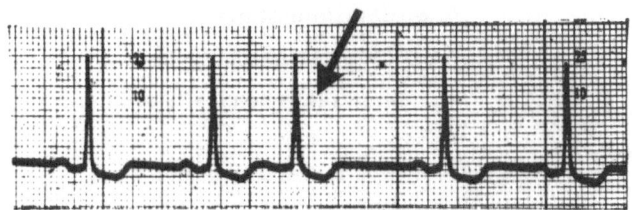

Fig. 13.2b *ECG showing supraventricular (atrial) ectopic beat (arrowed)*

atrial tachycardia (AT)
(Fig. 13.2c)
	• heart rate 140–220/min
	• rhythm regular
	• P usually abnormal
	    may be inverted
	    may follow QRS (nodal tachycardia)

- QRST often normal
- QRST may be bizarre due to inability of a-v node to conduct rapid beats '

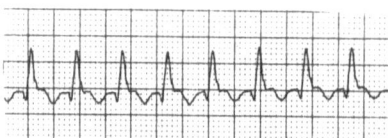

Fig. 13.2c   *ECG showing atrial tachycardia with heart rate of 150/min*

atrial flutter
(Fig. 13.2d)

- heart rate 100 or 150/min
- rhythm regular
- P wave usually upright and occurring at 100 or 150/min due to 3:1 or 2:1 a-v block which almost invariably accompanies atrial flutter
- QRS may be bizarre
- carotid sinus massage

    slows ventricular rate

    allows P to be clearly seen at 250–300/min

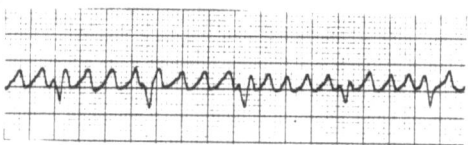

Fig. 13.2d   *ECG showing atrial flutter with varying atrio-ventricular block*

atrial fibrillation
(Fig. 13.2e)

- heart rate variable – may be 100–200/min or more
- rhythm totally irregular
- no P waves seen
- QRST usually normal unless distorted by underlying heart disease, e.g. ischaemia → BBB

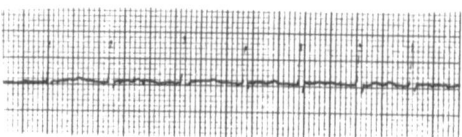

Fig. 13.2e   *ECG showing atrial fibrillation with rapid irregular heart rate (approximately 150/min) and no P waves*

ventricular ectopic beats
(Figs. 13.2f, 13.2g)

- heart rate normal except where altered by the ectopic beat
- rhythm basically regular unless multiple ectopic beats → irregular irregularity
- P wave absent
- QRS bizarre – widened, notched
- T always in opposite direction to QRS
- compensatory pause afterwards
- in acute myocardial infarction the dangerous ectopic beats are:

    frequent (> 1:10)

    multifocal

    occur in salvos

    R-on-T most hazardous because it may cause ventricular fibrillation

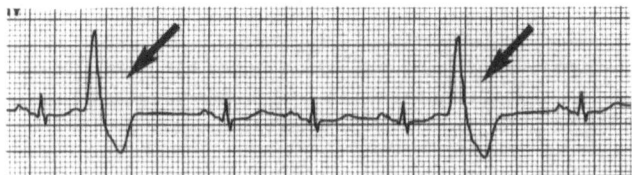

Fig. 13.2f *ECG showing ventricular ectopic beats (arrowed)*

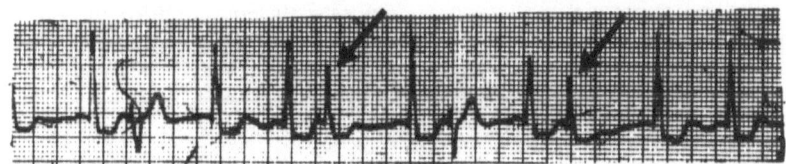

Fig. 13.2g *ECG showing R-on-T ventricular tachycardia (arrowed)*

ventricular tachycardia
(Fig. 13.2h)

- heart rate 140–220/min
- rhythm regular
- P waves not usually seen – if they are, they are unrelated to QRS complexes
- QRS broad and bizarre
- T in opposite direction to main QRS
- may be difficult to distinguish from atrial tachycardia with aberrant conduction

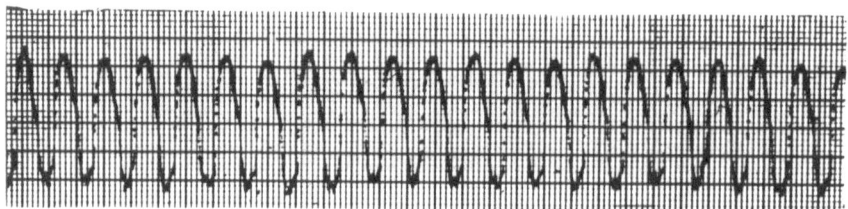

Fig. 13.2h   *ECG showing ventricular tachycardia*

AT with aberrant conduction	Ventricular tachycardia
absolutely regular	slightly irregular
first few beats may be normal QRS then they become aberrant	QRS may resemble previous ventricular ectopic beat
P waves (usually abnormal) may be seen with same frequency as QRS and precedes QRS	capture beats (normal QRS) or fusion beats (irregular QRS) diagnostic

atrioventricular block
(Fig. 13.3)

- heart rate slow
- rhythm regular
- P waves completely dissociated from QRS – normal atrial rate
- QRS bizarre and slow
- QRS may be normal rate and shape if pacemaker high in a-v bundle

340

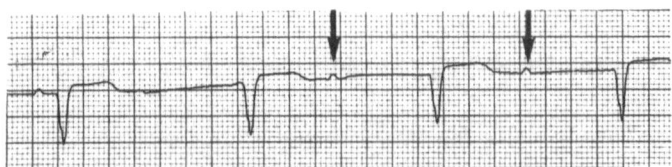

Fig. 13.3 *ECG showing complete heart block with complete dissociation of the P waves (arrowed) and the QRS*

Other investigations

His bundle electrocardiography

this is a technique of recording the ECG from inside the right atrium and right ventricle, using special electrode catheters

mainly used in the diagnosis of conduction disturbances but can also help in the differentiation of supraventricular and ventricular arrhythmias

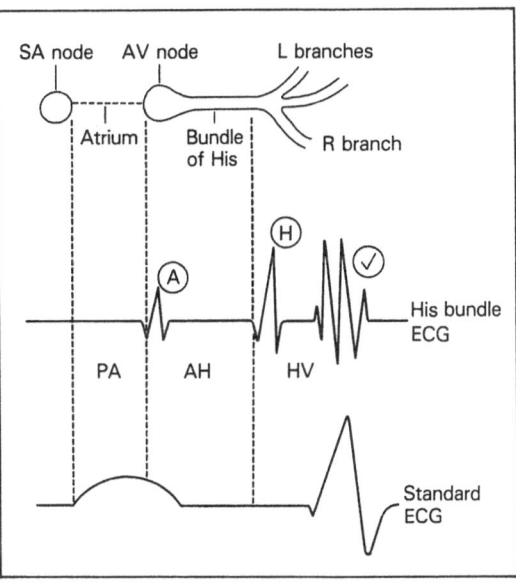

PA intra-atrial conduction time

AH nodal conduction time

HV intraventricular conduction time

341

24 hour ambulatory tape monitoring

this may be helpful in picking up a cardiac arrhythmia at the time of the attack of palpitations

facilities are available for the patient to record an event (attack) on to the tape recorder

indications
- document suspected rhythm disturbance
- correlate rhythm disturbance with symptoms
  palpitations
  syncope
  chest pain
  dyspnoea
- efficacy of anti-arrhythmic therapy
- pacemaker function
- recording ST–T changes in:
  Prinzmetal's angina
  atypical chest pain
- records 1000 times as many complexes as a routine ECG

chest X-ray
- of limited help in diagnosing the cause of palpitations
- may show a mitral contour (Figs. 13.4, 13.5)
- may show non-specific cardiac enlargement
  hypertension
  myocarditis
  cardiomyopathy
- may show overfilled lungs
  atrial septal defect

Blood tests
- thyroid function tests – thyrotoxicosis
- serum potassium – hypokalaemia
- serum magnesium – hypomagnesaemia
- liver function (especially gamma-GT) – alcoholism
- digitalis blood level – digitalis intoxication
- virus antibodies – myocarditis

342

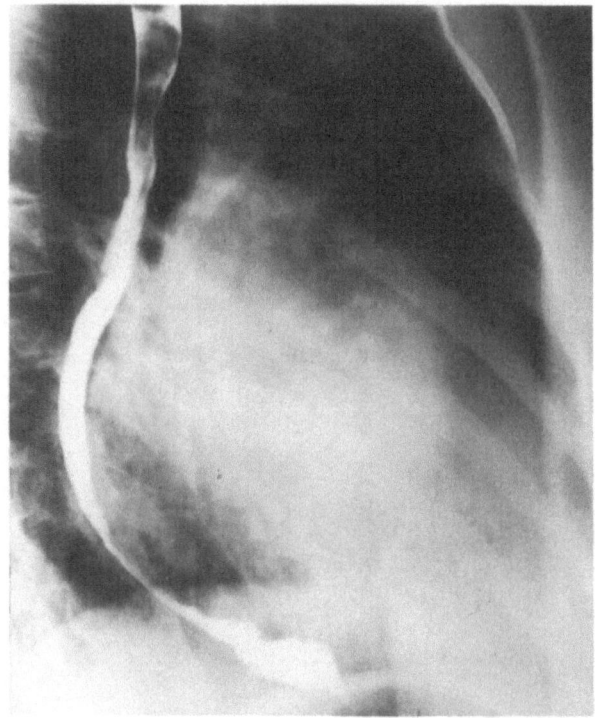

Fig. 13.4 *Right lateral chest X-ray with barium swallow showing marked dilatation of the left atrium in mitral stenosis displacing the oesophagus backwards*

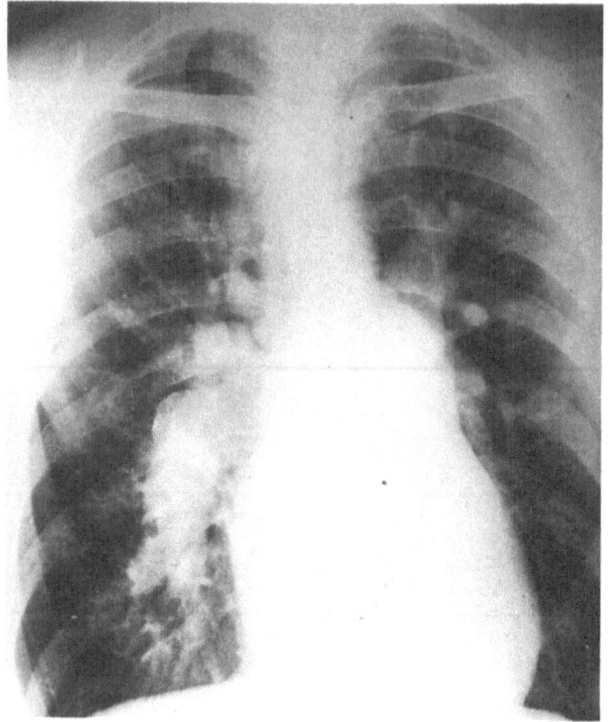

Fig. 13.5 *Chest X-ray showing grossly overfilled lungs and marked prominence of the pulmonary artery in atrial septal defect*

Specific conditions

Sinus tachycardia

- causes

    exercise

    emotional stress

    fever

    thyrotoxicosis

    early heart failure

    drugs

        nicotine (smoking)

        caffeine (coffee, tea)

        β-agonists, e.g. salbutamol

        xanthines, e.g. aminophylline

344

Palpitations

- heart rate 90–140/min
- examination
    may be no signs
    may be LVF
        dyspnoea
        gallop rhythm
        fine pulmonary crepitations
    thyrotoxicosis
        hot sweaty skin
        exophthalmos, other eye signs
        fine finger tremor
        systolic murmur in heart
        vascular goitre
- tests
    ECG
        rapid heart rate
        P–QRST normal
    chest X-ray – LV failure
        congestion upper lobe veins
        basal congestion
        hilar flare
        cardiac enlargement
    thyroid function test – thyrotoxicosis

Ectopic beats (atrial and ventricular)

- causes
    may be idiopathic
    ischaemic heart disease
    hypertensive heart disease
    drugs
        digitalis
        sympathomimetic
            β-agonists

345

xanthines

tricyclic antidepressants

smoking

cardiomyopathy/myocarditis

mitral valve prolapse

- significance

atrial – may herald other atrial arrhythmias:

tachycardia

flutter

fibrillation

ventricular – may herald other ventricular arrhythmias:

tachycardia

fibrillation

in myocardial infarction the myocardium is especially prone to serious ventricular arrhythmias and the types of ventricular ectopic beats which may herald these are:

frequent unifocal

multifocal

in salvos

R-on-T especially dangerous

- ECG (Fig. 13.6)

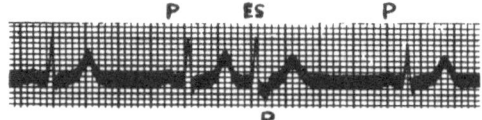

Fig. 13.6   *ECG showing nodal ectopic beats (ES)*

atrial ectopic

abnormal P wave

may precede or follow QRS or may be buried in QRS

QRS normal

ventricular ectopic

       bizarre ventricular complex

       T in opposite direction to main QRS

       no P wave

       compensatory pause

- exercise – may abolish ectopic beats

Atrial tachycardia

- causes

       ischaemic heart disease

       thyrotoxicosis

       digitalis intoxication especially with hypokalae-
       mia

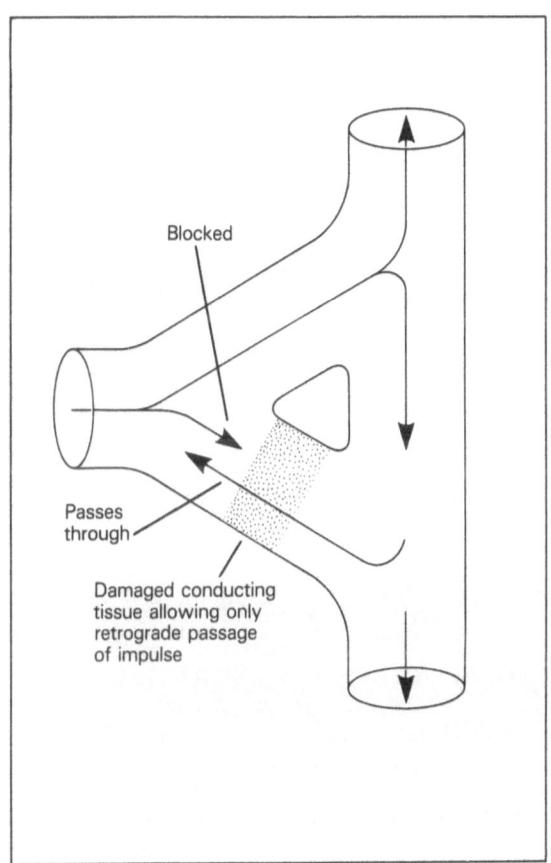

Mechanism of re-entrant tachycardia

- mechanism – usually a circus movement (re-entrant tachycardia) – caused by impairment of conduction through one path of a circuit allowing only retrograde passage of the impulse (see diagram) so setting up a circus movement with activation of the ventricle each time the impulse passes round the circuit.

- clinical

    abrupt onset

    rate 140–220/min

    rhythm regular

    duration – minutes to hours

- adverse effects

    increased ischaemia → angina

    breathlessness → LV failure

    dizziness/syncope – inadequate cerebral flow from reduced cardiac output

- ECG

    regular at 140–220/min

    P usually abnormal – depends on site of origin of tachycardia

    high atrial   – narrow pointed P – short P–R interval (Fig. 13.7)

    high a-v node – P buried in QRS

    low a-v node – inverted P after QRS

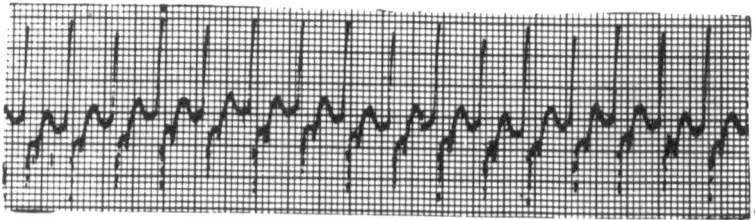

Fig. 13.7   *ECG showing atrial tachycardia originating in the a-v node (inverted P superimposed on S-T segment)*

- QRS

  usually normal with 1:1 response

  may show 2:1 response in digitalis intoxication

  may show bundle-branch block pattern – simulates ventricular tachycardia

Pre-excitation syndromes

- best known is Wolff–Parkinson–White syndrome
- due to presence of accessory a-v bundle (bundle of Kent) bypassing normal a-v nodal conduction – the accessory bundle conducts faster than normal a-v node
- in ¾ there is no associated organic heart disease though more likely in children (congenital or rheumatic heart disease)
- patients susceptible to recurrent attacks of re-entrant (circus) type of atrial tachycardia: less commonly paroxysmal atrial fibrillation will occur
- ECG (Fig. 13.8)

  type A – less common

  accessory path connects left atrium to left ventricle

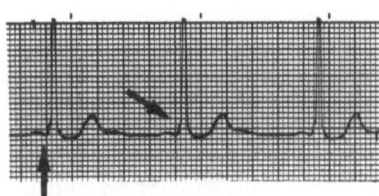

Fig. 13.8   *ECG in Wolff–Parkinson–White syndrome showing short P-R interval (arrowed) and a slurred delta wave (arrowed)*

  short P–R interval

  slurred upstroke of R in V1 (delta wave)

  type B – more common

  accessory path from right atrium to right ventricle

  short P–R

  slurred upstroke of R in V6

- if atrial fibrillation occurs digoxin is contraindicated as it accelerates a-v conduction through the accessory pathway

Atrial fibrillation

- causes

    ischaemic heart disease (in 15% of cases)

    rheumatic heart disease especially mitral stenosis

    thyrotoxicosis

    hypertensive heart disease

    idiopathic (lone fibrillation)

    young adults

        active rheumatic carditis

        atrial septal defect

        constrictive pericarditis (in 1/3)

- symptoms

    palpitations

    dizziness/syncope especially with aortic stenosis

    angina if associated coronary disease

    breathlessness due to heart failure

- signs

    completely irregular heart with pulse deficit

    first and second heart sounds vary in intensity

    apical diastolic rumble if due to mitral stenosis – the presystolic murmur due to atrial contraction is lost

    signs of thyrotoxicosis if this is the cause

    if ventricular rate slow

        elderly patient

        patient having digoxin

        aneurysmal left atrium

        'lone' atrial fibrillation

- ECG (see Fig. 13.2e)

    heart totally irregular

    rate 60–200/min

    pulse rate < apex rate (pulse deficit)

    no P waves seen

    fine fibrillatory waves may be seen

    QRST usually normal unless altered by associated disease or BBB

- complications

    emboli

    pulmonary – from R atrium

    systemic from L atrium

    brain

    limbs

    any organ

    may precipitate heart failure

Ventricular tachycardia

- very serious cardiac arrhythmia because:

    it may herald ventricular fibrillation

    it is associated with adverse haemodynamic results

    heart failure

    shock

    myocardial ischaemia

- causes

    ischaemic heart disease, especially acute myocardial infarction associated with ventricular aneurysm

    hypertensive heart disease

    cardiomyopathy/myocarditis

    drugs

    digitalis intoxication especially in the presence of hypokalaemia

    sympathomimetics

    tricyclic antidepressants

> > prolonged QT interval in ECG
> >
> > > congenital
> > >
> > > antiarrhythmic drugs

- clinical

  > heart rate 150–200, regular
  >
  > abrupt onset
  >
  > associated symptoms
  >
  > > angina
  > >
  > > breathlessness
  > >
  > > dizziness/syncope
  > >
  > > mental confusion

- ECG (see Fig. 13.2h)

  > looks regular but slightly irregular if checked carefully
  >
  > bizarre broadened QRS – resembles left bundle branch block most often
  >
  > P waves difficult to see but if seen have no relation to the ventricular complexes
  >
  > capture beats (normal QRS) may be seen
  >
  > fusion beats (tending to normal QRS) are also present

Atrioventricular block

- causes

  > ischaemic heart disease – especially acute myocardial infarction
  >
  > hypertensive heart disease
  >
  > digitalis intoxication
  >
  > myocarditis
  >
  > cardiomyopathy

- types

  first degree (Fig. 13.9a)

  prolonged P–R interval

  no symptoms/signs

  only diagnosable on ECG

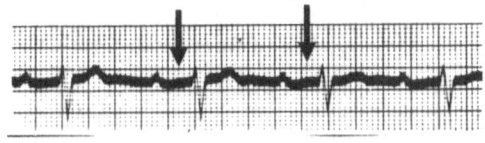

Fig. 13.9a *ECG showing first degree heart block (prolonged P-R interval)*

  second degree

  Wenckebach (Fig. 13.9b) – progressive lengthening of P-R interval ending with dropped beat and recovered P–R interval: benign

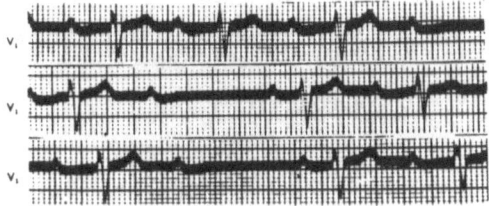

Fig. 13.9b *ECG showing Wenckebach phenomenon (progressive lengthening of P-R ending in dropped beat)*

  Möbitz (Fig. 13.9c)

  normal P–R

  dropped QRS

  may be 2 : 1 or 3 : 1

  may herald complete a-v block

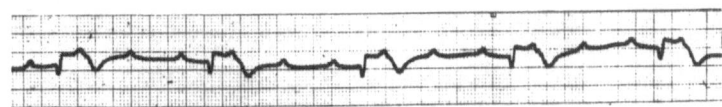

Fig. 13.9c *ECG showing Möbitz type of second degree heart block (normal P-R with dropped beats)*

complete a-v block

chronic or intermittent

if intermittent may lead to Stokes–Adams attack due to transient complete ventricular asystole

chronic heart block may lead to

excessive fatigue

dizziness

breathlessness

ECG

dissociation between P and QRS

P waves normal rate

QRS slow – 40/min

QRS bizarre

ventricular rate higher and QRS narrower if ventricular pacemaker is in bundle of His below the a-v block

● clinical diagnosis

slow pulse – usually 40/min

cannon (giant) waves seen over jugular veins as atrial and ventricular contractions coincide

may get systolic murmur due to increased stroke volume

Pitfalls in diagnosis

- It is easy to misdiagnose paroxysmal atrial tachycardia as due to an anxiety state.
- Thyrotoxicosis is often overlooked as a cause of atrial fibrillation especially in the elderly where clinical manifestations may be minimal ('masked' thyrotoxicosis).
- An attack of loss of consciousness, especially in the elderly, may easily be diagnosed as epilepsy due to cerebrovascular disease, and the possibility of a Stokes–Adams attack overlooked.
- It is easy to miss a cardiac arrhythmia as a cause of dizziness or syncope if a specific enquiry is not made for associated palpitations.
- If the heart rate is slow it is easy to miss atrial fibrillation – prolonged palpation of the pulse or auscultation of the heart sounds will help.

Useful practical points

- Paroxysmal atrial tachycardia is rarely the result of organic heart disease.
- The two commonest triggers of paroxysmal atrial tachycardia are cigarette smoking and anxiety.
- Passing profuse amounts of urine after an attack of palpitations indicates that the diagnosis is likely to be atrial tachycardia.
- Atrial ectopic beats may presage atrial fibrillation and ventricular ectopic beats, ventricular tachycardia or, more seriously, ventricular fibrillation, especially if they occur in the course of an acute myocardial infarction.
- A systolic ejection click on auscultation suggests mitral valve prolapse which may be a cause of a variety of arrhythmias, as well as atypical chest pain.
- Ectopic beats, atrial or ventricular, which are chronic are unlikely to cause any adverse complications and need not be treated.
- The only clue to a diagnosis of masked thyrotoxicosis in an elderly patient may be bright eyes (thyroid 'glitter') due to conjunctival oedema.

Case challenge

A 63-year-old female patient presented with a 4 month history of palpitations. She did not think that the palpitations occurred in specific attacks though sometimes she noticed them more than others, for example in bed at night when she would feel her heart thumping rapidly for prolonged periods until she fell asleep. She could not say whether the palpitations were regular or irregular. During the bad bouts she would feel a tightness in her chest going down the left arm, she would also feel breathless and often dizzy. She thought that the palpitations tended to get worse if she exerted herself. She thought she had lost a little weight recently but had not noticed any indigestion, bowel upset or change in appetite.

In the past history she had rheumatic fever as a child and had been told that her heart was affected but had no symptoms until a few months ago when the palpitations and breathlessness developed.

The findings on examination are shown in Fig. 13.10.

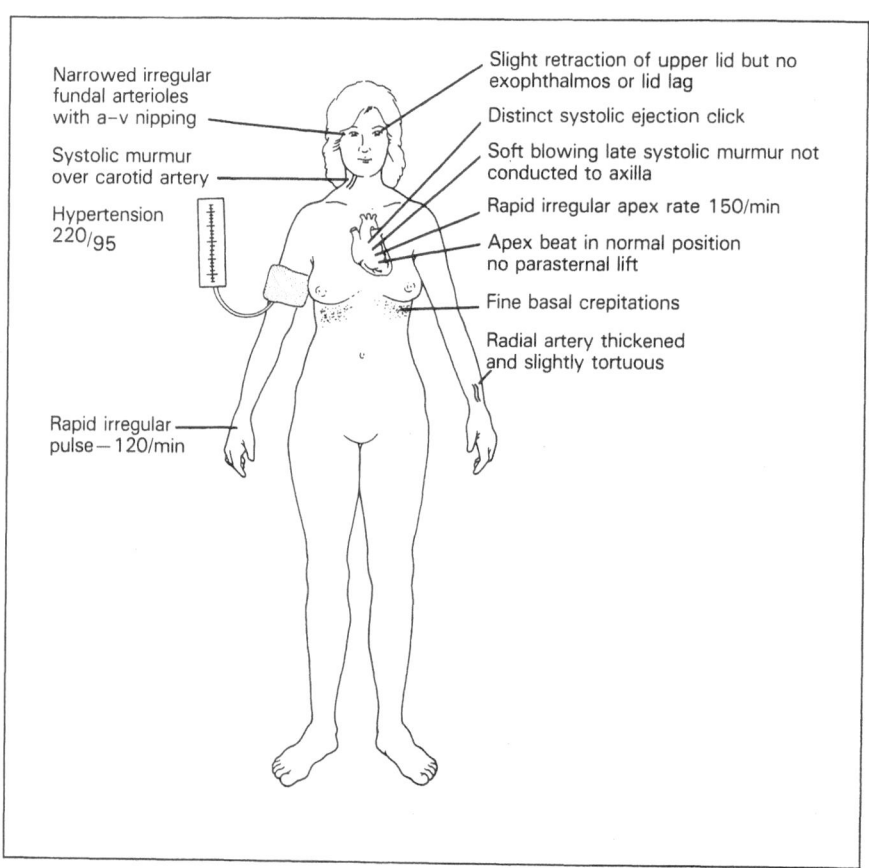

Narrowed irregular fundal arterioles with a-v nipping

Systolic murmur over carotid artery

Hypertension 220/95

Rapid irregular pulse — 120/min

Slight retraction of upper lid but no exophthalmos or lid lag

Distinct systolic ejection click

Soft blowing late systolic murmur not conducted to axilla

Rapid irregular apex rate 150/min

Apex beat in normal position no parasternal lift

Fine basal crepitations

Radial artery thickened and slightly tortuous

Fig. 13.10   *Examination findings in case challenge*

Questions

What is the cardiac arrhythmia?

Give four possible diagnoses

How would you distinguish between them?

Cardiac arrhythmia

● *atrial fibrillation* because

the heart is irregularly irregular

there is a well-marked pulse deficit

- *multiple ectopic beats* is another possibility but is much less common and is distinguished by periods of regular rhythm between the irregularities, i.e. it is a regular, as opposed to an irregular, irregularity.

Possible diagnoses

- rheumatic heart disease
- ischaemic heart disease
- mitral valve prolapse
- thyrotoxicosis

Rheumatic heart disease

For   history
- previous rheumatic fever
- told that her heart was affected

              exam
- systolic murmur which might represent mitral incompetence
- signs of basal pulmonary congestion which could be a complication of mitral valve disease

Against   history
- unusual for atrial fibrillation to develop for the first time as a result of rheumatic heart disease at this age

              exam
- there was no evidence of either left or right ventricular hypertrophy
- the systolic murmur did not have the characteristics of significant mitral regurgitation

    not pansystolic

    not conducted to axilla

- pure mitral incompetence is an uncommon manifestation of rheumatic heart disease
- no evidence of mitral stenosis which is much more likely to be associated with atrial fibrillation than mitral incompetence.

Tests
- ECG

    confirms atrial fibrillation

    shows left and/or right ventricular hypertrophy with mitral valve disease
- chest X-ray – may show a mitral contour
- echocardiogram – definitive test for mitral valve disease

Ischaemic heart disease

For	history	• the right age
		• gets angina at times
	exam	• evidence of atherosclerosis
		• fundal arteries affected
		• thickened radial artery
		• carotid atheroma with systolic murmur
		• hypertension → arterial disease
Against	history	• nil
	exam	• nil
Tests		• ECG – may show old ischaemic damage

- coronary arteriography – definitive test but there is no indication in this patient since the test carries a risk of morbidity and mortality, especially in an elderly patient

Mitral valve prolapse

- a comparatively recently recognized condition which may be associated with a variety of complications

    arrhythmias

    chest pain – non-anginal

    emboli

    infective endocarditis

Palpitations

For	history	• palpitations
	exam	• systolic ejection click
		• late systolic murmur
Against		• the arrhythmias associated with mitral valve prolapse are usually benign – atrial fibrillation is unusual as a complication
Tests		• echocardiography is very helpful in showing prolapse, usually affecting the posteror leaflet of the mitral valve
		• angiocardiography is the definitive test

Thyrotoxicosis

For	history	• weight loss with normal appetite
	exam	• lid retraction
Against		• no other symptoms or signs of thyrotoxicosis but could be 'masked'
Tests		• thyroid function

Actual diagnosis:

Thyrotoxicosis – shown by an increased serum thyroxine (T4) level in the thyroid function test.

Treatment

She declined an 18/12 course of antithyroid tablets so was treated with radioactive iodine: the atrial fibrillation persisted after she became euthyroid and was controlled by digoxin.

14 Dizziness, Giddiness, Vertigo

Introduction

Dizziness, giddiness and vertigo are subjective sensations capable of differing interpretations by sufferers.

It is up to the physician to try and translate vague feelings into a diagnosis following discriminating assessment

Generally benign but within the spectrum of possible causes there are some possible serious diseases.

Definitions

- dizziness

  light-headedness

  faintness

- giddiness

  unsteadiness

  loss of balance

- vertigo

  patient spins

  surroundings spin

  feeling of impulsion – being pulled to the ground or to the side

- a faint (vasovagal attack)

  sensation of impending loss of consciousness

  associated sweating, nausea

  dimness of vision

  rapid recovery on lying down

Causes of dizziness

General medical

cardiovascular

    cardiac
- arrhythmias
- Stokes–Adams attack
- aortic/pulmonary stenosis

    vasomotor
- vasovagal attack
- prolonged standing
- postural hypotension
  - drugs
  - old age

    respiratory
- cough epilepsy
- involuntary Valsalva manoeuvre
  - micturition
  - weight lifting
  - trumpeting

    metabolic
- hypoglycaemia
  - spontaneous
  - insulin therapy
  - insulinoma
- hyperventilation–anxiety state

    haematological
- anaemia
- polycythaemia
  - rubra vera
  - secondary
    - chronic lung disease
    - congenital cyanotic heart disease

Neurological
- epilepsy
- basilar migraine
- vertebro-basilar insufficiency
- multiple sclerosis
- posterior fossa tumours
- acoustic neuroma

Dizziness

- autonomic neuropathy
    diabetes
    peripheral neuropathy
      alcohol
      porphyria
      Guillain–Barré
      amyloidosis
- Shy–Drager syndrome

Otological

- Ménière's disease
- vestibular neuronitis
- infection middle/inner ear
- otosclerosis
- Paget's disease
- benign positional vertigo
- drugs
    salicylates
    phenytoin
    quinine
    streptomycin
    gentamicin

Psychiatric

- anxiety/depression

Grades of severity

MODERATE

benign positional vertigo

vestibular neuronitis

acute otitis media

hypoglycaemia

multiple sclerosis

epilepsy

cervical spondylosis

polycythaemia

MINOR

anxiety neurosis

motion sickness

ear wax

barotrauma

faint (vasovagal attack)

cough syncope

hyperventilation

vertigo in children

SEVERE

acoustic neuroma

labyrinthitis
(chronic suppurative otitis
media)

brain tumours (1° and 2°)

other causes of raised ICP

ALL GRADES

Ménière's syndrome

head injury
('compensation neurosis')

high blood pressure

cardiac arrhythmias

cerebrovascular accidents

vertebro-basilar occlusion

intoxications (aspirin,
salicylates, streptomycin,
gentamicin, quinine,
phenytoin, antihypertensives)

Age incidence

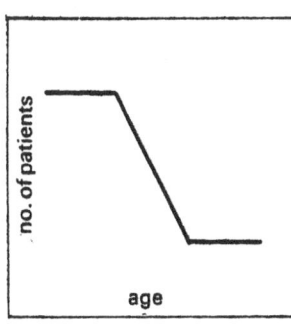

- acute otitis media
- migraine
- epilepsy (petit mal)
- brain tumour

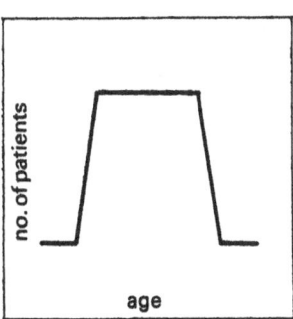

- benign positional vertigo
- vestibular neuronitis
- anxiety neurosis
- ear wax
- migraine
- auditory neuroma
- Ménières

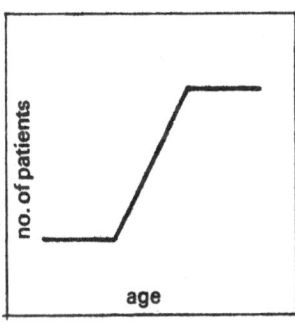

- cerebrovascular disease
- high blood pressure
- cervical spondylosis
- brain tumours (1° and 2°)

Frequency

Annual prevalence in a population of 2500	
Minor dizziness–giddiness	25
Benign positional vertigo and vestibular neuronitis	7
Ménière's syndrome	1
Cerebrovascular	1 every 2 years
Chronic otitis media (labyrinthitis)	1 every 5–10 years
Acoustic neuroma	1 every 25 years
Others	< 1

Diagnostic approach

History

Define precise nature of the complaint

- dizziness – light-headed
- giddiness – loss of balance
- vertigo

    spinning of self/surroundings

    impulsion to one side or to floor

    other helps in identifying vertigo

        can't walk during an attack

        tendency to incline towards one side

        worse during travel in a car/bus

        improves if head in a special position

- impending faint
- other vague feelings

    swaying

    swimming sensation

    walking on air

    queer feelings in the head

    (these symptoms are usually due to anxiety)

Onset

an acute onset of *true vertigo* may be due to:

young patient (< 40 y)   • vestibular neuronitis

older patient (> 40 y)   • vascular lesion

        vertebral artery

        basilar artery

        posterior inferior cerebellar artery

        labyrinthine artery

        Ménière's disease

an acute onset of *non-vertiginous dizziness* may be due to:

- cardiac arrhythmia, e.g. paroxysmal tachycardia
- Stokes–Adams attack
- vasovagal attack
- involuntary Valsalva
  - micturition
  - weight lifting
  - playing of trumpet
- epilepsy especially temporal lobe
- hypoglycaemia
- hyperventilation due to anxiety

Single attack or recurrent attacks of vertigo/dizziness

single episode

labyrinthine lesion
- vestibular neuronitis
- sudden vascular destruction

vascular lesion affecting the brain stem

recurrent episodes
- Ménière's disease
- benign positional vertigo
- chronic otitis media
- vertebro-basilar ischaemia
- epilepsy
- migraine
- multiple sclerosis
- paroxysmal cardiac arrhythmias
- anaemia
- hypotensive drugs especially in the elderly

chronic unremitting
- acoustic neuroma
- cerebello-pontine angle tumour

Dizziness

- drugs

    streptomycin

    gentamicin

    salicylates

    phenytoin

    quinine, e.g. for leg cramps

Aggravating factors

head position, e.g. lying
down →   • benign positional vertigo

movement head/neck →   • vertebro-basilar ischaemia

straining, e.g. micturition,
weight lifting, trumpet
playing →   • syncopal attack

coughing – 'cough
epilepsy' →   • syncopal attack

standing up →   • postural hypotension

     hypotensive drugs

     autonomic neuropathy, e.g. diabetes

     elderly arteriosclerotic

emotional crisis →   • hyperventilation

vigorous use of an arm →   • subclavian steal syndrome associated with vertebro-basilar ischaemia

Associated symptoms

sweating, vomiting →   • labyrinthine lesion (not brain stem)

deafness and tinnitus →   • labyrinthine lesion

     • acoustic neuroma

ear discharge →   • chronic otitis media

persistent inco-
ordination →   • brain stem lesion

     • cerebellar lesion

taste/smell hallucination
sinking feeling in
epigastrium   } → • temporal lobe epilepsy

palpitations →   • cardiac arrhythmia

angina/claudication →
- vertebro-basilar ischaemia
- cardiac arrhythmia

thumping headache ⎫
fortification spectra ⎭ →
- migraine

tingling in extremities ⎫
left mammary pain ⎬ →
lump in throat ⎭
- anxiety state

cough ± haemoptysis →
- brain metastases from cancer lung

hot flushes →
- menopausal women

glove/stocking numbness → • peripheral neuropathy with autonomic involvement

thirst, polyuria, loss of
weight →
- diabetes with autonomic neuropathy

sweating, malaise,
myalgia →
- virus infection leading to vestibular neuronitis

breathlessness ⎫
excessive fatigue ⎬ →
ankle swelling ⎭
- anaemia

double vision/speech
difficulty →
- brain stem ischaemia

Past history

Relevant factors of diagnostic help include:

ear disease in childhood → • chronic otitis media

alcoholism →
- Wernicke's encephalopathy
  vertigo
  ataxia
  nystagmus

head injury →
- may lead to non-specific dizziness for weeks, months or years especially if compensation involved

epileptic fits

psychiatric problems →
- especially anxiety/depression

menopause →
- dizziness common at this time

Family history
- migraine
- epilepsy

Drug history – a variety of drugs may cause dizziness or vertigo
- hypotensives especially in the elderly
- antibiotics
    streptomycin
    gentamicin
- salicylates
- quinine/quinidine
- tranquillizers
- antihistamines
- diuretics – if excessive volume depletion especially in the elderly

Examination

examination must be directed especially towards
- ear disease
- eye movements for nystagmus
- cranial nerves
- disturbance of cerebellum or its connections
- cardiovascular system for atherosclerosis

possible findings are shown in Fig. 14.1

nystagmus is a very helpful diagnostic sign
- labyrinthine
    conjugate
    horizontal or rotatory
    increases on looking away from lesion
- cerebellar
    wider amplitude
    increases looking towards lesion
    horizontal only

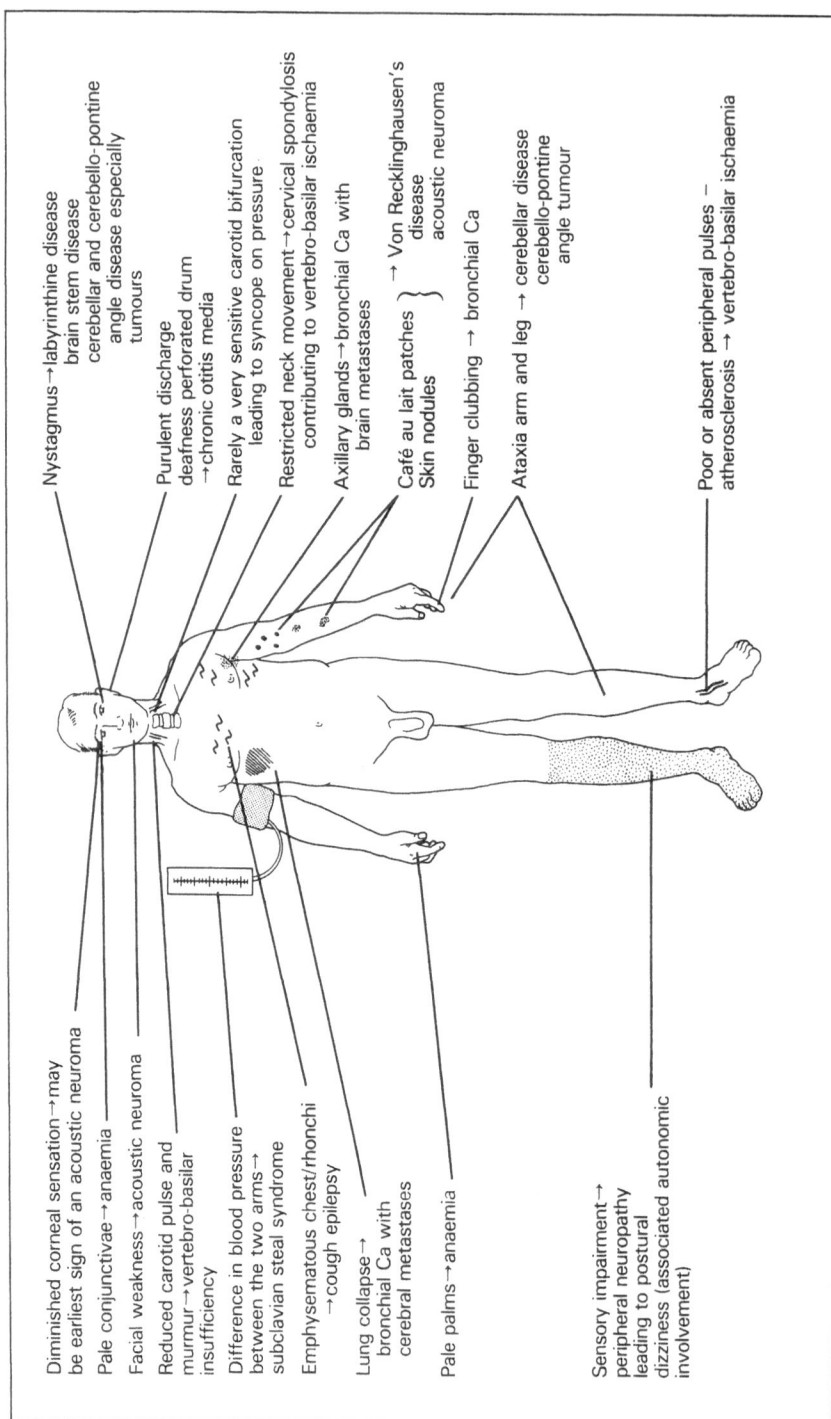

Nystagmus→labyrinthine disease
brain stem disease
cerebellar and cerebello-pontine
angle disease especially
tumours

Purulent discharge
deafness perforated drum
→chronic otitis media

Rarely a very sensitive carotid bifurcation
leading to syncope on pressure

Restricted neck movement→cervical spondylosis
contributing to vertebro-basilar ischaemia

Axillary glands→bronchial Ca with
brain metastases

Café au lait patches ⎱ → Von Recklinghausen's
Skin nodules   ⎰   disease
                         acoustic neuroma

Finger clubbing → bronchial Ca

Ataxia arm and leg → cerebellar disease
cerebello-pontine
angle tumour

Poor or absent peripheral pulses –
atherosclerosis → vertebro-basilar ischaemia

Diminished corneal sensation→may
be earliest sign of an acoustic neuroma

Pale conjunctivae→anaemia

Facial weakness →acoustic neuroma

Reduced carotid pulse and
murmur→vertebro-basilar
insufficiency

Difference in blood pressure
between the two arms→
subclavian steal syndrome

Emphysematous chest/rhonchi
→cough epilepsy

Lung collapse →
bronchial Ca with
cerebral metastases

Pale palms→anaemia

Sensory impairment→
peripheral neuropathy
leading to postural
dizziness (associated autonomic
involvement)

Fig. 14.1   *Possible findings in a patient with dizziness/vertigo*

- brain stem

  horizontal or vertical

  may be ataxic

  increased in abducting eye

  almost pathognomonic of multiple sclerosis

- local eye disease

  pendular

  symmetrical horizontal oscillation on either side of the mid-line

ear examination

- purulent discharge
- filled with wax
- perforated drum
- loss of hearing
- Weber and Rinné tests

	Weber	Rinné
middle ear disease	better affected side	bone > air
inner ear (labyrinthine) disease	better on normal side	air > bone but both reduced

Investigations

Audiometry

- helps to differentiate cochlear from eighth nerve lesions
- loudness recruitment (affected ear gains in loudness as the loudness of the stimulus increases) indicates cochlear disease, e.g. Ménière's disease
- reduction in speech discrimination indicates an eighth nerve lesion
- pure tone decay indicates an eighth nerve lesion

Caloric testing

- irrigation of ear canal with cold and warm water
- a normal ear reacts with nystagmus
- if vestibular disease is present nystagmus is reduced

Electronystagmography	• gives record of eye movements on paper
	• can help to distinguish central (brain stem or cerebellar) lesion from peripheral (labyrinthine) lesion
Lumbar puncture	• multiple sclerosis
	mild lymphocytosis (10–15/mm^3)
	mild protein increase (40–80 mg%)
	increase in γ globulin
	paretic Lange curve
	• acoustic neuroma – increased protein ($>$ 100 mg%)
Radiology	• chest X-ray – for bronchial carcinoma
	• cervical spine X-ray
	cervical spondylosis
	calcified carotid arteries
	• skull X-ray – petrous temporal bone and internal auditory meatus for erosion due to acoustic neuroma
	• CT scan for posterior fossa tumours
Electroencephalogram	• for epilepsy
Blood tests	• blood count – Hb – for anaemia
	• WBC
	for leukaemia
	leucocytosis – ear infection
	• raised ESR in neoplasia
	• blood sugar for hypoglycaemia

Specific conditions

Vestibular neuronitis

- characterized by single attack of vertigo without associated tinnitus and deafness
- mainly young adults – no sex difference
- sometimes occurs in small local epidemics
- preceding upper respiratory tract infection common
- abrupt onset with vertigo, nausea, vomiting
- usually lasts several days but may go on for weeks
- examination

    nystagmus – quick component away from side of lesion

    no hearing loss
- tests – caloric stimulation confirms impaired vestibular function

Benign positional vertigo

- at all ages
- episodic attacks of vertigo with certain positions of the head

    lying down in bed

    tilting the head backwards

    changing from recumbent to a sitting position
- recurs periodically for several days or for many months with no other symptoms
- examination

    vertigo produced by lying patient down with head back and tilted to the side

    latent period of a few seconds before vertigo

    accompanying nystagmus

    rotatory

    horizontal

    mixed

    slow phase towards dependent ear

    response 'fatigues' – absent after 3 or 4 consecutive tests
- cause unknown

Ménière's disease

- attacks most frequent between 40 and 50 years – no sex difference
- characterized by

  paroxysmal attacks of vertigo and tinnitus

  progressive deafness
- dilatation of endolymphatic system – cause unknown
- abrupt onset – patient may fall
- associated symptoms

  nausea and vomiting

  sweating
- attack lasts minutes to hours
- examination

  nerve deafness

  Weber→good ear

  Rinne – air > bone but both reduced

  rotatory nystagmus in an attack
- tests

  caloric – impaired vestibular function

  audiometry

  impaired hearing

  loudness recruitment

Acoustic neruoma

- may occur as

  an isolated lesion

  part of Von Recklinghausen's disease – might be bilateral
- adult men and women – no sex difference

- symptoms

    early

    progressive deafness

    tinnitus

    vertigo

    later

    paraesthesiae in one side of the face

    twitching of one side of the face

    inco-ordination of homolateral arm and leg

    post-auricular or suboccipital pain

    end stage

    severe headache and vomiting associated
    with raised intracranial pressure

    dementia

- signs – the possible findings are shown in Fig. 14.2
- tests

    audiometry – shows nerve lesion

    CSF analysis – high protein (up to 300 mg%)

    X-ray skull – widened internal auditory meatus

    CT scan – best test to show tumour

Pitfalls in diagnosis

- Diagnosing vertebro-basilar ischaemia on the basis of X-ray changes of cervical spondylosis; these are frequently present in asymptomatic middle-aged and elderly subjects.
- Forgetting about cardiac arrhythmias as a cause of dizzy attacks.
- Forgetting to consider anticonvulsant drugs such as phenytoin as a cause of dizziness in an epileptic patient.
- If the clinical picture suggests a brain tumour in a patient with progressive vertigo it is easy to forget that the commonest brain tumour is a metastatic deposit from carcinoma of the lung.
- Omitting to look into the ears in a dizzy patient with deafness – the cause may be nothing more complicated than obstruction with wax.

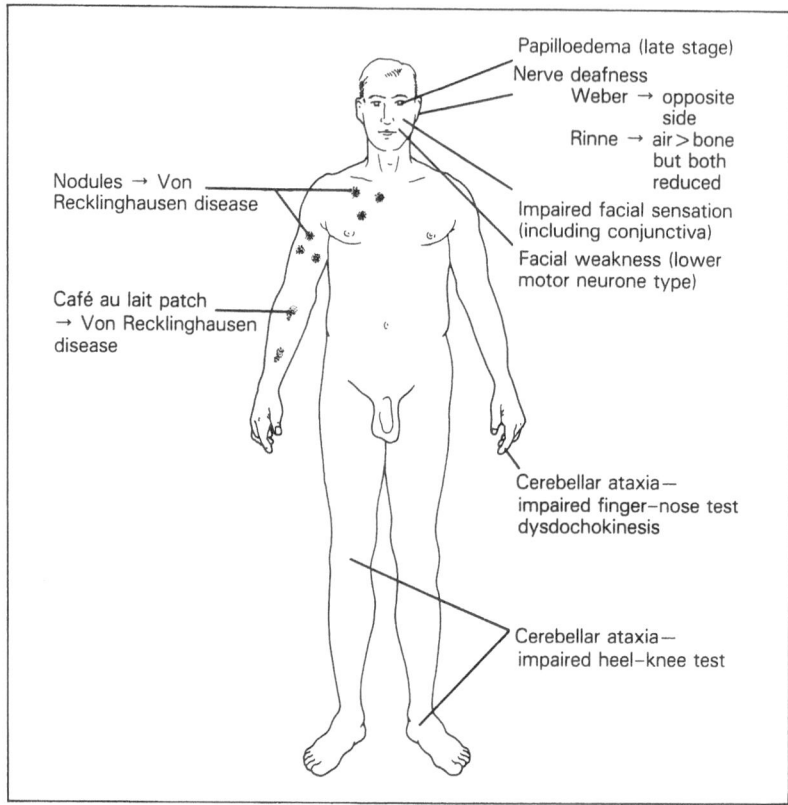

Papilloedema (late stage)

Nerve deafness
Weber → opposite
side
Rinne → air > bone
but both
reduced

Nodules → Von
Recklinghausen disease

Impaired facial sensation
(including conjunctiva)

Facial weakness (lower
motor neurone type)

Café au lait patch
→ Von Recklinghausen
disease

Cerebellar ataxia—
impaired finger–nose test
dysdochokinesis

Cerebellar ataxia—
impaired heel–knee test

Fig. 14.2   *Possible findings in acoustic neuroma*

Useful practical points

- Always ask about any palpitations associated with an attack of dizziness – the cause could be a cardiac arrhythmia.

- Don't forget about chronic otitis media as a cause of vertigo – a past history of recurrent ear infections in childhood is a helpful pointer.

- The first diagnostic step in a patient with true vertigo is to decide whether the lesion is in the ear, in the eighth nerve or in the brain stem; tinnitus and deafness associated with the vertigo indicates labyrinthine or nerve disease while focal neurological signs such as dysphagia, diplopia and dysarthria indicate the brain stem.

- Recurrent attacks of vertigo severe enough to cause the patient to fall are most likely to be due to Ménière's disease.

- Vertical nystagmus indicates central disease – it never occurs in a peripheral labyrinthine disorder.

Case challenge

A 63-year-old lady presented with a two-year history of recurrent attacks of dizziness which were getting progressively worse. She had noticed two kinds of dizziness; one type occurred when she got out of bed in the morning or turned her head rapidly – she described this as a feeling of light-headedness or faintness, and the second type which would occur any time and in which the room seemed to spin and was associated with ringing in her left ear, and in the more severe attacks, sweating and nausea or vomiting – this attack would last for about an hour at a time.

On direct enquiry other symptoms included occipital headache and creaking in her neck on movement of the head. She also thought her left hand was getting rather clumsy but found this a bit difficult to assess since she had a mild stroke affecting her left side 3 years previously which had left her slightly disabled – this had been attributed to hypertension from which she had suffered for 10 years and for which she was taking tablets.

Finally, in the past history she had a lot of ear trouble affecting both sides when she was a child and had a mastoidectomy carried out on the left side when she was 8 years old.

The examination findings are shown in Fig. 14.3.

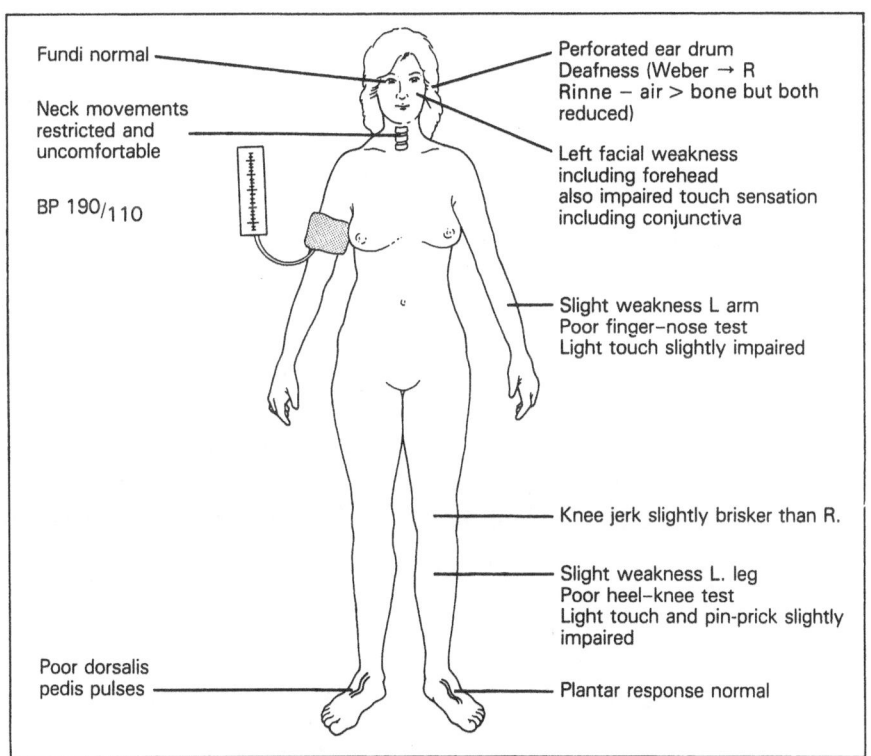

Fundi normal

Neck movements restricted and uncomfortable

BP 190/110

Poor dorsalis pedis pulses

Perforated ear drum
Deafness (Weber → R
Rinne – air > bone but both
reduced)

Left facial weakness
including forehead
also impaired touch sensation
including conjunctiva

Slight weakness L arm
Poor finger–nose test
Light touch slightly impaired

Knee jerk slightly brisker than R.

Slight weakness L. leg
Poor heel–knee test
Light touch and pin-prick slightly
impaired

Plantar response normal

Fig. 14.3 *Examination findings in case challenge*

Questions

Name four possible diagnoses

How would you distinguish between them?

Possible diagnoses

- vertebro-basilar ischaemia
- chronic otitis media with labyrinthine involvement
- Ménière's disease
- acoustic neuroma

Vertebro-basilar ischaemia

For   history

- dizziness on standing or head movement
- occipital headache and neck creaking indicates cervical spondylosis which is a frequent cause of vertebro-basilar ischaemia
- previous stroke indicating cerebrovascular disease

exam

- limited uncomfortable neck movement
- hypertension predisposing to atherosclerosis
- poor foot pulses suggesting generalized atherosclerosis

Against   history

- tinnitus associated with vertigo in the second type of attack

exam

- nil

Tests

- X-ray neck

  may show calcified carotid arteries

  will confirm cervical spondylosis which is a contributory factor

- arteriography – this is the definitive test but completely unnecessary in this type of problem: the only indication for this test is a carotid artery lesion which is being seriously considered for surgery

Chronic otitis media

For	history	• past history of chronic ear disease and mastoidec-tomy
	exam	• deafness
		• perforated eardrum confirming previous middle ear disease
Against	history	• can only account for the vertiginous attacks and not the other kind of dizziness
	exam	• Weber test referred to opposite side
		• Rinné test A>B – should be the reverse in chronic middle ear disease
Tests		• audiometry
		to detect hearing loss
		to establish conductive deafness
		• swab for bacterial culture if active discharge
		• X-ray skull for sclerosis or erosion of mastoid

Ménière's disease

For	history	• right age
		• symptoms of vertigo, tinnitus, sweating, nausea/vomiting are very typical of Ménière's disease
	exam	• nerve type deafness
Against	history	• nil
	exam	• nil

Acoustic neuroma

For	history	• attacks of tinnitus and vertigo is a common presentation
	exam	• signs of 5th and 7th nerve involvement in the face: although there are residual left-sided signs from the previous stroke, the involvement of the left frontal area in the facial weakness indicates that the origin is lower motor neurone (as in acoustic neuroma) and not upper motor neurone (as in the usual type of stroke)
Against	history	• nil
	exam	• nil

Tests

- audiometry – to establish nerve deafness
- X-ray of internal auditory meatus for erosion
- CT scan to show the tumour

Actual diagnosis:

Vertebro-basilar ischaemia – neck X-ray confirmed spondylosis and carotid calcification

Acoustic neuroma – shown on CT scan

Treatment and outcome

The acoustic neuroma was treated by surgical excision but unfortunately left the patient deaf: there was also a transient weakness of the facial nerve postoperatively which cleared within a month.

15   Sudden Loss of Vision

Introduction
Alarming symptom but if unilateral may not be noticed immediately.
Many possible causes related to the process of vision.
Early diagnosis may save eyesight.

Causes of blindness

Eye disease
- cataract
- glaucoma
- vitreous haemorrhage
- retinal

  detachment

  senile macular degeneration

  retinitis pigmentosa

  chloroquine toxicity

Optic nerve
- optic neuritis
- papilloedema
- toxic

  methyl alcohol

  quinine

  ethambutol (for tuberculosis)

  tobacco

  lead poisoning
- Leber's hereditary optic atrophy

Neurological
- chiasma
  - tumours
    - pituitary adenoma
    - craniopharyngioma
    - meningioma
    - aneurysm of carotid artery
- geniculate ganglia/optic radiation/occipital cortex
  - vascular
    - thromboembolic
    - haemorrhage
  - tumours
  - trauma

Vascular
- retinopathy
  - hypertension
  - diabetes
- retinal artery blockage
  - emboli
  - thrombosis
- retinal vein thrombosis
- cranial arteritis
- migraine

Hysterical

Grades of severity

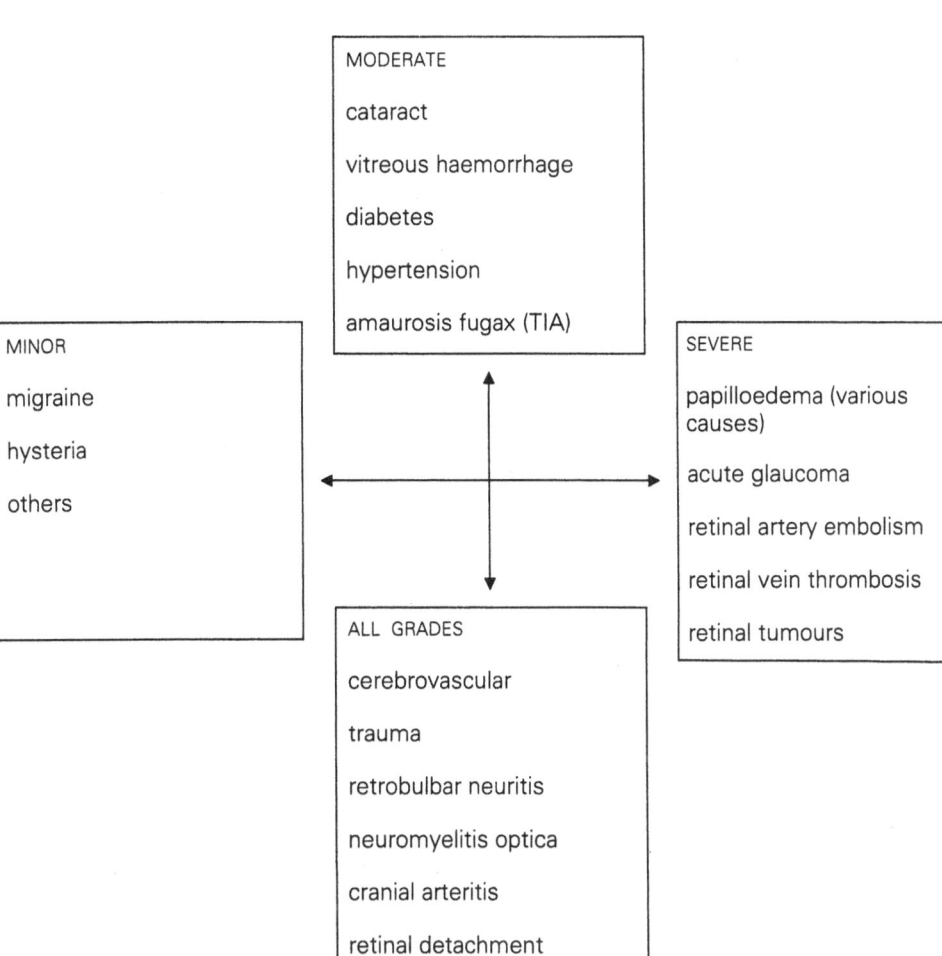

MODERATE

cataract

vitreous haemorrhage

diabetes

hypertension

amaurosis fugax (TIA)

MINOR

migraine

hysteria

others

SEVERE

papilloedema (various
causes)

acute glaucoma

retinal artery embolism

retinal vein thrombosis

retinal tumours

ALL GRADES

cerebrovascular

trauma

retrobulbar neuritis

neuromyelitis optica

cranial arteritis

retinal detachment

toxic/drugs
   methyl alcohol
   quinine
   chloroquine
   ethambutol
   lead

Frequency

Annual prevalence of sudden loss (disturbance) of vision in a population of 2500

Cataract	2
Migraine	2
Diabetes	1
High blood pressure	1
Retinal vessels	1 in 2 y
Glaucoma	1 in 3 y
Retrobulbar neuritis (MS)	1 in 3 y
Retinal detachment	1 in 5 y
Amaurosis fugax (TIA)	1 in 7 y

Age incidence

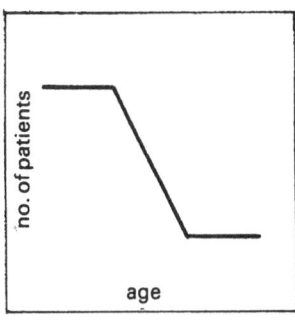

- retinoblastoma
- trauma

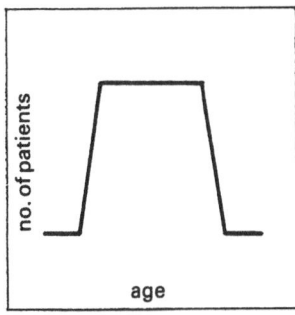

- retinal detachment
- diabetes
- migraine
- retrobulbar neuritis

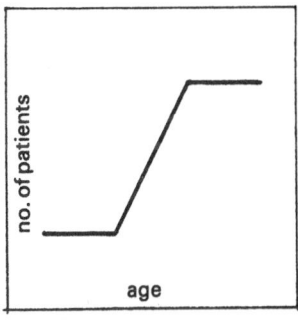

- cerebrovascular
- cataract
- retinal vessels
- glaucoma

Diagnostic approach

History

The 2 basic facts to establish are

- is the loss of vision unilateral or bilateral?
- is it an acute onset or gradual and progressive?

Acute onset

one eye

- retinal vein thrombosis
- retinal artery obstruction

    embolus

    thrombosis

- vitreous haemorrhage
- retinal haemorrhage
- retinal detachment
- optic neuritis – multiple sclerosis
- ischaemic optic neuropathy

    temporal arteritis

    atheroma

- thrombosis of internal carotid artery
- trauma – haemorrhage optic canal

both eyes

- bilateral optic neuritis

    neuromyelitis optica

    toxic

        methyl alcohol

        quinine

        tobacco

        ethambutol

        lead

- bilateral occipital lobe ischaemia – basilar artery thrombosis
- trauma to both occipital lobes
- cerebral oedema
- uraemia
- migraine

Sudden loss of vision

- hysteria
- homonymous hemianopia – vascular lesion

Gradual progressive onset
    one eye

- cataract
- refractive errors
- uveal tract inflammation
    iritis
    uveitis
    choroiditis
- glaucoma
- vitreous haemorrhage
- tumours
    orbital
    optic nerve
- dislocation of lens
- progressive optic atrophy

    both eyes

- all above causes may affect the second eye
- senile macular degeneration
- retinal disease
    hypertensive retinopathy
    diabetic retinopathy
    retinitis pigmentosa
    choroido-retinitis
        toxoplasmosis
        TB
        syphilis
- Leber's optic atrophy
- toxins
    tobacco
    ethambutol
    lead poisoning
    quinine

Other relevant symptoms

visual

  coloured haloes around lights → glaucoma

    worse in dim light

- vitamin A deficiency
- retinitis pigmentosa
- syphilitic retinitis
- hysteria

general

- symptoms of anaemia → optic neuritis
- vitamin B1 deficiency → optic neuritis
  paraesthesiae in limbs
  weakness of limbs
  oedema
- diabetes
  thirst
  polyuria
  loss of weight
- hypopituitarism (pituitary adenoma)
  amenorrhoea
  loss of libido
  hypothyroidism
  adrenal deficiency
- cardiac arrhythmia → retinal emboli
  palpitations
- temporal arteritis (see Fig. 15.1)
- general arterial disease – emboli/thrombosis
  angina
  claudication
  brain stem ischaemia
    dizziness
    diplopia
    dysarthria
    dysphagia

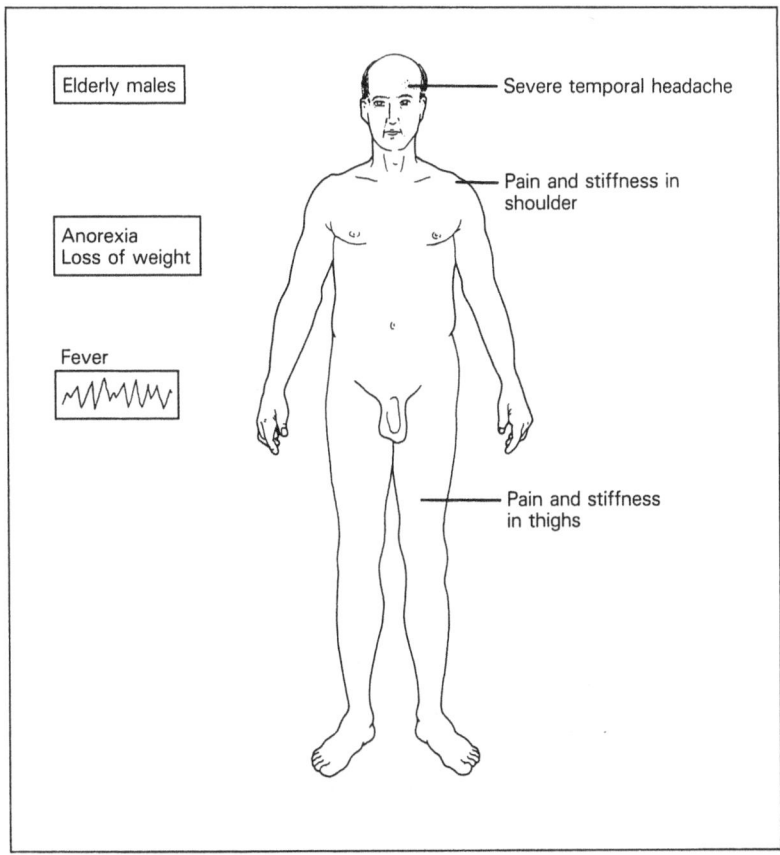

Elderly males

Severe temporal headache

Pain and stiffness in shoulder

Anorexia
Loss of weight

Fever

Pain and stiffness in thighs

Fig. 15.1   *Symptoms of cranial (temporal) arteritis*

- hysteria
  bizarre sensory loss
  bizarre fits
  bizarre speech disturbances

Past history
- symptoms of multiple sclerosis:
  previous temporary loss of vision
  transient focal sensory signs
  transient focal motor signs
  temporary incoordination
- migraine
- tuberculosis (ethambutol)

- rheumatoid arthritis (chloroquine)
- alcoholism
- contact with lead, e.g. making batteries

Family history
- hypertension
- diabetes
- migraine
- Leber's optic atrophy
- amaurotic familial idiocy
- Schilder's disease (diffuse sclerosis)

Examination

Eye

proptosis
- Graves' disease
- 1° or 2° tumour
- vascular tumour → pulsation
- aneurysm in cavernous sinus
- leukaemic infiltration
- granuloma, e.g. histiocytosis

cornea
- inflammation
- ulceration
- cloudy/oedematous → glaucoma

anterior chamber
- tension raised→ glaucoma
- pus/blood → iridocyclitis

iris
- fixed irregular (Argyll–Robertson) → syphilis (can affect retina also)
- tremulous iris → dislocated lens (e.g. myotonia dystrophica)

vitreous
- haemorrhage

fundus

retina
- retinopathy
  diabetic
  hypertensive
- senile macular degeneration
- choroido-retinitis

Sudden loss of vision

- detachment
- retinitis pigmentosa
- retinal tumours

retinal artery obstruction

central retinal vein thrombosis

optic nerve
- neuritis
- papilloedema
- atrophy

pupils

  shape

    abnormal if
- disease of iris
- disease of 3rd cranial nerve

    normal if disease of afferent visual pathway

  reflexes – indicates disease of anterior visual pathway
- retrobulbar neuritis
    no direct light reaction
    consensual reaction present
- Argyll–Robertson
    pupils unequal, irregular
    loss of light reaction
    preservation of accommodation
- Holmes–Adie (myotonic pupil)
    large pupils
    very sluggish reaction to light
    very slow reaction to accommodation
    of no significance
- optic atrophy
    consensual reflex present
    lack of direct light reflex in affected eye
    lack of consensual reflex in good eye
    accommodation reaction preserved

visual acuity

    check with Snellen or Jaeger chart

    if unable to see charts check

        finger counting

        hand movements

        light perception

    little affected in papilloedema

    severely affected   ● optic neuritis

                                ● ischaemic optic neuropathy

                                ● tumours of optic nerve

visual fields

    can be assessed simply by the confrontation technique with a coloured pin

    provides very useful information about the site of a lesion of the visual pathways (Fig. 15.2)

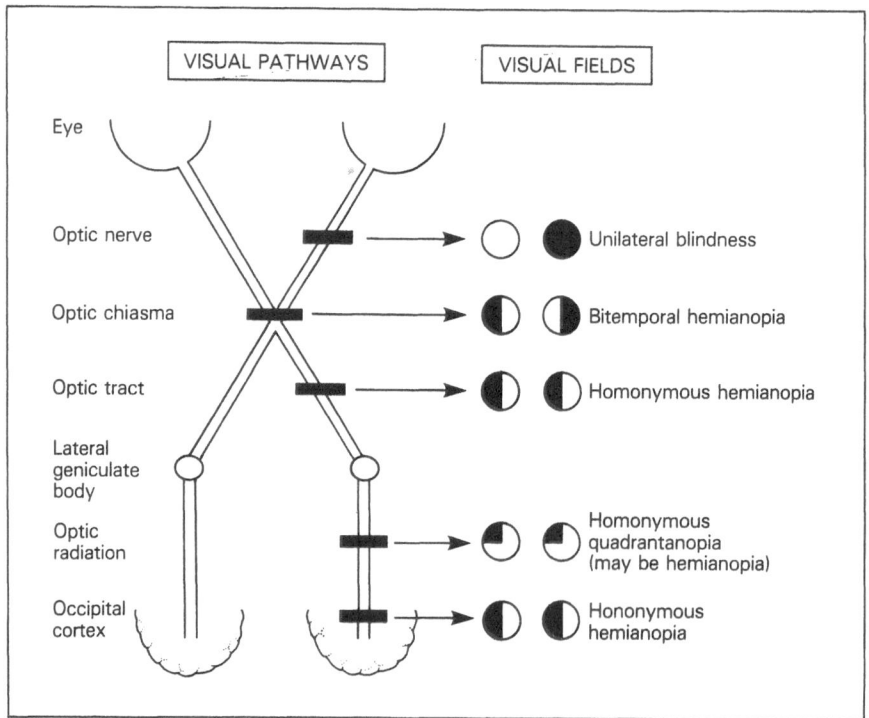

Fig. 15.2   *Disturbance of visual fields related to site of lesion along visual pathways*

General examination

A general examination should pay particular attention to

- general observations
- nervous system
- cardiovascular system
- endocrine system

Some possible findings are shown in Fig. 15.3.

Investigation

Perimetry – accurate picture of visual fields

central scotoma →

- optic neuritis
- optic atrophy
- retinal macular disease
- occipital lobe lesion

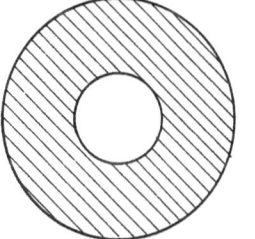

peripheral concentric →

- chronic papilloedema scotoma (tunnel vision)
- retinal disease
- retinitis pigmentosa
- choroido-retinitis
- cortical blindness
- hysteria

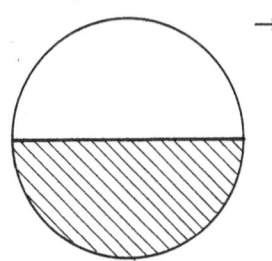

altitudinal (horizontal demarcation)

→
- optic neuritis
- ischaemic optic neuropathy
- hereditary atrophy (Leber)
- toxic optic neuropathy

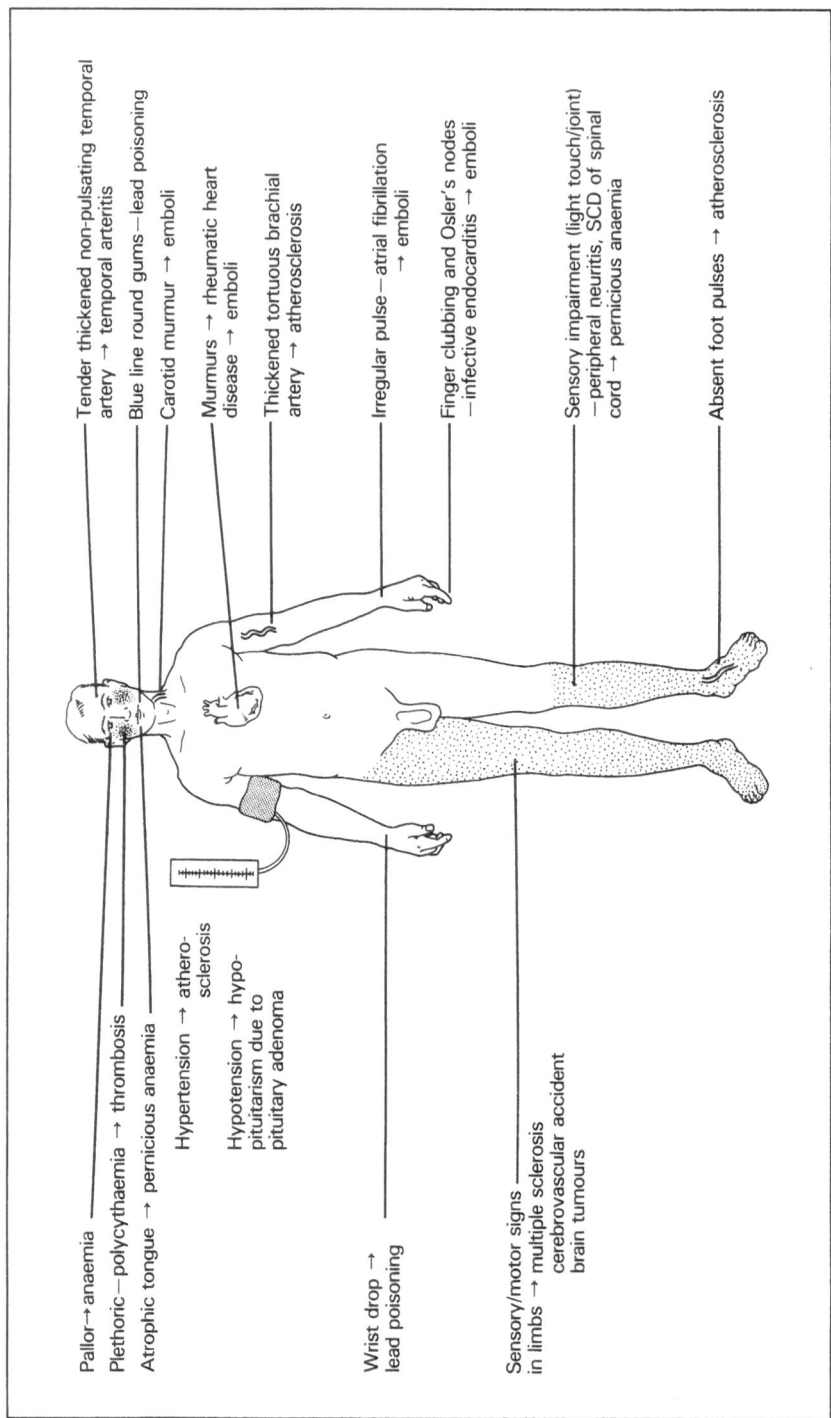

Fig. 15.3   *Possible general findings in patients with loss of vision*

bitemporal hemianopia →   • chiasmal lesion

homonymous hemianopia

                →   • optic tract lesion

                    • cerebral lesion

homonymous quadrantanopia

                →   • lesion of optic radiation, e.g. temporal lobe tumour

Fluorescein angiography   • retinal vascular obstruction

                    • diabetic retinopathy

                    • retinal vascular tumours

                    • detection of doubtful papilloedema

Radiology

  X-ray skull   • orbital tumours

                    • brain tumours

                        meningioma

                        metastases

                        angioma

                        craniopharyngioma

                    • pituitary tumours – eroded sella turcica

                    • acoustic neuroma – eroded internal auditory canal

  tomography of orbit   • for tumours

  carotid arteriography   • carotid atheroma (→ emboli)

                    • brain tumour

                        vascular

                        avascular

  CT scan – best test   • cerebrovascular accident

                    • optic nerve lesions

                    • brain tumour

                    • other space-occupying lesions

  chest X-ray   • for rheumatic heart disease

Lumbar puncture	• for multiple sclerosis
	protein ↑
	lymphocytosis
	γ-globulin ↑
	Lange 1st zone curve
	• for acoustic neuroma – high protein (up to 300 mg %)
Visual evoked reflex	• for demyelinating disease
Blood tests	
blood sugar	• diabetes
blood urea	• uraemia (causes amaurosis)
vitamin B12 level	• for pernicious anaemia (causes optic neuritis)
blood cortisol level	• for pituitary adenoma
ESR	• very high in temporal arteritis
Hb	• for anaemia
WBC	• for leukaemia
Temporal artery biopsy	• for temporal arteritis

Specific conditions

Retrobulbar neuritis	• causes
	multiple sclerosis – commonest
	neurosyphilis
	diabetes
	vitamin deficiency – B1
	B12
	toxins – alcohol
	tobacco
	lead
	quinine
	neuromyelitis optica
	• loss of vision in hours to days
	• pain on eye movement frequent

- examination

  visual acuity severely impaired

  loss of direct light reflex if nerve severely damaged

  fundus

  papillitis with blurred disc margins if anterior part of optic nerve affected

  optic disc may be normal if retrobulbar neuritis

  other neurological signs if multiple sclerosis is the cause: one third of patients with optic neuritis go on to develop clinical features of MS

- optic atrophy may follow
- tests

  CSF analysis for multiple sclerosis

  raised protein

  raised γ-globulin

  lymphocytosis

  paretic (1st zone) Lange curve

  visual-evoked reflex for subclinical optic neuritis

  nuclear magnetic resonance may be an important diagnostic tool in the future.

Amaurosis fugax

- transient episode of loss of vision affecting one eye
- causes

  platelet embolus from atheromatosis carotid artery in the neck is commonest cause

  emboli from heart

  atrial fibrillation

  rheumatic valve disease

  infective endocarditis

  atrial myxoma

  mitral valve prolapse

  benign intracranial hypertension

  temporal arteritis

- mechanism is transient occlusion of a retinal artery
- other symptoms of cerebral ischaemia may accompany loss of vision, e.g. transient numbness or weakness
- examination (see Fig. 15.4)

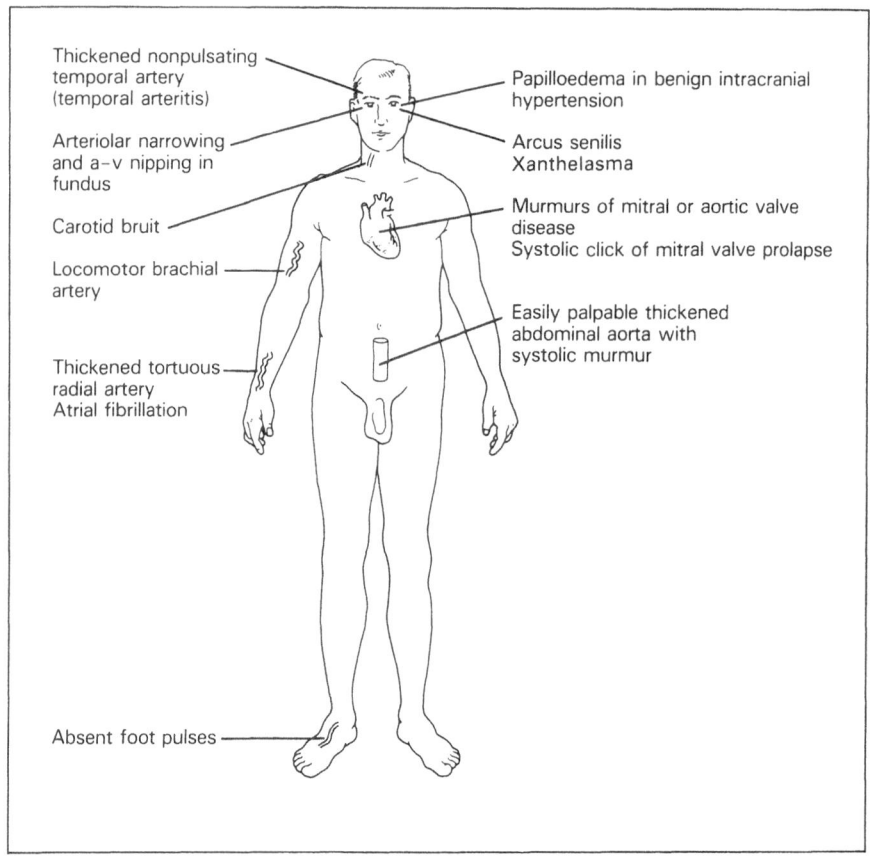

Thickened nonpulsating temporal artery (temporal arteritis)

Arteriolar narrowing and a–v nipping in fundus

Carotid bruit

Locomotor brachial artery

Thickened tortuous radial artery
Atrial fibrillation

Absent foot pulses

Papilloedema in benign intracranial hypertension

Arcus senilis
Xanthelasma

Murmurs of mitral or aortic valve disease
Systolic click of mitral valve prolapse

Easily palpable thickened abdominal aorta with systolic murmur

Fig. 15.4   *Possible signs in amaurosis fugax*

signs of atherosclerosis especially carotid artery in neck

signs of heart disease

signs of temporal arteritis

Fundus:

gray platelet embolus in retinal arteriole

yellow atheromatous material in retinal arteriole .

white fibrous scars along course of arteriole

no abnormality – commonest

- tests

ophthalmodynamometry may help to detect
blockage in the ophthalmic artery

fluorescein angiography

for temporal arteritis

ESR

temporal artery biopsy

CT scan for benign intracranial hypertension

angiography for carotid artery disease – only if
operation contemplated

echocardiogram

mitral valve disease

mitral valve prolapse

atrial myxoma

Glaucoma

- may be acute or chronic
- causes

trauma to eye

ocular inflammation – uveitis

iritis

choroido-retinitis

vascular occlusion   – diabetes

retinal vein thrombosis

carotid thrombosis

retinal disease

malignant disease of eye

- acute glaucoma – sudden onset over few days
- chronic glaucoma – slow and insidious – `may not
be appreciated by victim

- symptoms

    coloured haloes round lights

    severe pain in the eye or headache above the eye

    vision impaired

    vomiting may occur

- signs

    conjunctival injection

    increased tension over the eyeball

    haziness of the cornea

    visual acuity impaired

    visual field shows peripheral constriction (tunnel vision)

    pupil irregular or dilated – fixed

    cupping of the optic disc

- differential diagnosis

    conjunctivitis

    iritis/iridocyclitis

    keratitis

    scleritis

- total and permanent loss of vision can occur if untreated

- tests

    direct intraocular pressure measurement (tonography)

    gonioscopy – measures angle of anterior chamber

Retinal detachment

- causes

    severe myopia

    eye operations

    trauma

    advanced diabetic retinopathy

    choroidal tumours, e.g. haemangioma

Sudden loss of vision

- symptoms
  - unilateral
  - visual impairment
    - grey cloud
    - black spot
    - shadow or curtain ascending or descending
    - flashes or twinkling lights
- fundal examination
  - part of retina
    - grey or white
    - wrinkled
    - hole occasionally
    - vessels dark and tortuous
  - visual field
    - scotoma
    - central vision lost if macula involved

Pitfalls in diagnosis

- Using drops to dilate the pupil prior to fundal examination without first checking eyeball tension for glaucoma.
- Misinterpreting the coloured haloes of glaucoma as the eye manifestations of migraine.
- Not realizing the need for urgent treatment in retinal detachment where visual impairment may be only slight.
- Not thinking of temporal arteritis as a cause of sudden deterioration of vision in an elderly patient, especially if temporal headache is present.
- Not appreciating the urgency of steroid treatment in a patient with temporal arteritis and deterioration of vision.
- Misdiagnosing glaucoma as acute conjunctivitis since both conditions cause pain in the eye and conjunctival redness.
- Missing serious retinal disease because adequate fundal examination is precluded by senile cataract.
- Omitting a urine check for sugar in any patient with cataract.

Useful practical points

- A past history of transient visual disturbance with pain behind the eye is virtually diagnostic of multiple sclerosis.
- In a patient with monocular visual impairment the presence of neurological manifestations of spinal cord involvement is highly suspicious of multiple sclerosis.
- The Holmes–Adie (myotonic) pupil – very sluggish response to light/accommodation often with absent knee jerks – is of *no* clinical significance.
- Pupillary reactions are normal in cortical blindness.
- Vision is only minimally affected even in severe papilloedema – the reverse is true for optic neuritis.
- Always dilate the pupil for an adequate fundal examination – but don't forget to check eyeball tension for glaucoma first.
- Frequent requests for a change of glasses may be the first indication of glaucoma.

Case challenge

A 63-year-old overweight male patient with a 10-year history of Type B (maturity-onset) diabetes, controlled on oral hypoglycaemic drugs alone, presented with a 3 months history of deterioration of vision. He had worn spectacles for reading since his early fifties and had changed them every 2–3 years: however, in spite of a recent 'updating' of his spectacles he was finding it increasingly difficult to read a daily newspaper – he could start the line of print all right but found it an effort to follow the print.

On direct enquiry he admitted other interesting symptoms: he had developed chest pain on effort over the previous 2–3 years; he was getting pain in the right calf on walking uphill and this was getting worse; he had noticed some recent headache in the left fronto-temporal area; he was tending to become a little clumsy, e.g. when pouring he would occasionally miss the cup and he had also noticed a tendency to bump into things on his right hand side.

He was a moderately heavy smoker, 25 cigarettes a day for about the past 40 years, and was quite fond of drinking beer, perhaps 4–5 pints a night 3–4 times a week and he had done this for some years.

He was taking glibenclamide 10mg/day for his diabetes and quinine 300 mg once or twice a day for the pain in his right calf.

The *examination* findings are shown in Fig. 15.5.

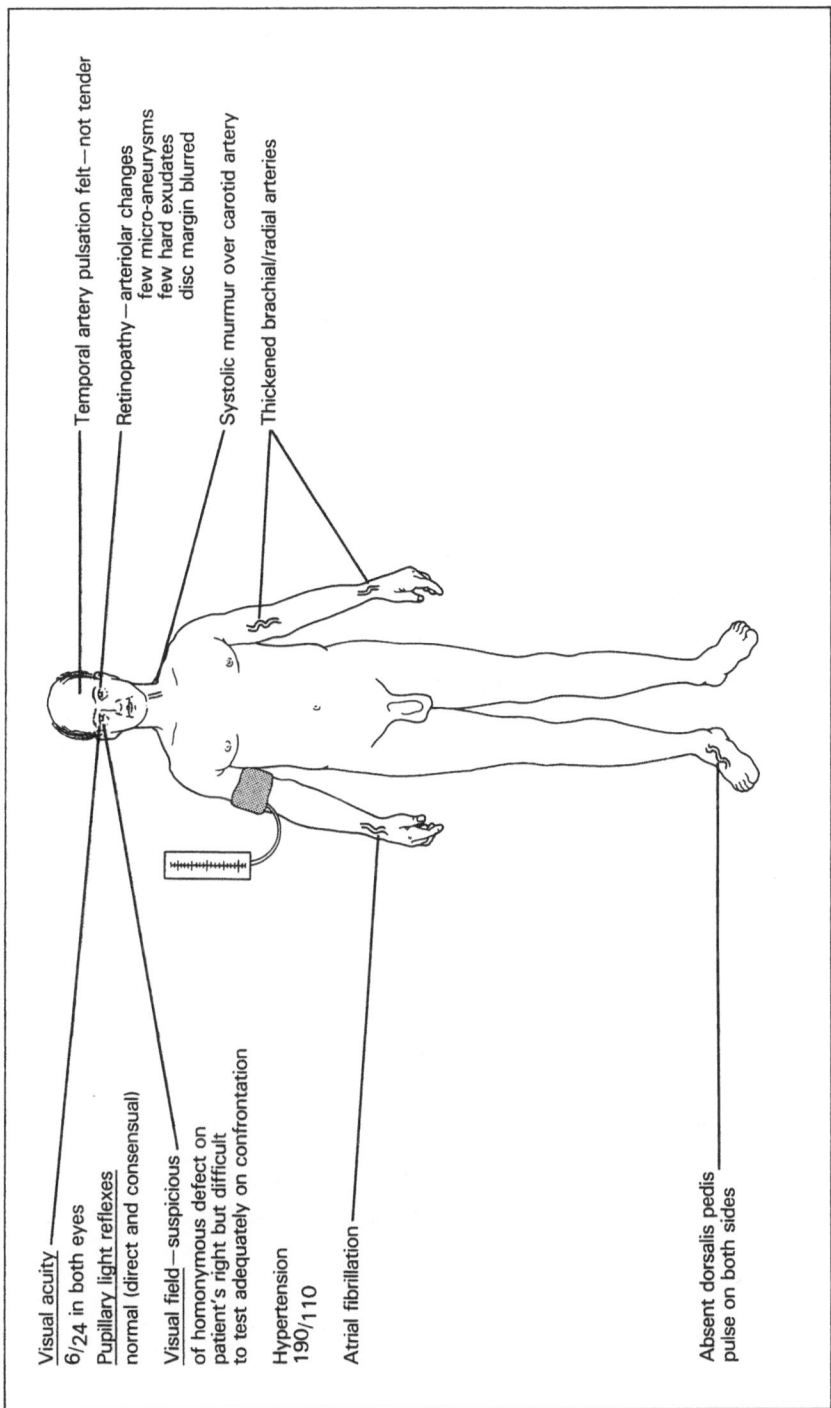

Visual acuity
6/24 in both eyes
Pupillary light reflexes
normal (direct and consensual)

Visual field—suspicious
of homonymous defect on
patient's right but difficult
to test adequately on confrontation

Hypertension
190/110

Atrial fibrillation

Absent dorsalis pedis
pulse on both sides

Temporal artery pulsation felt—not tender

Retinopathy—arteriolar changes
few micro-aneurysms
few hard exudates
disc margin blurred

Systolic murmur over carotid artery

Thickened brachial/radial arteries

Fig. 15.5 *Examination findings in case challenge*

Questions		What are the possible diagnoses?
		How would you distinguish between them?

Possible diagnoses

- presbyopia
- diabetic retinopathy
- retinal artery emboli
- temporal arteritis
- toxic damage to optic nerve

    tobacco

    alcohol

    quinine

- brain tumour

Presbyopia

For	history	• right age
		• has had to change glasses regularly
	exam	• refraction difficult to check on clinical examination but one useful test is to see whether vision improves on looking through a pin-hole in a dark card
		• impaired visual acuity in both eyes
Against	history	• nil
	exam	• visual field defect does not fit
		• looking through a pin-hole did not improve newspaper reading
Tests		• requires full assessment of refraction by optician/ophthalmologist

Diabetic retinopathy

For	history	• fairly long history of diabetes
	exam	• features of diabetic retinopathy seen

Sudden loss of vision

Against	history	• unusual to get such rapid deterioration of vision in a Type B diabetic
	exam	• blurred disc margin on left
		• no evidence of retinitis proliferans which is most likely to cause rapid deterioration of vision in a diabetic
		• visual field defect atypical
Tests		• fluorescein angiography will help to establish full extent of the retinopathy

Retinal artery emboli

For	history	• visual disturbance in a patient with obvious symptoms of atherosclerotic disease (angina/claudication)
	exam	• evidence of carotid artery disease – the most frequent source of retinal emboli
		• evidence of peripheral vascular disease in legs confirming the widespread nature of the arterial disease
		• fundal arteriolar changes making them susceptible to blockage
Against	history	• atypical – usual presentation is amaurosis fugax – transient visual disturbance
	exam	• homonymous field defect – retinal emboli tend to produce a unilateral altitudinal (horizontal) field defect
		• blurred right disc margin
Tests		• fluorescein angiography if it can be carried out soon after the onset of the visual impairment – may sometimes show the embolus

Temporal arteritis

For	history	• elderly male patient
		• recent frontotemporal headache
	exam	• blurred right disc might be due to ischaemic optic neuropathy

Against	history	• progressive deterioration of vision over 3 months – in temporal arteritis visual loss is much more rapid
		• no polymyalgia
	exam	• normal temporal arteries on palpation
Tests		• ESR – should be very high, e.g. > 50 mm
		• temporal artery biopsy best test

Toxic damage to optic nerve

For	history	• toxins evident – tobacco alcohol quinine
	exam	• blurring of optic disc – may indicate damage
Against	history	• usually heavy pipe, not cigarette, smoking
		• quinine small dose and only recent
	exam	• homonymous field defect atypical for optic nerve damage – should be altitudinal
		• no loss of direct consensual pupillary light reflex – expected in optic nerve damage where afferent pathway is impaired
Tests		• nil

Brain tumour

For	history	• nature of visual deterioration suggests right homonymous defect which could be due to a left cerebral tumour
		• recent left frontotemporal headache
		• clumsiness involving right side suggests possible left cerebral lesion or could be due to right homonymous field defect
	exam	• homonymous field defect would fit in
		• blurred left disc would fit in
Against	history	• nil
	exam	• nil

Tests

- perimetry – would establish a more accurate picture of visual fields

- CT scan – best test for tumour; supersedes all other tests

Actual diagnosis:

L. temporal lobe glioblastoma

perimetry showed a right homonymous upper quadrantanopia

CT scan showed the tumour in the left temporal lobe

burr biopsy confirmed the nature of the tumour

Treatment and outcome

The extent and malignancy of the tumour rendered it inoperable.

The patient was treated with a combination of radiotherapy and carmustine as specific treatment for the tumour itself, and also with dexamethasone 4mg/day to control the raised intracranial pressure.

He survived for only 7 more months.

16 'Funny Turns'

Introduction

Subjective sensations that are frightening, unknown and inexplicable to the patient. The physician is presented with a package of symptoms that test his clinical acumen. Disturbances of many systems can produce 'funny turns'.

Causes of 'funny turns' (light-headedness)

Syncope

cardiac
- arrhythmia
  - tachy – atrial fibrillation, paroxysmal tachy-cardia
  - brady – sinus bradycardia, Stokes–Adams attack
- outflow obstruction
  - aortic or pulmonary stenosis
  - hypertrophic cardiomyopathy

vasomotor
- vasovagal attack (faint)
- prolonged standing
- autonomic neuropathy
  - diabetes
  - alcoholism
  - malignancy
- hypotensive drugs

cough and micturition syncope

Cerebrovascular

transient ischaemic attacks   ● carotid artery disease

                                   ● cardiac

                                          mitral/aortic valve disease

                                          atrial fibrillation

                                          mitral valve prolapse

                                          atrial myxoma

vertebro-basilar ischaemia   ● basilar migraine

Blood   ● anaemia

                                     ● polycythaemia

                                          primary – rubra vera

                                          secondary

                                             chronic lung disease

                                             cyanotic heart disease

                                     ● hyperviscosity – myelomatosis

Hypoglycaemia   ● spontaneous

                                   ● insulin treatment of diabetic

                                   ● insulinoma in pancreas

Epilepsy   ● temporal lobe

                                   ● petit mal

Hyperventilation/anxiety

Grades of severity

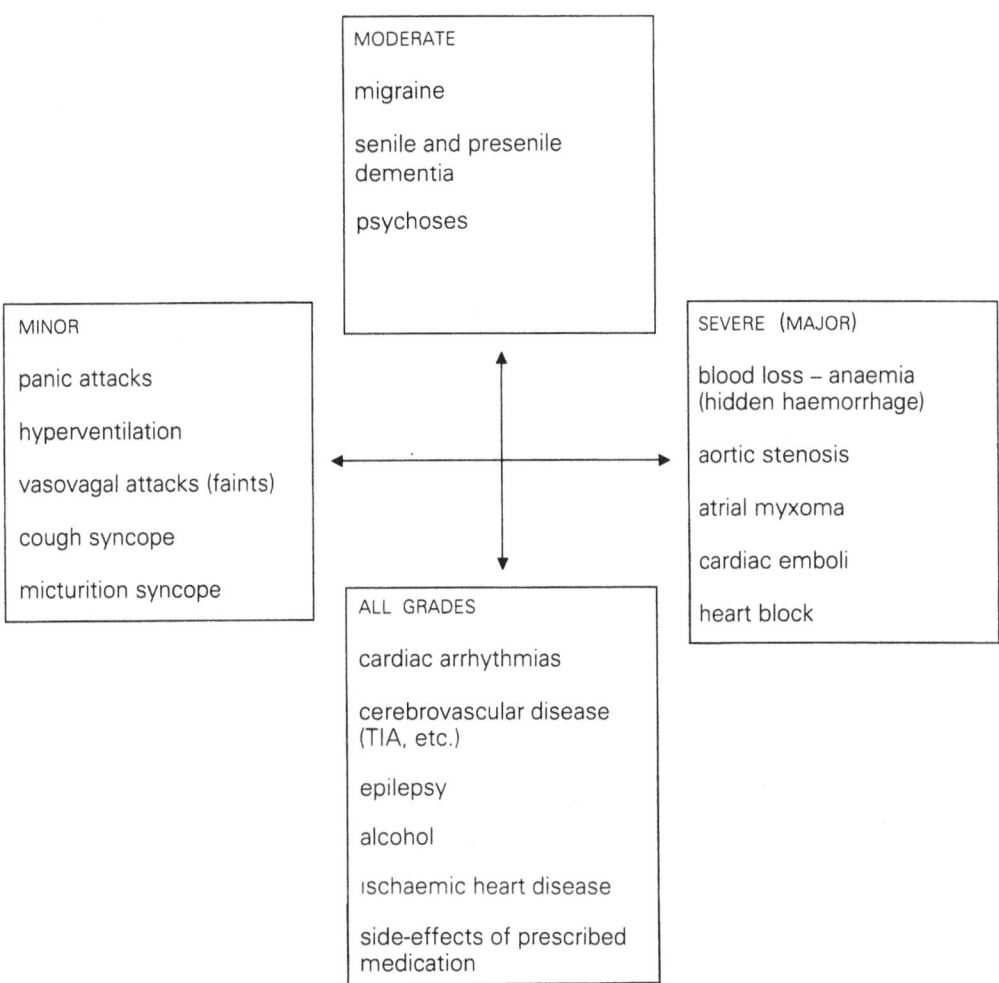

MODERATE

migraine

senile and presenile dementia

psychoses

MINOR

panic attacks

hyperventilation

vasovagal attacks (faints)

cough syncope

micturition syncope

SEVERE (MAJOR)

blood loss – anaemia (hidden haemorrhage)

aortic stenosis

atrial myxoma

cardiac emboli

heart block

ALL GRADES

cardiac arrhythmias

cerebrovascular disease (TIA, etc.)

epilepsy

alcohol

ischaemic heart disease

side-effects of prescribed medication

Frequency

'Funny turns' presenting in a general practice population of 2500 in a year	
Anxiety, panics, hyperventilation etc.	10
Vasovagal faints	5
Arrhythmias	5
Vertigo etc.	3
Epileptic phenomena	2
Migraine phenomena	2
Cerebrovascular: TIA etc.	2
Drug side-effects	2
Cardiac: IHD and aortic stenosis etc.	1 in 2 y
Blood loss: anaemia +	1 in 5 y

Age incidence

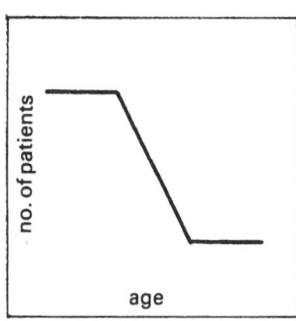

- epilepsy (petit mal)
- anxiety

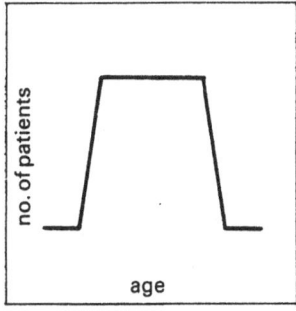

- hyperventilation
- panic attacks
- faints
- migraine
- epilepsy (temporal lobe)

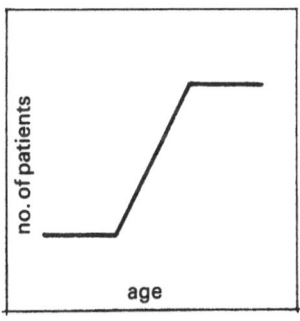

- cerebrovascular (TIA etc.)
- cardiac (arrhythmias etc.)
- side-effects of drugs

Diagnostic approach

History

It is necessary first to obtain as clear a description as possible of what the patient means by 'funny turn'

- most often the symptom means 'light-headedness'
- if the patient rotates or the surroundings rotate he has *vertigo* which is discussed in detail in Chapter 14
- if he is complaining of unsteadiness of gait he may well have disease of the nervous system
- if he complains of vague and bizarre symptoms – 'swimming sensation', 'walking on air', 'queer feelings in the head' he is likely to have an anxiety state

Onset – an acute onset of light-headedness may be due to

- paroxysmal tachycardia
- Stokes–Adams attack
- vasovagal attack
- cough/micturition syncope
- epilepsy
- transient ischaemic attack

Precipitating factors
- stress → hyperventilation
- exertion → aortic stenosis
- head movement → vertebro-basilar ischaemia
- coughing bout → cough syncope
- micturition → micturition syncope
- standing up → postural hypotension

Associated symptoms

feelings of panic →
breathing problems
- anxiety state

breathlessness
can't take deep breath } → • anxiety state

palpitations →
- paroxysmal arrhythmia with syncope

visual disturbances

teichopsia →
- migraine

transient blindness/
blurring →
- transient ischaemic attack

diplopia →   ● transient ischaemic attack (brain stem)

thumping headache →   ● migraine

taste/smell
hallucination →   ● temporal lobe epilepsy

sinking feeling in
epigastrium →   ● temporal lobe epilepsy

left inframammary pain → ● anxiety state

tingling in extremities → ● hyperventilation

tremor, sweating,
feeling of hunger →   ● hypoglycaemia

slurred speech →   ● transient ischaemic attack

Drug history – the drugs which may cause light-headedness

peripheral vasodilators   ● hydrallazine

     ● prazosin

     ● minoxidil

     ● captopril

adrenergic neuron-
blockers   ● guanethidine

     ● bethanidine

     ● debrisoquine

anti-epileptic drugs

tranquillizers and other psychotropic drugs

Past history   ● migraine

     ● epilepsy

     ● angina/claudication → vertebro-basilar ischaemia

     ● rheumatic heart disease → transient ischaemic attacks

     ● alcoholism → autonomic neuropathy with postural hypotension

     ● psychiatric disease

     ● peptic ulcer/piles → anaemia

Family history   ● migraine

     ● epilepsy

     ● hypertension

     ● ischaemic heart disease

Examination

Assess mental state especially the presence of anxiety

- anxious demeanour
- tachycardia
- sweating
- overbreathing
- trembling

Some of the physical signs which may be present are shown in Fig. 16.1

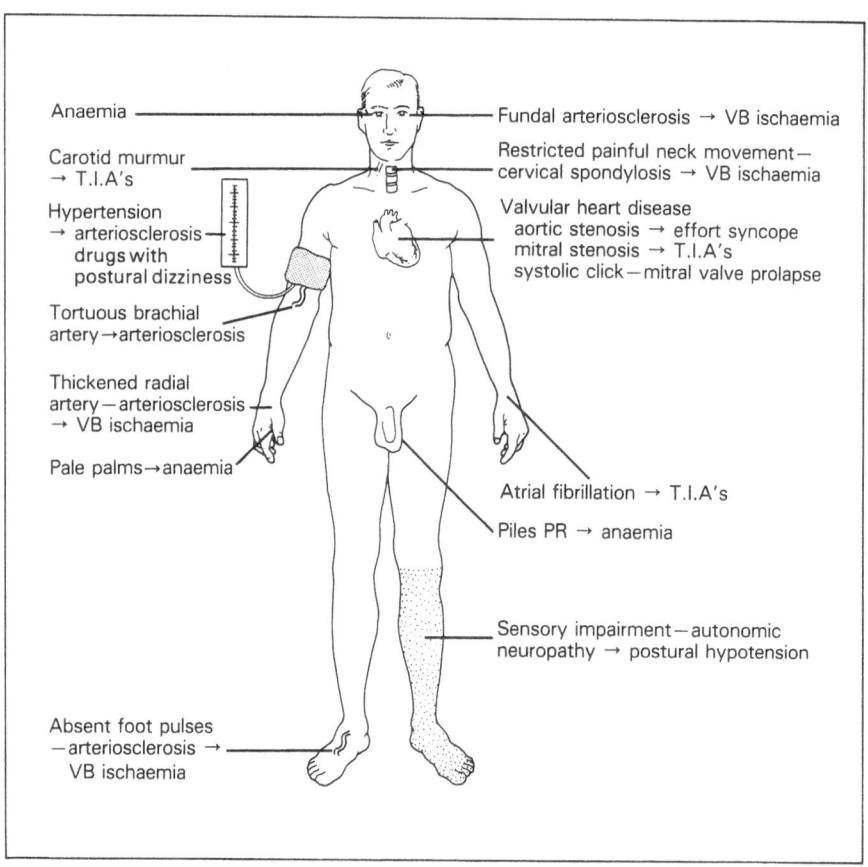

Fig. 16.1 *Physical signs in light-headedness*

Investigations

The purpose of investigating 'funny turns' is:

to confirm organic disease if present

to reassure the patient if organic disease absent and the symptoms are likely to be due to anxiety – this may be of therapeutic benefit

Blood tests
- anaemia

  hypochromic → blood loss

  macrocytic → pernicious anaemia
- polycythaemia

  primary – WBC and platelets also increased

  secondary – only RBC increased
- blood sugar

  diabetes

  hypoglycaemia – may need to fast first
- vitamin B12 level → pernicious anaemia
- immunophoresis for myelomatosis

Urine
- glycosuria → diabetes
- Bence Jones protein → myelomatosis

ECG
- atrioventricular conduction defect (heartblock)
- arrhythmia, e.g. atrial fibrillation
- Wolff–Parkinson–White syndrome (see Fig. 13.8)

  short P–R interval

  slurred upstroke of R in V6
- mitral stenosis (Fig. 16.2)

  bifid P wave

  right ventricular hypertrophy

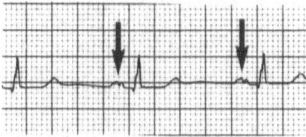

Fig. 16.2 *ECG showing bifid P wave (arrowed) indicating left atrial hypertrophy in mitral stenosis*

- aortic stenosis – LV strain (Fig. 16.3)

    tall R V6

    ST–T ↓ V6

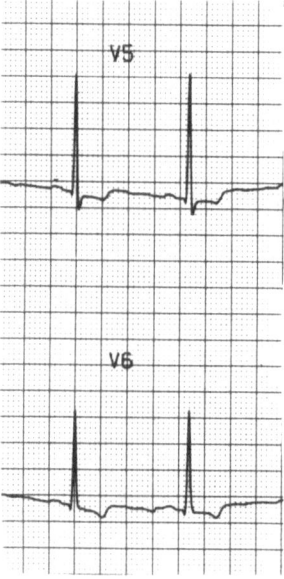

Fig. 16.3 *ECG showing left ventricular hypertrophy (tall R wave) and strain (S-T depression with T inversion)*

Radiology

chest X-ray
- mitral contour in mitral stenosis (see Fig. 13.4)
- boot-shaped (LV+)

    aortic stenosis (Fig. 16.4)

    hypertension
- chronic obstructive lung disease
- secondary polycythaemia
- cough syncope

neck X-ray (Fig. 16.5)
- cervical spondylosis
- carotid calcification

skull X-ray
- for myelomatosis (Fig. 16.6)

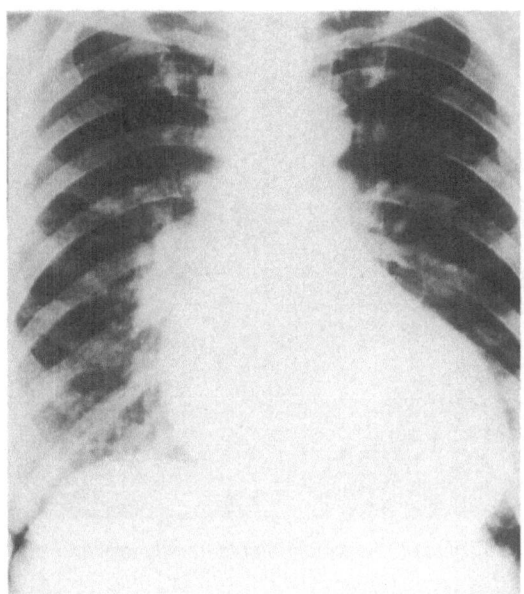

Fig. 16.4   *Chest X-ray showing 'boot-shaped' heart in left ventricular enlargement*

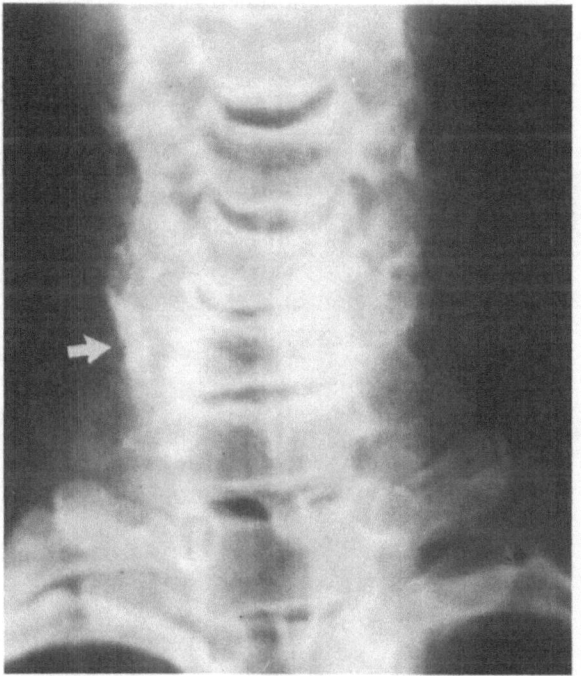

Fig. 16.5   *X-ray of neck showing cervical spondylosis and carotid calcification (arrowed)*

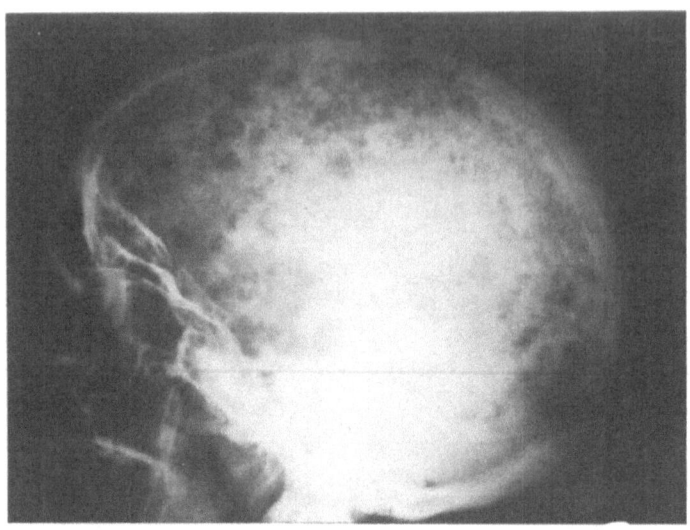

Fig. 16.6   *X-ray of skull showing multiple translucent areas due to myelomatous deposits*

Echocardiogram

- typical changes in mitral stenosis (Fig. 16.7)

  thickened anterior leaflet

  slow closure

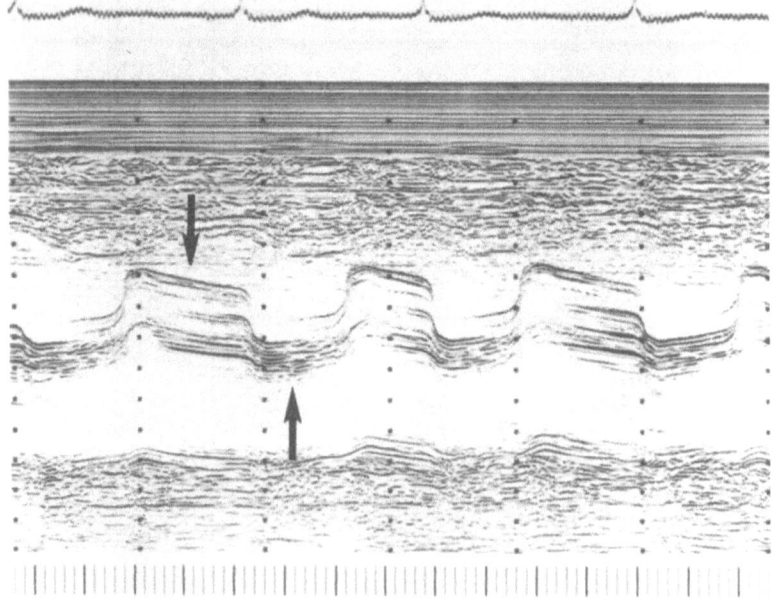

Fig. 16.7   *Echocardiogram in mitral stenosis showing thickened mitral valve leaflets (arrowed) and a slow closure rate*

Funny turns

- typical changes in aortic stenosis

  thickened valves

  impaired opening
- changes in atrial myxoma

Electroencephalogram for epilepsy

Carotid arteriography
- for carotid disease in the neck as a source of TIAs
- not justified unless surgery is contemplated

Specific conditions

Panic attacks
- manifestation of an anxiety neurosis
- familial tendency
- F : M   2 : 1 – most 20–60 years
- probably follows emotional trauma in formative years

  insecurity

  unloved

  unwanted

  broken marriage

  school trauma

  trauma in adolescence, e.g. love affair
- attacks of overwhelming panic or even terror for which there is no apparent reason
- somatic symptoms common

  light-headed ('funny turns')

  left inframammary pain

  palpitations

  sweating

  breathlessness

  can't swallow ('lump in the throat')

  tension headache

- signs

    nervousness

    tremor

    tachycardia

    hyperventilation

    systolic hypertension

    general tenseness of muscles and inability to relax, e.g. for abdominal examination

- tests – only indicated to reassure the patient that there is no organic disease

Epilepsy
Temporal lobe

- commonest type of focal epilepsy
- may be momentary or last several minutes
- manifestations

    subjective:

    hallucinations – smell

    taste

    visual

    sounds

    vertigo

    illusions – objects/persons shrink or expand

    dyscognitive – déjà vu (familiarity)

    jamais vu (strangeness)

    vivid memory

    affective – epigastric feeling

    fear

    anxiety

    rage/anger – rare

    objective:

    lip-smacking

    sucking/chewing/swallowing

    automatic behaviour

    unresponsive to question/commands

    may proceed to grand mal (2/3 of patients)

Funny turns

- tests – EEG

Petit mal
- typically affects children from 4 years up to puberty
- may be very numerous during the day
- often occurs during periods of inattention in the classroom
- no warning
- brief interruption of consciousness
    - motionless
    - sudden stare
    - sudden stop in conversation
- signs
    - sometimes clonic movements
        - eyelids
        - face
        - arms
        - fingers
    - lip-smacking or chewing
    - fumbling movements of fingers
    - mild vasomotor upset – flushing/pallor
- only lasts a few seconds – usually < 10 seconds
- tests – EEG
    - classically 3/s wave and spike
    - occasionally multiple sharp waves
    - may be normal

Aortic stenosis
- causes
    - rheumatic heart disease – commonest
    - congenital
    - old age – atheroma

- symptoms

  syncope – especially on effort due to inadequate cardiac output

  angina

  reduced coronary filling pressure

  increased demand from hypertrophied left ventricle

  breathless – due to LV failure

- signs – see Fig. 16.8

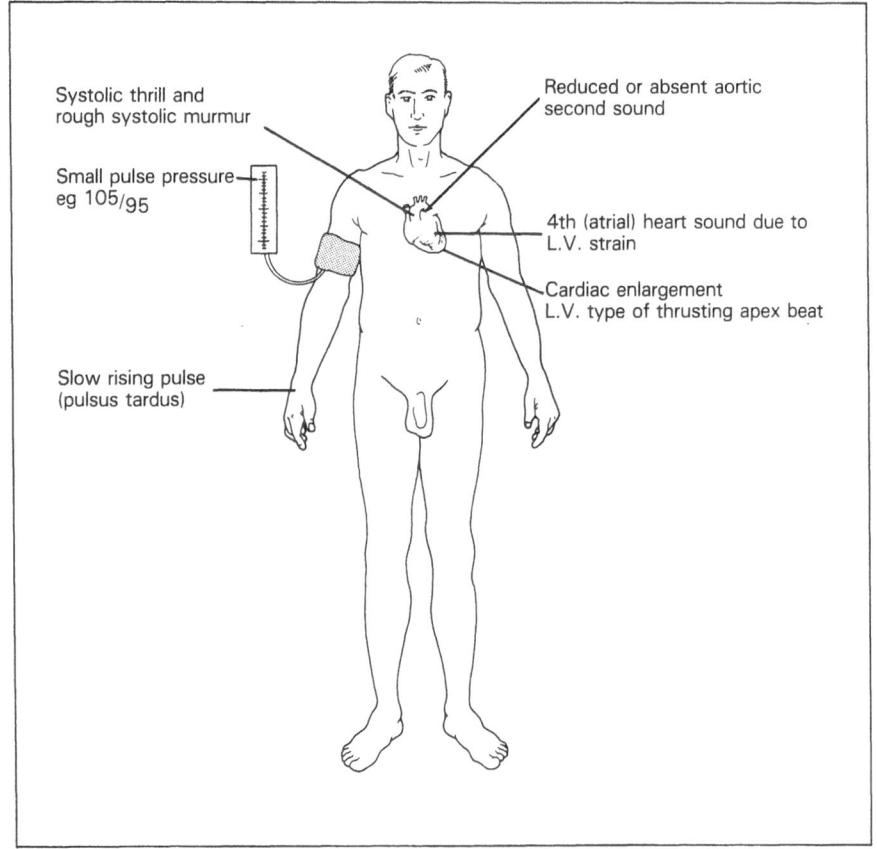

Fig. 16.8 *Signs in aortic stenosis*

Funny turns

- tests

    chest X-ray

    cardiac enlargement boot-shaped (LV) (see Fig. 16.4)

    may see calcified aortic valve

    ECG – LV hypertrophy often with strain (see Fig. 16.3)

Pitfalls in diagnosis

- Mistaking a faint with a few involuntary movements for an epileptic attack.
- Expecting a positive EEG before diagnosing epilepsy; it is a clinical diagnosis based on an adequate history – the EEG is very frequently normal anyway in a confirmed epileptic.
- Omitting to lean a patient with suspected aortic stenosis forwards in full expiration in order to listen for an aortic murmur.
- Omitting to record the *standing* blood pressure in an elderly patient complaining of light-headedness to pick up the very frequent cause of postural hypotension due to cerebrovascular disease.
- Forgetting the possibility of heart block in an elderly patient with recurrent dizziness especially if it is not postural.

Useful practical points

- Be wary of diagnosing epilepsy on the basis of one atypical attack, e.g. fainting/ flushing in adolescence.
- The more bizarre the description of a 'funny turn' the more likely it is to be functional.
- Be very careful in giving an elderly patient with mild, or even moderate, hypertension a potent hypotensive drug, especially a peripheral vasodilator; if there is no target organ damage treatment is unlikely to be necessary at all.
- If a mitral stenotic murmur seems to come and go always think of an atrial myxoma; diagnosis will depend then on a high ESR, altered serum proteins and an echocardiogram which shows a classical picture.

Case challenge

A 55-year-old male patient with a 10-year history of hypertension presented with recurrent attack of light-headedness over the previous 3 months. The attacks would occur without warning and were not particularly related to standing up, to move-

ments of the head and neck, or to exercise. On one occasion he had lost consciousness for a few minutes only and had not bitten his tongue or been incontinent.

On direct enquiry he admitted to some mild chest pain on exertion over the last
few months but it had never lasted more than a few minutes at a time.

His doctor was treating his hypertension with methyldopa 500 mg tds and Navi-
drex K 0.25 mg daily. He smoked 20 cigarettes a day for at least 25 years.

The examination findings are shown in Fig. 16.9.

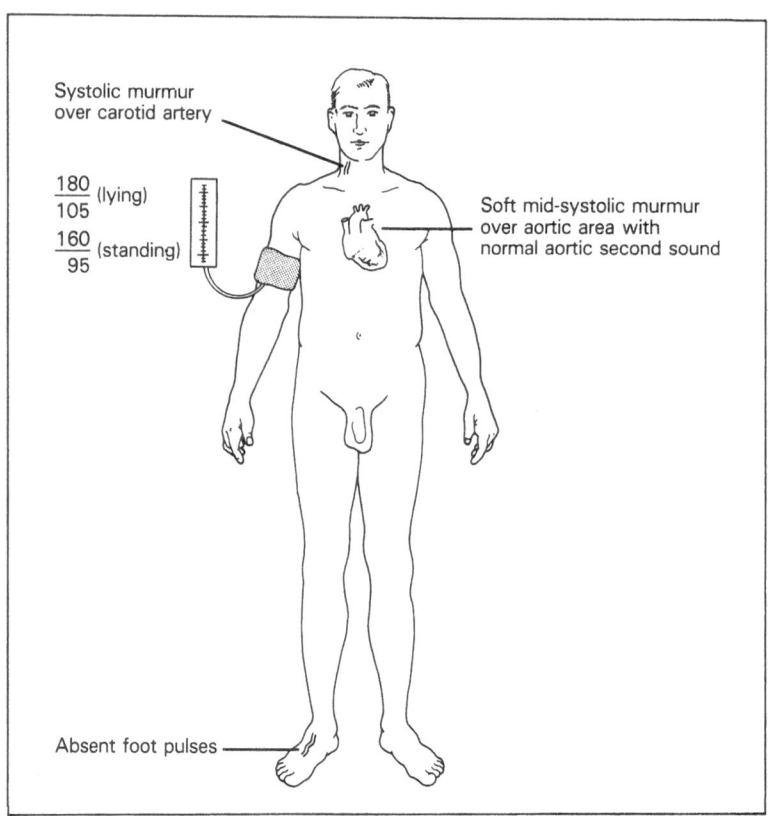

Fig. 16.9   *Examination findings in case challenge*

Questions   Suggest four possible diagnoses

                             How would you differentiate between them?

Possible diagnoses   • iatrogenic postural hypotension

                             • aortic stenosis

                             • carotid stenosis with transient ischaemic attacks

                             • heart block due to ischaemic heart disease

Postural hypotension

For	history	• he was on hypotensive treatment
	exam	• there was some evidence of postural hypotension
Against	history	• the dizziness is not related to standing up
		• the hypotensive regime (Aldomet and Navidrex K) is one that is unlikely to produce any significant postural hypotension
	exam	• the level of the standing blood pressure is not likely to cause cerebrovascular insufficiency
Tests		• none except repeated recording of the *standing* blood pressure to see if any more substantial falls occur

Aortic stenosis

For	history	• pre-syncopal attacks can occur in aortic stenosis if the restriction on cardiac output is severe enough
	exam	• he has a basal systolic murmur
Against	history	• the dizziness has no relation to exercise which is typical in aortic stenosis
	exam	• the normal aortic second sound excludes significant aortic stenosis: the murmur is more likely to be due to aortic sclerosis since the absent foot pulses indicate extensive atherosclerotic disease
Tests		• chest X-ray
		left ventricular enlargement
		calcified aortic valve
		• ECG – left ventricular hypertrophy ± strain
		• echocardiogram – typical changes in aortic stenosis
		• the definitive test is angiocardiography – this would only be justified if valve replacement is being considered

Carotid stenosis/TIAs

For	history	• TIAs can cause transient dizziness with or without loss of consciousness
	exam	• systolic murmur over the carotid artery

Against	history	• there are no other manifestations of TIAs, e.g. transient blindness, dysarthria, diplopia, limb weakness or paraesthesia
	exam	• the systolic murmur could be conducted up from the atherosclerotic aortic valve
Tests		• carotid angiography but only justified if carotid endarterectomy is being considered

Heart block

For	history	• he has a history of angina indicating ischaemic heart disease which is the usual basis for heart block
		• the attacks of light-headedness occur for no obvious reason
	exam	• evidence of widespread atherosclerosis confirming the likelihood of associated coronary disease
Against	history	• nil
	exam	• no evidence of heart block on examination of CVS i.e. no bradycardia, no widely split heart sounds indicative of bundle-branch block
Tests		• ECG

resting record

may show ischaemia

may show a-v block or bundle-branch block

24 h tape – this is more likely to show up a transient conduction disturbance

---

Actual diagnosis:

Stokes–Adams attacks which showed on the 24 hour ambulatory ECG

Treatment and outcome

He was treated by implantation of an 'on demand' permanent pacemaker. He immediately lost his attacks of lightheadedness, had no further loss of consciousness and also found that his angina improved.

17 Swollen Legs

Introduction

Everyone has 'swollen legs' at some time – even if it is only after a long plane or coach journey.

Swollen legs are often the result of a vascular condition but there are other causes.

It must not be assumed that all swollen legs need intensive investigation and treatment, many do not.

Significance of swollen legs is very different at various ages.

Mechanism of oedema is different in different conditions (Fig. 17.1)

- local obstruction
- cardiac oedema – increased hydrostatic pressure at venous end of capillaries
- renal disease

  acute nephritis – generalized capillary damage (auto-immune inflammatory reaction)

  nephrotic syndrome – loss of albumin in urine → reduced plasma osmotic pressure
- hepatic disease – defective synthesis of albumin → reduced plasma osmotic pressure

Causes of oedema

Physiological

- prolonged standing
- prolonged sitting

  old people

  long journeys

  hospital patients

431

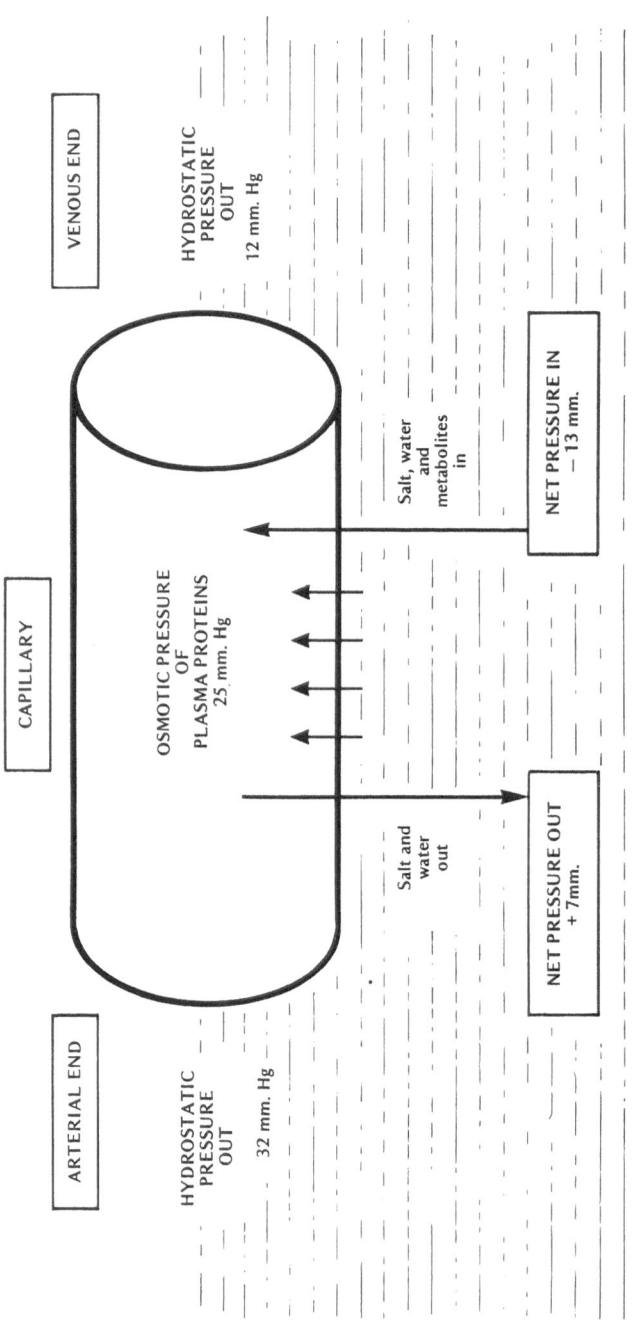

Fig. 17.1 *Swollen legs – formation of tissue fluid*

Swollen legs

- pregnancy
    normal
    toxaemia
- hot weather

Local disease

Local tissue involvement

skin
- inflammation
- burns
- trauma
- allergy

underlying arthritis → peri-articular oedema
post-traumatic

Local vascular obstruction (Fig. 17.2)

venous
- varicose veins with incompetent valves
- thrombosis

lymphatic
- primary
    congenital
    Milroy's disease
- secondary
    recurrent lymphangitis
    neoplasia
      infiltration
      lymph node compression

Generalized disease (Fig. 17.2)

right ventricular failure
- chronic lung disease
- chronic left ventricular failure
- congenital heart disease
- idiopathic pulmonary hypertension
- pulmonary thromboembolic disease

kidney disease
- acute nephritis
- nephrotic syndrome

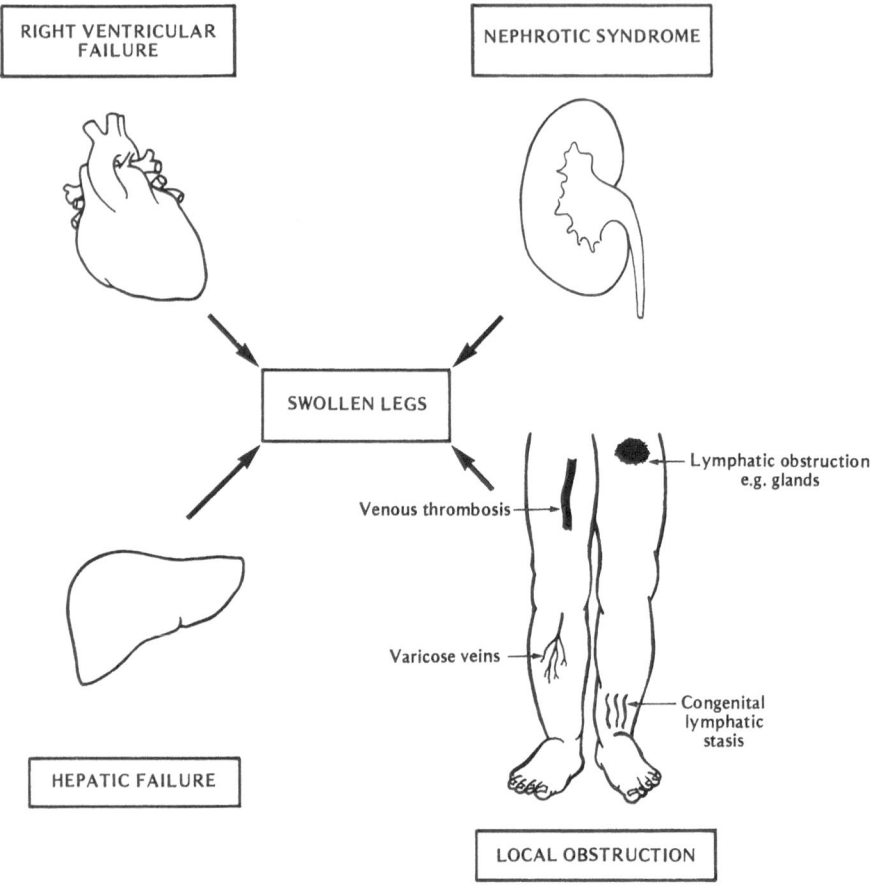

Fig. 17.2   *Causes of swollen legs*

liver disease	• chronic hepatitis
	• cirrhosis
Drugs	• oestrogens
	• vasodilator antihypertensives

liver disease
- chronic hepatitis
- cirrhosis

Drugs
- oestrogens
- vasodilator antihypertensives
    - hydrallazine
    - nifedipine
    - minoxidil
    - diazoxide
- steroids – prednisolone
- non-steroidal anti-inflammatory drugs (NSAIDs)

Swollen legs

Miscellaneous
- pre-tibial oedema in treated thyrotoxic patients
- anaemia
- 'idiopathic' oedema – no cause found

Grades of severity

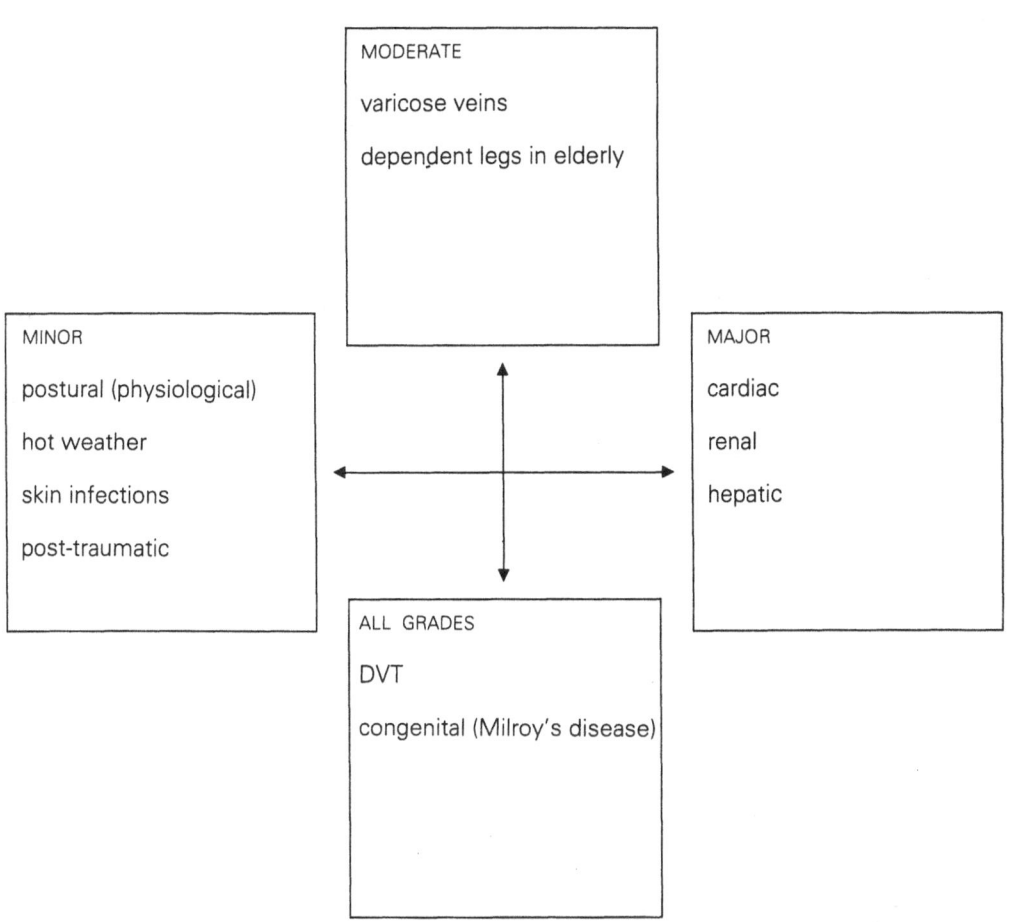

MODERATE

varicose veins

dependent legs in elderly

MINOR

postural (physiological)

hot weather

skin infections

post-traumatic

MAJOR

cardiac

renal

hepatic

ALL GRADES

DVT

congenital (Milroy's disease)

Age incidence

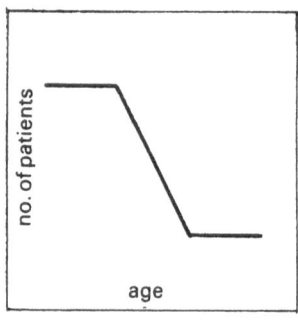

- congenital (Milroy's)
- nephrotic syndrome

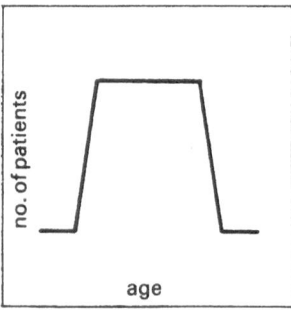

- varicose veins
- hepatic

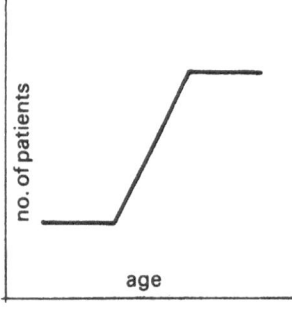

- dependent legs
- cardiac

Frequency

Annual prevalence in practice population of 2500	
Dependent legs (elderly)	20
Venous incompetence	15
Physiological	10
Cardiac	10
D V T	2
Hepatic	1 in 5 y
Renal	1 in 10 y
All	60

Diagnostic approach

History

Local oedema

unilateral (or asymmetrical if both legs are involved)

painful →	• acute inflammation of the tissues
	infection
	arthritis
	post-traumatic
	insect sting
	• acute venous thrombosis
painless →	• lymphatic obstruction
	• chronic venous obstruction
	varicose veins
	deep vein thrombosis
pruritus →	• local allergic reaction
underlying arthritis →	• peri-articular oedema
recent trauma to a leg	
intra-abdominal or pelvic malignancy →	• lymph node involvement
Generalized oedema →	• *RV failure*

                           past history of

                              chronic bronchitis

                              hypertension

                              ischaemic heart disease

                                angina

                                heart attack

                              rheumatic fever

                        if secondary to chronic left ventricular failure

                              progressive exertional dyspnoea

                              orthopnoea

                              paroxysmal nocturnal dyspnoea

                            abdominal swelling due to ascites

Swollen legs

- *renal disease*
    - acute nephritis
        - recent sore throat
        - fever, malaise
        - haematuria
        - oliguria/anuria
    - nephrotic syndrome
        - puffiness of face/eyes, especially early morning
        - past history
            - sore throat
            - kidney disease
            - diabetes
            - collagen disease
        - drugs
            - gold/penicillamine for rheumatoid arthritis
            - tridione for epilepsy
- *hepatic disease*
    - past history
        - jaundice
        - hepatitis
        - alcoholism
        - gallstones
        - drugs causing *chronic* hepatitis
            - isoniazid for tuberculosis
            - nitrofurantoin for urinary infection
            - dantrolene for spasticity
            - methyldopa for hypertension
    - symptoms of cirrhosis
        - may be asymptomatic
        - weakness
        - weight loss
        - anorexia, nausea, vomiting

 upper abdominal discomfort

  hepatomegaly

  splenomegaly

 if varices

  haematemesis/melaena

  symptoms of anaemia from GI blood loss

 bleeding tendency

  bruising

  nose bleeds

  menorrhagia

 if hepatic failure ensues

  drowsiness

  confusion

  difficulty in speaking

  unsteadiness

additional symptoms of chronic active hepatitis

 polyarthralgia

 dry eyes (Sjögren's syndrome)

 pleurisy

 precordial chest pain – pericarditis

Miscellaneous conditions – symptomatology

- anaemia

 breathlessness

 palpitations

 excessive fatigue

 dizziness

 pallor

- pretibial myxoedema – past history of treated thyrotoxicosis

- history of

  menopause – oestrogen treatment

  rheumatoid arthritis/chronic asthma treatment with steroids or NSAID

  hypertension – treatment with vasodilators producing oedema

Examination

Possible findings are shown in Fig. 17.3.

Investigations

Urine examination

red cells →	• acute nephritis
albumin	
mild →	• acute nephritis
> 3.5 g/24 h →	• nephrotic syndrome

Blood tests

anaemia

ESR ↑ →	• malignancy
	venous thrombosis
	obstruction by lymph nodes
	• acute nephritis
urea/creatinine ↑ →	• renal disease
serum albumin ↓ →	• nephrotic syndrome
	• chronic liver disease
liver function tests →	• chronic liver disease
	gamma G–T ↑
	alkaline phosphatase ↑
	bilirubin normal or slightly ↑
	other liver enzymes ↑
M band on electrophoresis →	• myeloma leading to amyloidosis and nephrotic syndrome

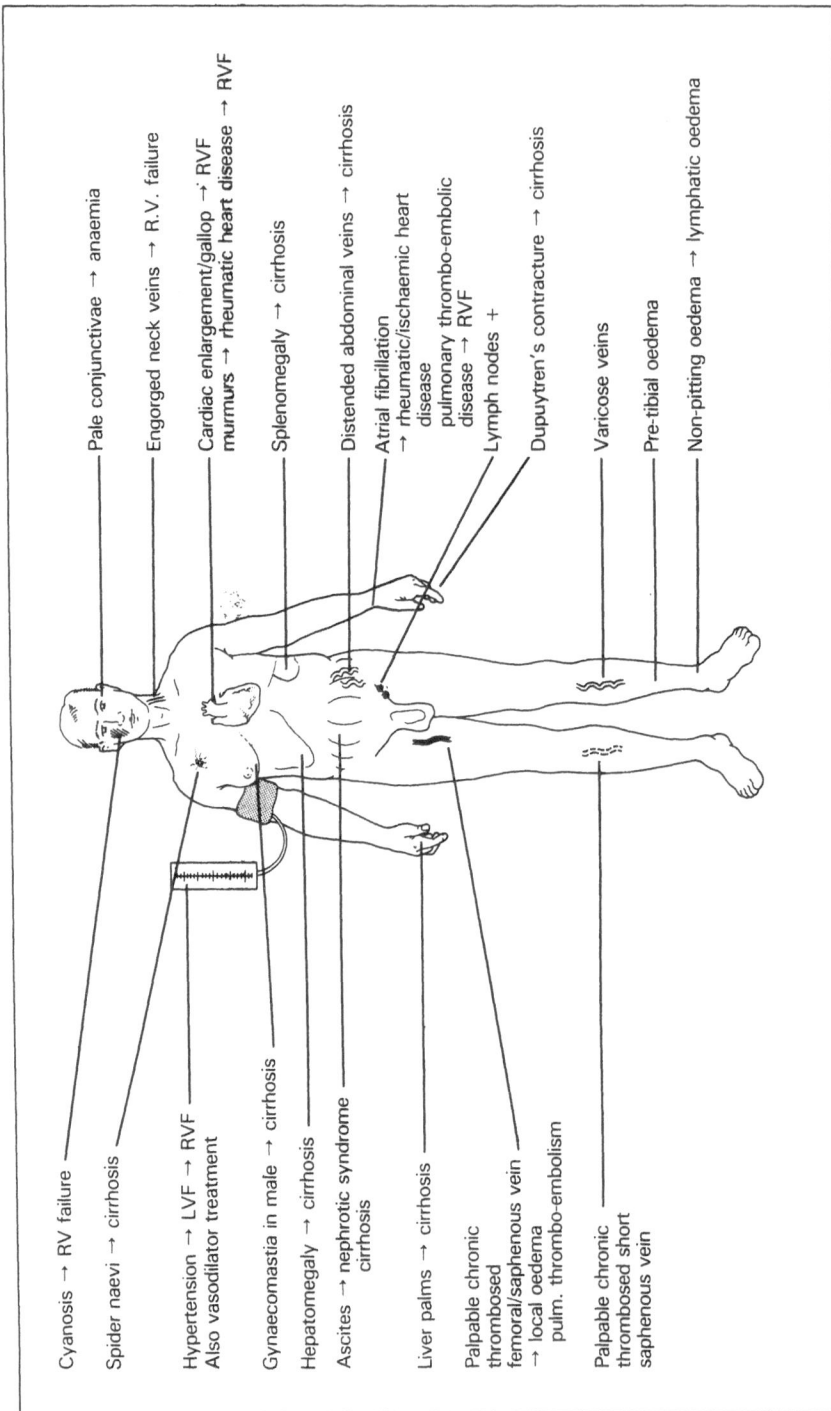

Cyanosis → RV failure

Spider naevi → cirrhosis

Hypertension → LVF → RVF
Also vasodilator treatment

Gynaecomastia in male → cirrhosis

Hepatomegaly → cirrhosis

Ascites → nephrotic syndrome
cirrhosis

Liver palms → cirrhosis

Palpable chronic
thrombosed
femoral/saphenous vein
→ local oedema
pulm. thrombo-embolism

Palpable chronic
thrombosed short
saphenous vein

Pale conjunctivae → anaemia

Engorged neck veins → R.V. failure

Cardiac enlargement/gallop → RVF
murmurs → rheumatic heart disease → RVF

Splenomegaly → cirrhosis

Distended abdominal veins → cirrhosis

Atrial fibrillation
→ rheumatic/ischaemic heart
disease
pulmonary thrombo-embolic
disease → RVF

Lymph nodes +

Dupuytren's contracture → cirrhosis

Varicose veins

Pre-tibial oedema

Non-pitting oedema → lymphatic oedema

Fig. 17.3   *Possible findings in swollen legs*

Radiology

phlebography   • deep vein thrombosis

chest X-ray   • chronic lung disease

     • cardiac enlargement

         hypertension – boot shaped

         rheumatic heart disease

           enlarged L. atrium

           enlarged L. ventricle

         pulmonary hypertension

           enlarged pulmonary conus

           Kerley B lines

         thromboembolic disease

         pulmonary plethora due to congenital septal defect

IVP   • may show large kidney in nephrotic syndrome

lymphangiogram   • Milroy's disease

     • secondary lymphatic obstruction

CT scan   • chronic liver disease

Electrocardiogram   • LV hypertrophy

         hypertension

         rheumatic heart

     • bifid P wave → mitral stenosis

     • ischaemic changes → RV failure

Ultrasound   • chronic liver disease

Biopsy   • liver – cirrhosis

     • kidney – nephrotic syndrome

Specific conditions

Idiopathic oedema

- common disorder
- exclusively in women
- no evidence of cardiac, renal or hepatic disease
- may be cyclical or persistent – often premenstrual
- may affect face and hands as well as feet
- may be accompanied by headache, irritability, depression
- often has postural factor – marked pitting oedema of legs when standing
- main abnormality is retention of salt of unknown cause – theories:

  undue postural fall of BP

  altered capillary permeability

  increased aldosterone secretion

  increased oestrogen/progesterone

  hypoproteinaemia

- treatment difficult
- diuretics can aggravate

  enhanced postural effects by fluid depletion

  potassium depletion → weakness

- mechanical support (stockings) best

Pitfalls in diagnosis

- Omitting to confirm deep vein thrombosis objectively with venography – clinical diagnosis is highly unreliable.
- Forgetting that a ruptured Baker's cyst produces identical symptoms and signs to an acute deep vein thrombosis.
- Overlooking drug therapy as a cause of leg oedema especially vasodilator antihypertensive drugs such as hydrallazine, prazosin and nifedipine (Adalat)
- Forgetting to look for the systemic signs of cirrhosis in patients with leg oedema such as liver palms, spider naevi, gynaecomastia, etc.
- Forgetting that recurrent venous thrombosis may be a manifestation of occult intra-abdominal malignancy especially carcinoma of the pancreas.
- Forgetting the possibility of amyloid nephrosis in a patient with chronic suppurative lung disease, e.g. bronchiectasis who develops leg oedema

Useful practical points

- If there is unilateral leg oedema or asymmetrical bilateral oedema, the cause is likely to be localized obstruction in the venous system from deep vein thrombosis.
- The important distinguishing feature between lymphatic and venous obstruction is that lymphatic obstruction is non-pitting.
- Remember to look for oedema over the sacrum rather than in the legs in a patient at prolonged recumbency.
- Puffiness in the face, especially round the eyes, on waking in the morning is suggestive of nephrotic syndrome.
- The essential requirements to diagnose nephrotic syndrome are generalized oedema, albuminuria > 3.5 g in 24 hours and hypo-albuminaemia (< 30 g/litre).

Case challenge

A 42-year-old housewife presented with a 3 month history of increasing swelling of the legs. She had not noticed any breathlessness, she denied any current urinary symptoms and apart from an increase in weight over the period of the leg swelling, there were no other relevant symptoms.

In the past history she had been prone to recurrent sore throat in childhood but denied rheumatic fever, growing pains or chorea. She had been excused sport at school as she was told she had a murmur but had not experienced any heart trouble since. Her periods were heavy and she had noticed some hot flushes for which her doctor had prescribed some 'hormone' tablets several months ago.

She did not smoke and drank alcohol on social occasions only.

The findings of examination are shown in Fig. 17.4.

Questions
: Give five possible diagnoses to account for the oedema.

  How would you distinguish between them?

Possible diagnoses
: - anaemia
  - venous insufficiency
  - rheumatic heart disease with heart failure
  - oestrogen therapy
  - nephrotic syndrome

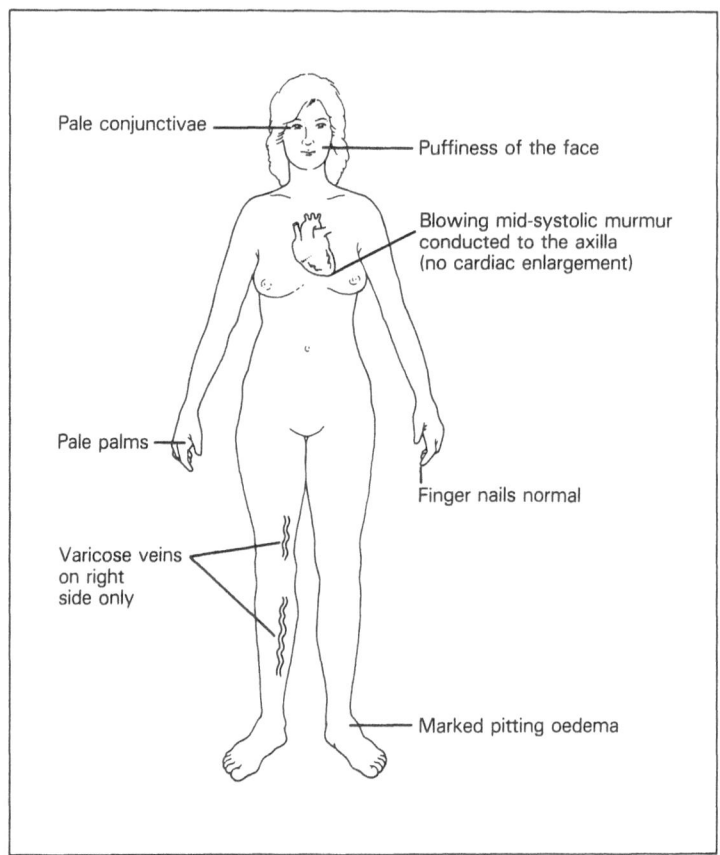

Fig. 17.4   *Examination findings in case challenge*

Anaemia

For	history	• menorrhagia
	exam	• anaemia found
		• systolic murmur (can occur in anaemia)
Against	history	• nil
	exam	• no koilonychia – oedema due to anaemia, usually occurs after long-standing anaemia (which often leads to koilonychia)
		• facial oedema is never due to anaemia
Tests		• a blood count will indicate the type and severity of the anaemia – if long standing it should show a microcytic hypochromic blood picture

Venous insufficiency

For	history	• nil
	exam	• varicose veins in right leg
Against	history	• no complaints which might indicate previous venous thrombosis
	exam	• the oedema is bilateral but the varicose veins are unilateral
Tests		• venography

        extent of varicosities

        presence of incompetent valves

        previous thrombosis

Rheumatic heart disease with heart failure

For	history	• recurrent sore throats
		• murmur in childhood
	exam	• murmur of mitral incompetence
Against	history	• no breathlessness
	exam	• no evidence of either left ventricular failure (crepitations, gallop rhythm), or right ventricular failure (cyanosis, distended jugular veins)
		• facial oedema unusual
Tests		• chest X-ray

        left atrial enlargement

        left ventricular enlargement

        pulmonary hypertension

• ECG

        bifid P wave (L atrial hypertrophy)

        left ventricular hypertrophy

• echocardiogram – typical echoes from a diseased mitral valve

Oestrogen therapy

For	history	• hot flushes
		• started on 'hormones' by GP
	exam	• there are no helpful signs of oestrogen therapy
Against	history	• nil
	exam	• nil
Tests		• there are no specific investigations
		• the best test is to stop the oestrogen and see what happens to the oedema

Nephrotic syndrome

For	history	• recurrent sore throats – could have led to the development of nephritis
		• absence of breathlessness excludes a cardiac cause and is typical of oedema due to nephrotic syndrome
	exam	• facial oedema – an important sign of 'renal' oedema
Against	history	• nil
	exam	• nil
Tests		• urine – heavy albuminuria > 3.5 g/24 h
		• serum albumin $\downarrow$ – below 30 g/1
		• renal biopsy – definitive test may show:

        minimal lesion (lipoid nephrosis)

        membranous glomerulo-nephritis

        membrano-proliferative nephritis

        focal proliferative nephritis

Actual diagnosis:

Nephrotic syndrome – confirmed by renal biopsy which showed membrano-proliferative glomerulonephritis.

Treatment and outcome

The patient was treated with

frusemide 40 mg/day and spironolactone 100 mg/day to provide control of oedema

prednisolone starting with 40 mg/day for 2 weeks reducing slowly to a maintenance dose of 7.5 mg/day

She rapidly became oedema-free and maintained control of oedema on long-term prednisolone.

18 Anorexia (Loss of Appetite)

Introduction

Personal and subjective.

Differentiate between

appetite – a pleasant sensation

hunger – unpleasant

not eating – a negative and wilful act

Capacities for eating have wide personal range.

Appetite may be affected by:

mood

health

sickness

Well-meaning relatives may over-stress importance of eating in health and in sickness.

Causes of anorexia

Organic

acute minor illnesses of all types, e.g. flu, gastroenteritis, migraine

gastrointestinal

- gastritis

    acute

        alcohol

        drugs

    chronic

- gastric ulcer
- carcinoma of stomach
- postgastrectomy syndrome

451

hepatic	• acute hepatitis
	• chronic hepatitis/cirrhosis
	• chronic pancreatitis
cardiorespiratory	• congestive failure
	• chronic lung disease
chronic renal failure	
endocrine	• Addison's disease
	• hypopituitarism
	• hyperparathyroidism
chronic infections (TB etc.)	
malignancy anywhere	

Functional
- depression
- anxiety
- psychoses
- dementias
- anorexia nervosa
- negative phase – 'not eating' in children

Others
- drugs
  - digitalis
  - alcohol
  - narcotics
- lead poisoning

Grades of severity

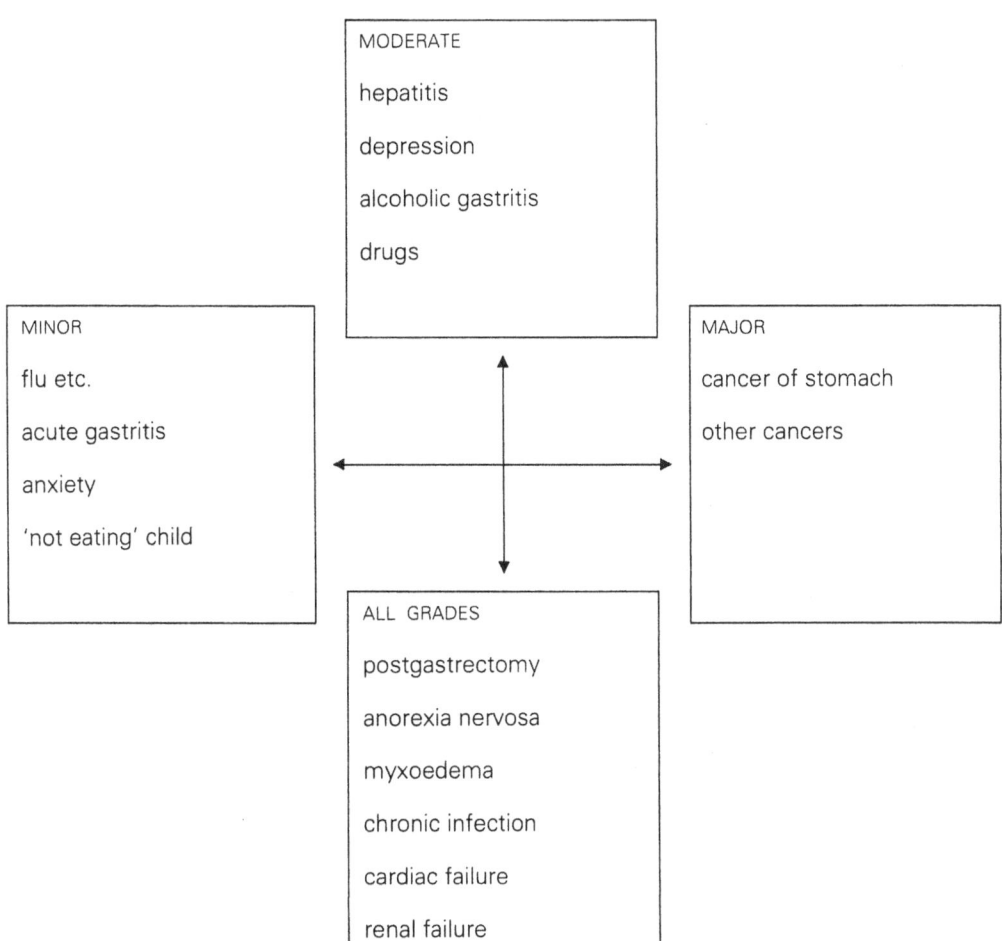

Frequency

Annual prevalence of 'anorexia' *in practice population of 2500*	
Acute minor (post-flu etc.)	25
Anxiety-depression	15
Alcohol	5
Cardiac	2
Hepatitis	1
Cancer of stomach	1 in 2 y
Anorexia nervosa	1 in 5 y
Other major illnesses	3
All	50

Age incidence

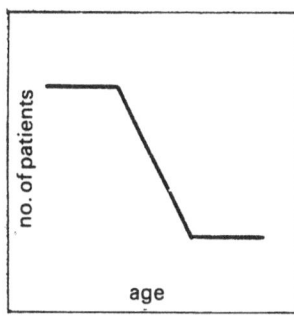

- not-eating child
- post-infections
- anorexia nervosa

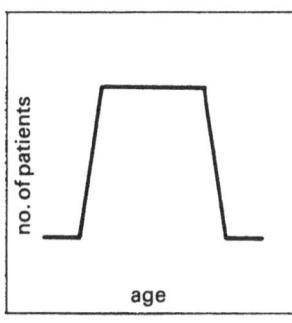

- depression
- alcohol
- hepatitis
- migraine

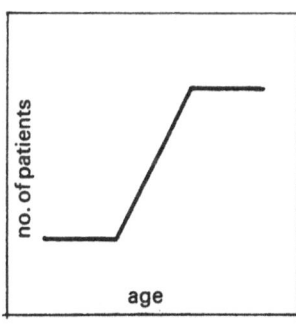

- cancer of stomach
- senile dementia
- gastric ulcer
- cardiac failure
- drugs

Diagnostic approach

History

Because anorexia may be a symptom of many diverse conditions the diagnostic approach through the history is based on the presence of associated and distinctive symptoms of the various conditions involved.

gastritis	• acute
	ingestion of
	aspirin
	non-steroidal anti-inflammatory drugs
	steroids
	alcohol
	epigastric pain/heartburn
	nausea
	• chronic
	often asymptomatic
	anorexia is a possible symptom
	symptoms of pernicious anaemia
	anaemia itself
	neurological
	paraesthesiae
	leg weakness
	leg inco-ordination
	cerebellar ataxia
	pseudo-dementia
gastric carcinoma	• epigastric discomfort unrelated to meals
	• vomiting if obstruction
	• loss of weight – prominent
	• symptoms of anaemia
gastric ulcer	• epigastric pain soon after eating
	• rapid relief with alkalis
	• vomiting frequent – relieves pain

postgastrectomy syndromes • 'small stomach'

        early distension after eating

        reduced food intake

        loss of weight

        anorexia most frequent

• dumping – post-prandial

        drowsiness

        weakness

        nausea

        flushing

        palpitations

• hypoglycaemia – post prandial

        faintness

        weakness

        tremor

acute hepatitis • general

        fever

        rigors

        headache

        malaise

• distaste for cigarettes in smokers

• nausea/vomiting

• upper abdominal discomfort

• jaundice

• pale stools/dark urine

chronic hepatitis • persistent

        fatty food intolerance

        discomfort over liver

• active

        jaundice

        fever

        arthralgia

        bleeding, e.g. epistaxis, easy bruising

        amenorrhoea

chronic pancreatitis	• epigastric pain radiating through to back
	• pain relieved by sitting up and crouching forward
	• diarrhoea due to malabsorption – stools pale, bulky, offensive, difficult to flush away
	• diabetes (1/5)
	thirst
	polyuria
	loss of weight
	• jaundice in some patients
cardiorespiratory disease	• heart failure
	breathlessness
	frothy sputum
	swelling of ankles/legs
	history of
	cardiac ischaemia
	hypertension
	rheumatic heart disease
	• chronic lung disease
	breathlessness
	chronic productive cough
	white/grey/green sputum
	wheezing
	often heavy smokers
chronic renal failure	• previous kidney disease
	• polyuria
	• drowsiness
	• hiccups
	• pruritus
	• diarrhoea
	• twitching
	• bleeding

endocrine
- Addison's disease
  - excessive fatigue
  - postural dizziness
  - constipation/diarrhoea
  - abdominal pain in crisis
- hypopituitarism
  - history of post-partum haemorrhage
  - loss of libido
  - amenorrhoea
  - symptoms of hypothyroidism
  - symptoms of adrenal deficiency
- hyperparathyroidism
  - renal
    - colic
    - dysuria
  - musculoskeletal
    - limb weakness
    - bone pain
  - psychiatric
    - depression
    - change in personality

Examination

The examination should be directed primarily to the abdomen but a general examination may also show some helpful pointers to the diagnosis.

Possible findings are shown in Fig. 18.1

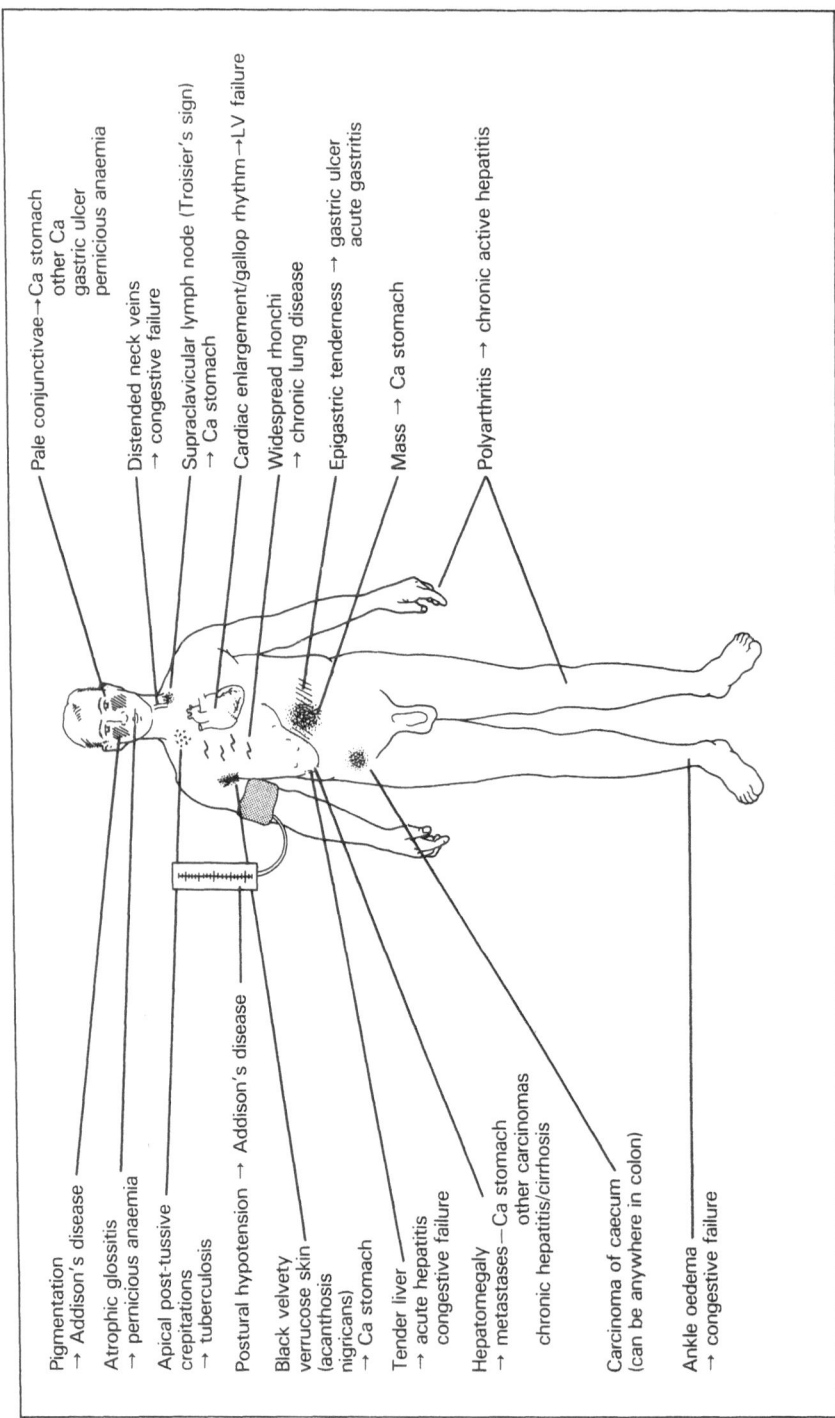

Fig. 18.1   *Possible findings on examination in patients with anorexia*

Investigation

Tests are always necessary to establish the diagnosis in a patient with anorexia

The most helpful investigation is *radiological* examination of the gastrointestinal tract

Barium meal
- gastric ulcer

  niche of barium in stomach wall

  sharply pinched out margins

  mucosal folds radiating to crater
  (Fig. 5.5a – page 113)
- carcinoma stomach

  filling defect antrum/body

  ulcer on greater curve with irregular margins

  rigid tube in diffuse scirrhus carcinoma
  (Fig. 5.5c – page 115)
- carcinoma of pancreas – widened duodenal loop
- chronic gastritis – absence of mucosal folds

Barium enema
- carcinoma of colon (Fig. 18.2)

  usually constricting lesion descending colon

  proliferative lesion

    ascending colon/caecum

    rectum

Intravenous cholangiography
- dilatation of biliary tree in carcinoma of pancreas

CT scan
- carcinoma of stomach
- carcinoma of pancreas
- chronic hepatitis/cirrhosis

The other invaluable test in the diagnosis of anorexia is *endoscopy* – the major advantage over barium studies is that a biopsy can be taken of any suspicious lesions.

Gastroscopy
- acute gastritis

  mucosal engorgement

  acute erosions

  acute haemorrhagic gastritis

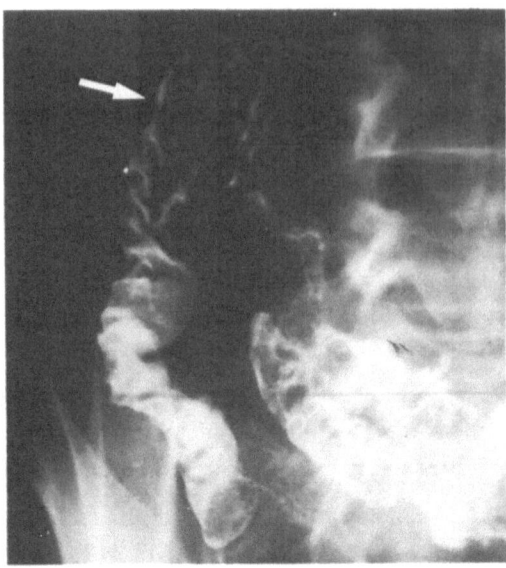

Fig. 18.2 *Barium enema showing filling defect in hepatic flexure of colon due to carcinoma (arrowed)*

- chronic gastritis
  - superficial gastritis
  - atrophic gastritis
- gastric ulcer
- gastric carcinoma
- carcinoma of pancreas – retrograde cholangio-pancreatography is carried out at gastroscopy

Colonoscopy   • carcinoma of colon

Ultrasound   • chronic pancreatitis
- carcinoma pancreas
- cirrhosis/chronic hepatitis

Radio-isotope scan   • chronic hepatitis/cirrhosis
- pancreatitis
- pancreatic carcinoma

Other relevant tests
  blood tests
    ESR ↑   • malignancy – non-specific test
    anaemia   • blood loss from cancer in gastrointestinal tract
                                 • chronic renal failure
                                 • malignancy anywhere
                                 • chronic infections, e.g. tuberculosis
                                 • lead poisoning
    liver function   • acute hepatitis
                                    SGPT ↑
                                    bilirubin ↑
                                    alkaline phosphatase slightly ↑
                                 • chronic hepatitis
                                    SGPT ↑
                                    γ-GT ↑
                                    alkaline phosphatase ↑
                                    bilirubin ↑
                                    albumin ↓
                                 • chronic pancreatitis – bilirubin ↑ if obstruction
    blood sugar ↑   • chronic pancreatitis
                                 • carcinoma of pancreas
              ↓   • hypopituitarism
    blood urea ↑   • chronic renal failure
    hepatitis A/B antigen/antibodies
    auto-antibodies   • chronic active hepatitis
      (types   • primary biliary cirrhosis
        smooth muscle
        antimitochondrial
        antinuclear)
    serum cortisol ↓   • Addison's disease
                                 • hypopituitarism
    serum calcium ↑   • hyperparathyroidism

alkaline phosphatase ↑	• hyperparathyroidism
	• hepatitis
Na ↑ / K ↓	• Addisonian crisis

urine tests

glycosuria	• chronic pancreatitis
	• carcinoma pancreas (1/5)
bile pigments	• hepatitis
	• pancreatitis
lead content ↑	• lead poisoning
protein/casts	• chronic renal failure

stool examination

occult blood	• gastric ulcer
	• carcinoma – stomach
	colon
bulky, offensive, floating	• chronic pancreatitis
clay coloured	• obstruction due to carcinoma pancreas
liver biopsy	• chronic active hepatitis
	infiltration lymphocytes/plasma cells
	hepatic cell regeneration (rosettes)
	fibrous bridges
	piecemeal necrosis

Specific conditions

Anorexia nervosa

- • mainly affects young girls
- • psychology
  - obsessive fear of being fat
  - fear of growing up and accepting responsibility
  - hostile relationship with family
  - emotional trauma in past
  - sometimes preoccupation with sex
- • symptoms
  - won't eat
  - may induce self-vomiting
  - amenorrhoea often

Anorexia

- signs

    gross emaciation

    bird-like 'twittering' activity

    pubic/axillary hair present (unlike hypopituitarism)

- tests

    urinary gonadotrophin ↓ (LH, FSH)

    thyroid function

        thyroxine level normal

        tri-iodothyronine level ↓

    growth hormone level and cortisol levels are normal or high – unlike hypopituitarism where both levels are low

Pitfalls in diagnosis

- The possibility of a gastric carcinoma developing in a patient with pernicious anaemia is often overlooked.
- Omitting to check-up by barium meal, or better, gastroscopy on whether a gastric ulcer has healed with treatment because it is difficult sometimes to distinguish between a benign and malignant ulcer.
- Forgetting that anorexia may be an important symptom in Addison's disease or hypopituitarism.
- Not thinking about chronic pancreatitis when a diabetic patient presents – offensive bulky stools will help in the diagnosis.

Useful practical points

- Anorexia and weight loss in a middle-aged patient should be regarded as stomach cancer until proved otherwise.
- Fluctuation of epigastric pain and relief with alkalis does not exclude the diagnosis of stomach cancer.
- The diagnosis of gastritis should only be made relative to ingestion of gastric irritants such as drugs and alcohol – it is not a diagnosis to be 'conjured up' to appease a patient with vague indigestion which cannot be explained otherwise.
- The presence of pubic and axillary hair helps to distinguish anorexia nervosa from hypopituitarism, since both produce amenorrhoea.
- Diabetes may be the initial presentation of carcinoma of the pancreas – it occurs in 20% of those patients.
- A change in the pattern of long-standing indigestion in gastric ulcer should suggest malignancy.

Case challenge

A 63-year-old lady presented with a 6 months history of increasing weakness, malaise, breathlessness, palpitations, anorexia and loss of weight. Other symptoms which emerged on direct enquiry included postural dizziness, pain in the neck, pins and needles and numbness in her feet ('as if I'm walking on air') and periodic upper abdominal discomfort not particularly related to meals.

She had a past history of gastric ulcer for which she had a year's course of cimetidine and she has had no recurrence of the ulcer symptoms since she finished treatment about 3 years previously. She had also been found to have high blood pressure 10 years earlier and had been on continuous treatment with Aldomet since. Finally there was a past history of pulmonary tuberculosis when she was 22, treated in a sanatorium for 1 year.

The findings of examination are shown in Fig. 18.3.

Questions

What are the possible diagnoses to account for the anorexia?

How would you distinguish between them?

Are there any supplementary diagnoses?

Possible diagnoses

- recurrence of gastric ulcer
- gastric carcinoma
- Addison's disease

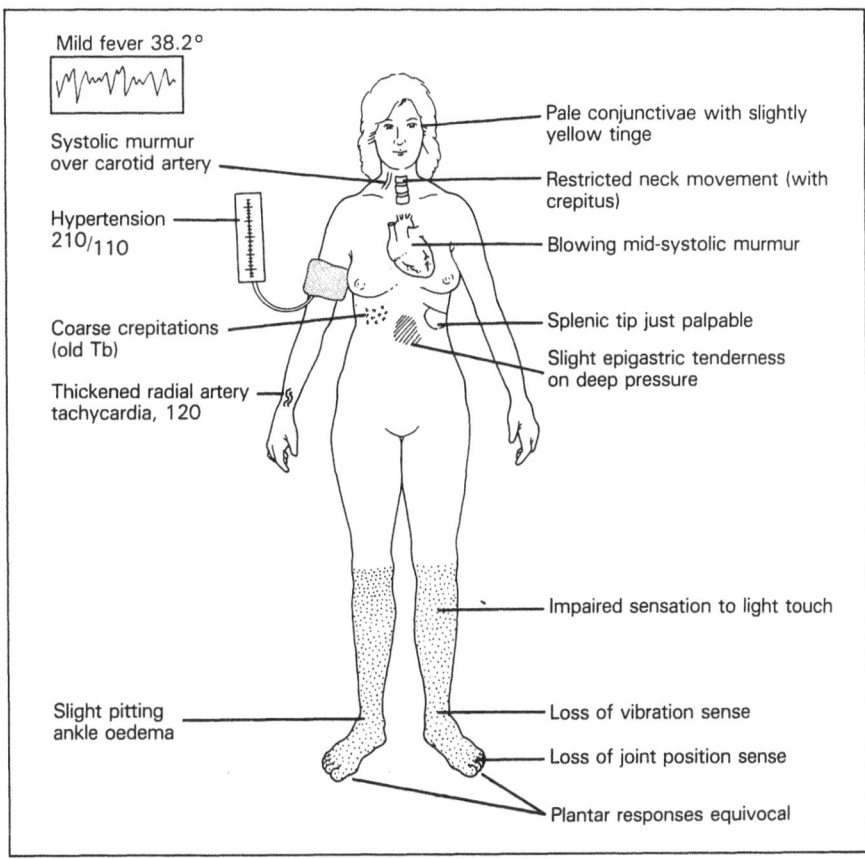

Fig. 18.3   *Signs in case challenge*

Recurrence of gastric ulcer

For	history	• previous gastric ulcer
		• upper abdominal discomfort has recurred
		• anorexia can result from gastric ulcer
	exam	• anaemic – could be blood loss from an ulcer
		• slight epigastric tenderness
Against	history	• no relationship of upper abdominal discomfort to meals
	exam	• nil

Tests
- barium meal
- gastroscopy – better than barium meal since more accurate and allows biopsy
- blood count for anaemia
- stool examination for occult blood

Gastric cancer

For   history
- anorexia
- loss of weight
- abdominal discomfort unrelated to meals

         exam
- anaemia – from occult blood loss
- fever – common in malignancy
- epigastric tenderness
- evidence of polyneuropathy – can be associated with carcinoma

Against   history
- perhaps rather long at 6 months for gastric cancer – progress is usually more rapid

         exam
- no abdominal mass
- no liver enlargement
- no supraclavicular lymph node (Troisier's sign)

Tests
- gastroscopy best – diagnostic
- barium meal – may show

    ulcer

    filling defect

    rigid 'tube'
- blood count – anaemia
- ESR ↑
- stool examination for occult blood

Addison's disease

For	history	• previous pulmonary tuberculosis – common cause of Addison's disease in the past
		• anorexia can be prominent symptom
		• fatigue is important symptom
		• postural hypotension occurs
	exam	• nil
Against	history	• hypertension (Addison's disease) leads to hypotension
	exam	• no pigmentation
		• no hypotension
Tests		• serum cortisol level with ACTH/Synacthen stimulation to decide whether primary or secondary
		• Na/K serum levels only relevant in Addisonian crisis when Na ↑ and K ↓
		• X-ray abdomen for adrenal calcification

Supplementary diagnoses

Vertebro-basilar ischaemia

causing postural dizziness

produced by
- cerebral ateriosclerosis resulting from hypertension
- carotid stenosis in the neck
- cervical spondylosis

Pernicious anaemia

- anaemia
- icteric tinge in conjunctivae
- peripheral neuropathy
- early subacute combined degeneration of spinal cord

    posterior column involvement

    pyramidal involvement (equivocal plantars)

- splenomegaly
- fever – if not due to cancer
- tests

    serum vitamin B12 level

    bone marrow examination for megaloblastic change

    Schilling test for vitamin B12 absorption

Actual diagnoses:

Carcinoma of stomach – seen on gastroscopy and confirmed on biopsy

Pernicious anaemia – this condition predisposes to the development of gastric carcinoma

---

Treatment and outcome

An exploratory laparotomy was carried out, the diagnosis confirmed and the condition considered inoperable because of extensive involvement of lymph glands and two obvious metastases in the liver.

She survived only a further 3 months.

19 Jaundice

Introduction

Although not a common sign in practice jaundice raises many possible causes.

Early diagnosis of jaundice rests more on clinical acumen than on batteries of tests, which have to be complementary and supportive of clinical hypotheses.

Causes of jaundice (Fig. 19.1)

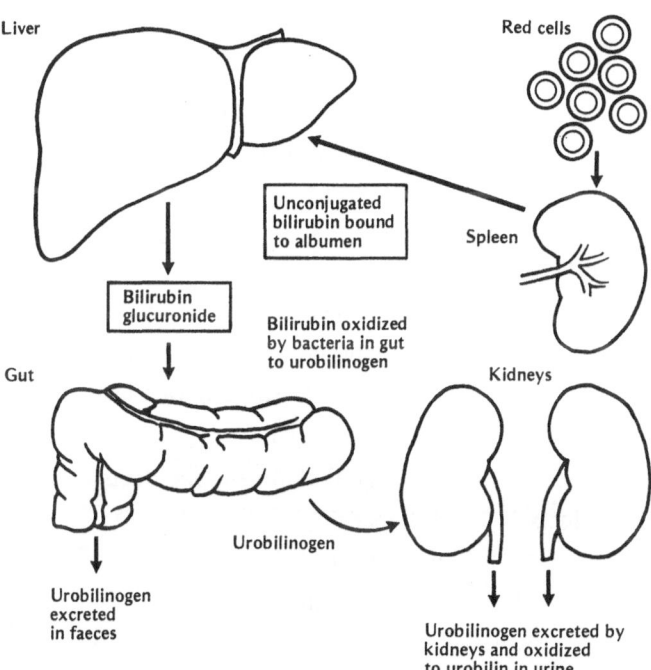

Fig. 19.1   *Jaundice – pathways in bile metabolism*

471

3 groups of common causes

- hepatocellular
- obstructive (cholestatic)
- haemolytic

Hepatocellular

- hepatitis – acute/chronic
- cirrhosis
- drugs

    mono-amine oxidase inhibitors, e.g. Nardil

    phenylbutazone (now withdrawn)/indomethacin

    hydrallazine

    phenytoin

    sulphonamides

    methyldopa

    nitrofurantoin

    isoniazid

    dantrolene

- infections

    glandular fever

    leptospirosis

- metabolic – Wilson's disease (hepato-lenticular degeneration)

Obstructive (cholestatic) jaundice

bile duct obstruction

- gallstones
- carcinoma head of pancreas
- carcinoma Ampulla of Vater
- enlarged glands
- congenital atresia bile ducts

intrahepatic cholestasis

- hepatitis
- cirrhosis

    alcoholic

    primary biliary

Jaundice

- drugs
    - tricyclic antidepressives
    - phenothiazines
    - benzodiazepines
    - gold salts
    - chlorpropamide
    - tolbutamide
    - oral contraceptives
- sclerosing cholangitis
- other
    - metastases
    - granuloma, e.g. sarcoid
    - amyloid
    - abscess

acute cholecystitis
Haemolytic jaundice
neonatal
hereditary

- congenital spherocytosis/ellipsocytosis
- thalassaemia
- sickle cell anaemia

acquired

- auto-immune disease
- drugs
    - methyldopa
    - quinine/quinidine
- cold haemoglobinuria
- hypersplenism – any cause
- mismatched blood transfusion
- infections, e.g. malaria

Grades of severity

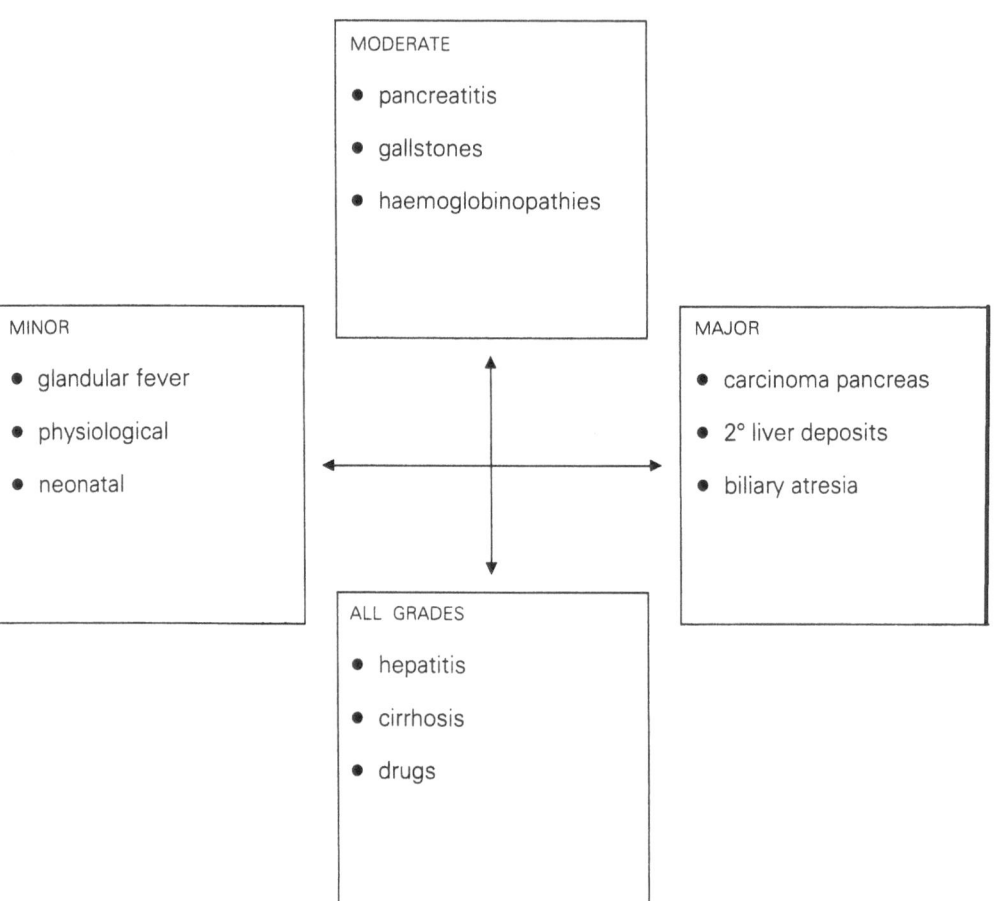

MODERATE

- pancreatitis
- gallstones
- haemoglobinopathies

MINOR

- glandular fever
- physiological
- neonatal

MAJOR

- carcinoma pancreas
- 2° liver deposits
- biliary atresia

ALL GRADES

- hepatitis
- cirrhosis
- drugs

Age incidence

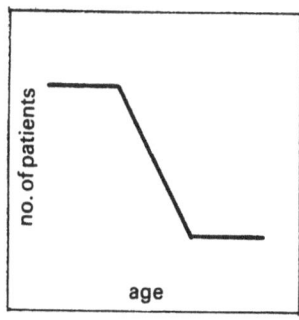

- physiological (neonatal)
- hypothyroid
- haemoglobinopathies
- biliary atresia
- (drugs)

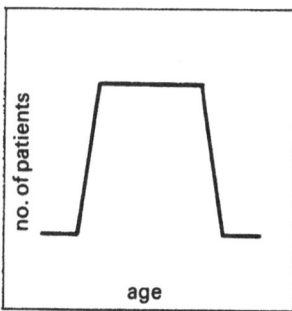

- hepatitis
- glandular fever
- gallstones
- cirrhosis
- pancreatitis
- (drugs)
- alcohol

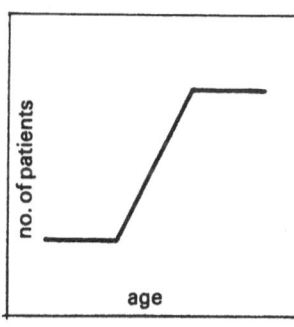

- carcinoma pancreas
- 2° deposits liver
- (drugs)

Frequency

Annual prevalence of jaundice in a general practice population of 2500 (by cause)	
Hepatitis	1–2 per year
Gallstones	1 every 3 years
Carcinoma pancreas	1 every 5 years
Cirrhosis	1 every 5 years
Pancreatitis	1 every 7 years
Drugs	1 every 10 years
All jaundice	2–3 cases

Diagnosis approach

History

Abdominal pain

   severe colicky pain in
R. hypochondrium →   • gallstones

   severe constant pain in
R.hypochondrium →   • gallstones

   pain in R.hypochondrium
to R.shoulder tip or
R.infrascapular area →   • cholecystitis

   dull upper abdominal
ache →   • acute hepatitis

   epigastric pain → back   • cancer pancreas

Colour of stools/urine

   pale (clay-coloured)
stools →   • obstructive jaundice

   dark urine →   • obstructive jaundice

Associated symptoms

   anorexia/nausea/
vomiting →   • hepatocellular disease

   fever →   • acute viral hepatitis

                  • drug induced hepatitis

   severe sore throat →   • infectious mononucleosis with hepatitis

   distaste for smoking → • acute viral hepatitis

   pruritus →   • cholestatic jaundice

   diarrhoea/blood in stools →• inflammatory bowel disease associated with chronic active hepatitis

   polyarthralgia }
dry eyes   } → • chronic active hepatitis

Past history – the relevant factors which suggest the possibility of viral hepatitis are:

- recent transfusions/inoculations
- contact with a jaundiced patient
- recent skin tattoos
- recent travel abroad to the Tropics suggests possible malaria
- any therapeutic drugs which may be hepatotoxic

Personal history

drug abuse →   • viral hepatitis

homosexuality →   • viral hepatitis

alcoholism →   • alcoholic cirrhosis

Occupation

medical/nursing →   • viral hepatitis

other contact with blood or blood products →   • viral hepatitis

sewage workers/farmers → • leptospirosis through contact with rats

Family history

haemolytic anaemia/jaundice →   • hereditary spherocytosis or haemoglobinopathies

splenomegaly from any cause

Examination

Possible examination findings are shown in Fig. 19.2

Investigations

Urine examination

examination for bile pigments is helpful in distinguishing the three types of jaundice –

	Haemolytic	Hepatocellular	Obstructive
Bilirubin	−	+ +	+ +
Urobilinogen	+ + +	+ +	−

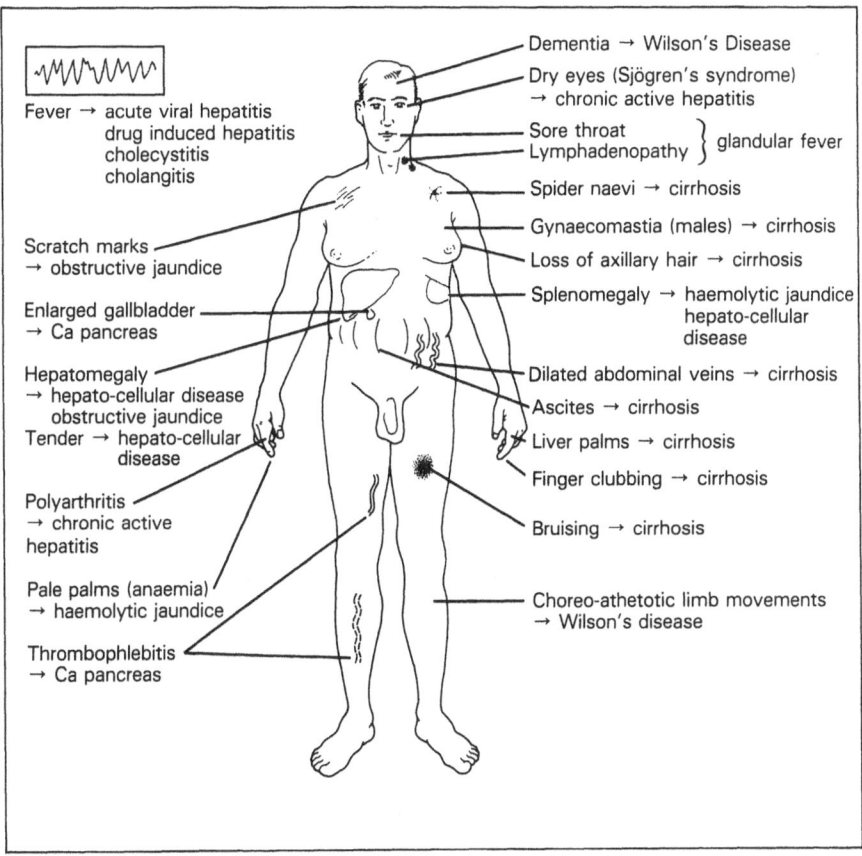

Fig. 19.2   *Possible findings on examination in jaundice*

Liver function tests

value of specific tests

- bilirubin – degree of jaundice
- akaline phosphatase – degree of obstruction
- transaminases – degree of liver cell damage
- albumin – productive capacity of the liver

	Haemolytic	Hepatocellular	Obstructive
Bilirubin	+ (unconjugated)	+ (mainly) conjugated)	+ + (mainly conjugated)
Alkaline phosphatase	normal	+	+ +
Transaminases (AST, ALT)	normal	+ +	+
Albumin	normal	reduced	normal

Differentiation between the three types of jaundice

Other blood tests

blood count

anaemia →
- marked in haemolytic disease
- mild in hepatocellular disease

leucocytosis →
- hepatocellular disease with active inflammation

leucopenia →
- hepatocellular disease with hypersplenism

thrombocytopenia →
- hepatocellular disease with hypersplenism

prothrombin time

reduced and not affected by vitamin K injections →
- severe hepatocellular disease

slightly reduced and improved with vitamin K →
- obstructive jaundice

serum auto-antibodies →
- in chronic liver disease

	Antinuclear	Antismooth muscle	Mitochondrial
Chronic active hepatitis	+ +	+ +	+
Primary biliary cirrhosis	+	+ +	+ + +
Alcoholic cirrhosis	±	−	−
Obstruction common bile duct	−	−	±

virus studies – antibody/antigen studies are helpful in detecting hepatitis A, B and non-A – non-B

Radiology

plain X-ray abdomen
- size of liver/spleen
- gallstones (10% opaque)
- ascites

chest X-ray – cancer lung (with liver metastases)

barium meal
- oesophageal varices due to cirrhosis
- widened duodenal loop – cancer pancreas
- carcinoma stomach (with liver metastases)

transhepatic percutaneous cholangiography
- dilated biliary tree in cholestasis
- site of obstruction

endoscopic retrograde cholangiopancreatography
- may show cancer pancreas

CT scan
- cirrhosis
- metastases in liver
- carcinoma pancreas
- bile duct obstruction

Ultrasound
- biliary dilatation
- cirrhosis
- metastases in the liver

Liver biopsy

this is the definitive test in deciding the nature of liver disease

hazardous in the severely jaundiced patient because of risk of bleeding (due to low prothrombin levels) – may or may not be correctable with vitamin K

detects
- chronic active hepatitis
  - infiltration lymphocytes/plasma cells
  - piecemeal necrosis
  - regeneration (rosettes)
  - fibrous bridges
- chronic persistent hepatitis
  - mainly portal involvement
  - slight fibrosis only

- primary biliary cirrhosis
    - periductal granulomata
    - proliferation of bile ducts
    - piecemeal necrosis
    - fibrosis
- alcoholic cirrhosis (micronodular)
    - multilobular involvement
    - regenerating nodules (1mm/size)
    - regular septa

Specific conditions

Viral hepatitis (types A and B)

Type A

- due to picornavirus group of enteroviruses
- highly infectious
    - spread from contaminated stools – oral route
    - also from homosexual practices
    - occasionally from blood transfusions
- children often affected – bad hygiene important
- incubation one month
- symptoms
    - prodromata few days to 2 weeks
        - headache, rigors, malaise
        - anorexia, nausea, vomiting, diarrhoea
        - distaste for cigarettes, pruritus
    - upper abdominal discomfort
    - jaundice
    - pale stools/dark urine
- signs
    - mild fever, e.g. 38.5°C
    - enlarged tender liver (50%)
    - palpable spleen (10–15%)

Jaundice

- tests

  urine: bilirubin +

                 urobilinogen +

  liver function: aminotransferase > 400 u/ml

                 bilirubin ↑

                 alkaline phosphatase slightly ↑

                 prothrombin ↓ severe cases

- hepatitis A-antibody is definitive test

Type B

- caused by DNA-containing virus
- spread

  blood transfusion

  inoculation

  tattooing

  acupuncture

  drug abuse – contaminated needles

  homosexual practices

  transplacental at childbirth

- incubation 3 months
- symptoms

  gastrointestinal symptoms similar to Type A

  transient rashes including urticaria

  polyarthralgia/myalgia

  jaundice

  pale stools/dark urine

- signs

  similar to type A

  lymphadenopathy may occur

- tests

  urine – as in type A

  liver function – as in type A

  hepatitis B surface antigen HB_s Ag is the definitive test

483

Gallstones

- common in N. America, Europe, Australia
- uncommon India, Africa, Far East
- M : F 3 : 1 under 40 years old equal in elderly
- types
    cholesterol (75%)
    calcium salts of bilirubin
    bilirubin
- predisposing factors
    cholesterol stones
        obesity – especially when dieting
        hyperlipidaemia
        clofibrate therapy
        malabsorption states
        oestrogen treatment
            contraceptive
            menopause
    pigment stones
        haemolytic conditions
            alcoholic cirrhosis
            biliary infection
- symptoms
    many are asymptomatic
    recurrent biliary colic
    jaundice with pale stools/dark urine if stone
    impacts in common bile duct
    colicky abdominal pain and vomiting if stone
    impacts in terminal ileum
- signs
    fever if associated cholecystitis
    tenderness over gallbladder with positive
    Murphy's signs
    jaundice if stone in common bile duct

- tests
    - plain X-ray abdomen – stone (10–30% opaque)
    - cholecystogram
        - non-opaque stones
        - non-functioning gallbladder
    - ultrasound – dilated bile ducts
    - transhepatic cholangiography
        - dilated ducts
        - site of obstruction
    - ERCP – if stone low in common bile duct
    - CT scan
        - dilated ducts seen in up to 90% of cases
        - may show stone
    - ultrasound
    - isotope scan

Cirrhosis

- causes
    - alcoholism
    - chronic active hepatitis
    - primary biliary cirrhosis
    - haemachromatosis
    - cryptogenic (no cause found)
- symptoms
    - anorexia, nausea, vomiting
    - abdominal swelling
    - swelling of legs
    - bleeding
        - spontaneous bruising
        - from bowel
    - if hepatic failure – drowsiness
                              confusion
                              coma
- signs – see Fig. 19.3

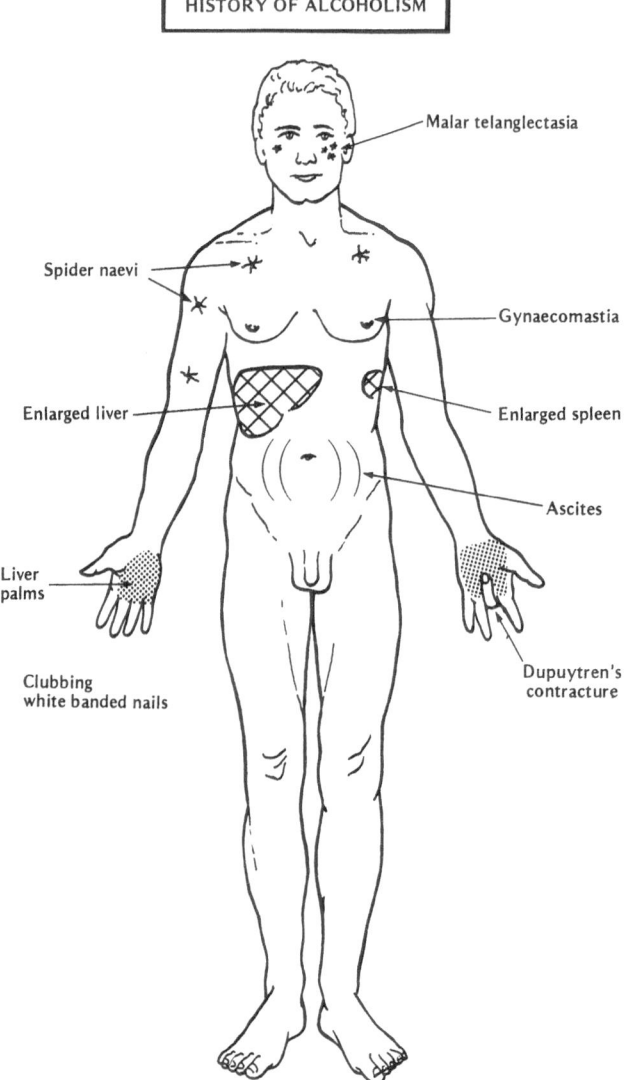

Fig. 19.3 *Features of cirrhosis*

Jaundice

- tests

urine:	urobilinogen +
	bilirubin ±
liver function:	aminotransferase +
	alkaline phosphatase +
	albumin ↓

  serum globulin ↑

  prothrombin ↓

  auto-antibodies may be found in

    chronic active hepatitis

    primary biliary cirrhosis

  liver biopsy – definitive test

  ultrasound

  CT scan

  isotope scan

  plain X-ray abdomen – stone (10% opaque)

  cholecystogram

    non-opaque stones

    non-functioning gall bladder

  ultrasound – dilated bile ducts

  transhepatic cholangiography

    dilated ducts

    site of obstruction

  ERCP – if stone low in common bile duct

  CT scan

    dilated ducts seen in up to 90% of cases

    may show stone

  liver biopsy – definitive test

Pitfalls in diagnosis

- Omitting to listen for a systolic murmur over the liver which may be heard in alcoholic hepatitis and hepatoma.
- Failing to register mentally that the patient has gynaecomastia indicative of cirrhosis – especially if he is obese and has a fat chest wall.
- Omitting to look for the flapping tremor indicative of developing hepatic failure, in a patient with jaundice – untreated the outcome is likely to be fatal.
- Excluding jaundice by looking at the conjunctivae in artificial light.

Useful practical points

- Always enquire for previous drug therapy in any patient with jaundice.
- Remember that most drugs affecting the liver produce only transient hepatotoxicity which disappears on stopping the drug but several drugs can produce permanent damage by inducing chronic active hepatitis – isoniazid, nitrofurantoin, dantrolene and methyl dopa.
- A distaste for smoking followed by jaundice suggests acute viral hepatitis.
- Hepatic failure can occur in a severe case of acute viral hepatitis.
- Diagnostic liver biopsy is essential in all patients with chronic hepatitis.
- The best test for hepatitis A is finding antibodies in the blood, and for hepatitis B finding the surface antigen (HB$_s$ Ag) in the blood.
- The conjunctivae in elderly patients often have an icteric tinge in the absence of jaundice.

Case challenge

A 59-year-old hypertensive salesman presented with a 2 months history of increasing jaundice. His appetite was poor and he had been losing weight. He had a long history of vague abdominal pain in varying parts of the abdomen, often on the left side, with rumbling, flatulence and occasional episodes of diarrhoea. Currently the stools were pale.

He had a past history of psychiatric problems and had also had problems with heavy drinking which he blamed on the pressure of his work. He had been hypertensive for about 10 years and had a variety of different drugs for treatment, but he had been on methyl dopa for the last 2 or 3 years which he thought suited him best.

He was a heavy smoker, 30+ cigarettes a day and admitted a smoker's cough but denied any recent exacerbation of his cough, or haemoptysis.

The findings of examination are shown in Fig. 19.4.

Questions

Give four possible diagnoses to account for the jaundice.

How would you decide the diagnosis?

Possible diagnoses

- cirrhosis
- drug-induced hepatitis
- liver metastases
- carcinoma of pancreas

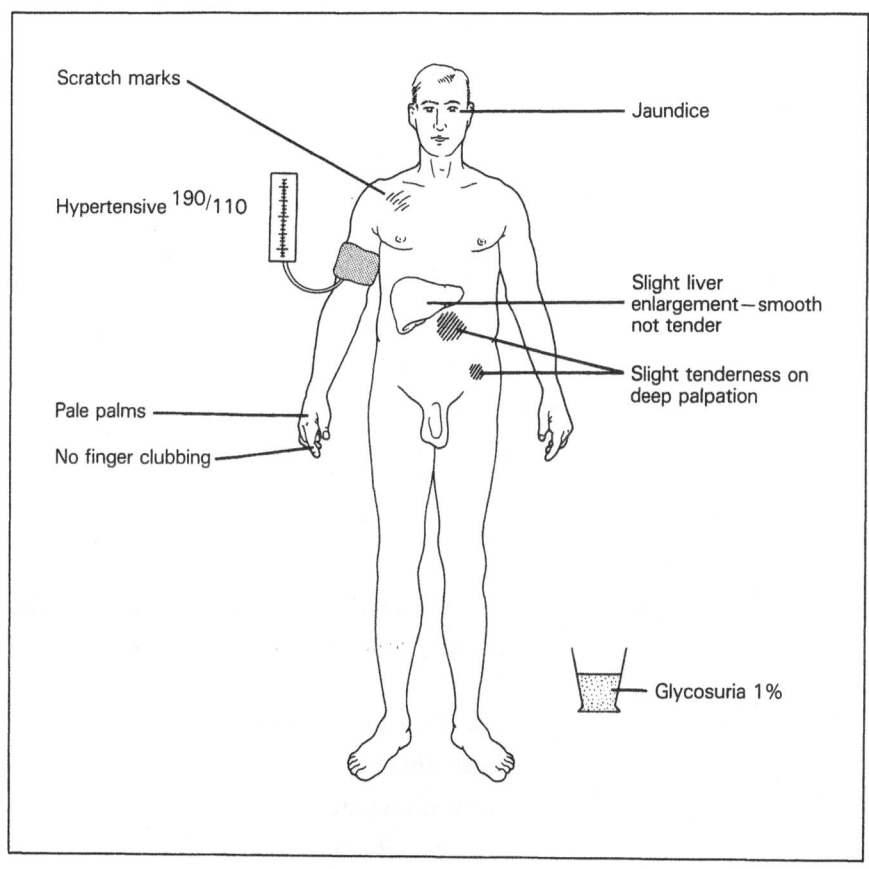

Scratch marks

Hypertensive 190/110

Pale palms

No finger clubbing

Jaundice

Slight liver enlargement—smooth not tender

Slight tenderness on deep palpation

Glycosuria 1%

Fig. 19.4   *Examination findings in case challenge*

Cirrhosis

For	history	• alcoholism
		• anorexia, loss of weight
	exam	• liver enlargement
Against	history	• no swelling abdomen/legs
		• no bleeding diathesis
	exam	• no signs of cirrhosis

        liver palms

        finger clubbing

        spider naevi

        gynaecomastia

        ascites

        dilated abdominal veins

    • no splenomegaly

Tests		• liver function

        AST/ALT $\uparrow$

        alkaline phosphatase slightly $\uparrow$

    • other blood tests

        albumin $\downarrow$

        globulin $\uparrow$

        prothrombia $\downarrow$

    • ultrasound

    • isotope scan

    • CT scan

Drug-induced hepatitis

For	history	• on methyl dopa → chronic aggressive hepatitis
		• previous psychiatric drugs which could be hepatoxic

        tricyclic antidepressants

        phenothiazines

        benzodiazepines

        MAO inhibitors

	exam	• nil specific

Jaundice

Against	history	• anorexia/loss of weight
	exam	• liver not tender
Tests		• liver function may show a slight rise in aminotrans-ferase and alkaline phosphatase but there are no specific tests

Liver metastases

For	history	• heavy smoker? cancer lung
		• abdominal pain/diarrhoea? cancer colon
		• anorexia, loss of weight
	exam	• liver enlargement
Against	history	• no increased cough or haemoptysis
		• abdominal pain/diarrhoea long standing – probably represents aspastic colon
	exam	• liver smooth, not irregular
		• nil to suggest cancer lung
		no glands
		no clubbing
		no lung signs
		• no mass to suggest cancer colon
Tests		• liver
		ultrasound
		isotope scan
		CT scan
		• for carcinoma lung
		chest X-ray
		bronchoscopy
		• for carcinoma colon
		sigmoidoscopy/colonoscopy
		barium enema

Carcinoma of pancreas

For	history	• anorexia, loss of weight
		• often no abdominal pain
		• jaundice clearly obstructive
	exam	• slight epigastric tenderness – non-specific
		• liver enlargement
		• glycosuria (25% of cases cancer pancreas)
Against	history	• nil
	exam	• no epigastric mass
Tests		• barium meal for widened duodenal loop
		• ultrasound
		• isotope scan
		• ERCP
		• CT scan
		• laparotomy

Actual diagnosis:
Carcinoma of head of pancreas

Treatment and outcome

An exploratory laparotomy was carried out because the diagnosis was uncertain (barium meal normal and ultrasound negative): an *inoperable carcinoma* was found in the head of the pancreas affecting also the portal lymph glands with multiple metastases in the liver. By-pass operation relieved symptoms.

He survived only 10 weeks.

Index